314
Current Topics in Microbiology and Immunology

D. B. Moody (Ed.)

T Cell Activation by CD1 and Lipid Antigens

With 25 Figures and 5 Tables

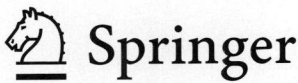 Springer

D. Branch Moody, M.D.

Brigham and Women's Hospital
Harvard Medical School
Smith 514
1 Jimmy Fund Way
Boston, MA 02115
USA
e-mail: bmoody@rics.bwh.harvard.edu

Cover Illustration:
The cover illustration is a computer generated (Maxon CINEMA 4D and Photoshop 3D) image of
the CD1b structure with a lipid antigen in the pocket. The model is rendered as a solid abstract
glass sculpture held in place by a metallic base depicting the heavy chain (red) and the light chain
(purple). An abstract glass model of a hypothetical T cell receptor with alpha and beta subunits is
suspended over the CD1. Illustration by Chris Dascher (www.cdascher.com).

Library of Congress Catalog Number 72-152360

ISSN 0070-217X
ISBN 978-3-540-69510-3 Springer Berlin Heidelberg New York

Springer is a part of Springer Science+Business Media
springer.com
© Springer-Verlag Berlin Heidelberg 2007

Editor: Simon Rallison, Heidelberg
Desk editor: Anne Clauss, Heidelberg
Production editor: Nadja Kroke, Leipzig
Cover design: WMX Design, Heidelberg
Typesetting: LE-TEX Jelonek, Schmidt & Vöckler GbR, Leipzig
Printed on acid-free paper   SPIN 11614562   27/3150/YL – 5 4 3 2 1 0

List of Contents

List of Contributors

(Addresses stated at the beginning of respective chapters)

Barral, D. C.   143
Behar, S. M.   215
Besra, G.   73
Blumberg, R. S.   113
Brenner, M. B.   143

Cerundolo, V.   325
Coquet, J. M. C.   293

Dascher, C. C.   3
DeKruyff, R. H.   269
Dougan, S. K.   113
Dover, L. G.   73

Godfrey, D. I.   293

Kaser, A.   113
Kronenberg, M.   165

Libero, G. De   51

MacDonald, H. R.   195

Meyer, E. H.   269
Miyake, S.   251
Mori, L.   51
Mycko, M. P.   195

Porcelli, S. A.   215

Salio, M.   325
Smyth, M. J.   293
Sugita, M.   143
Sullivan, B. A.   165
Swann, J. B.   293

Umetsu, D. T.   269

Willcox, B. E.   73
Willcox, C. R.   73
Wilson, I. A.   27

Yamamura, T.   251

Zajonc, D. M.   27

Section I
Molecular Biology

CTMI (2007) 314:3–26

Evolutionary Biology of CD1

C. C. Dascher

Center for Immunobiology, Mount Sinai School of Medicine, 1 Gustave Levy Place, Box 1630, New York , NY 10029, USA
christopher.dascher@mssm.edu

Abstract The recognition more than a decade ago that lipids presented by CD1 could function as T cell antigens revealed a startling and previously unappreciated complexity to the adaptive immune system. The initial novelty of lipid antigen presentation by CD1 has since given way to a broader perspective of the immune system's capacity to sense and respond to a diverse array of macromolecules. Some immune recognition systems such as Toll-like receptors can trace their origins back into the deep history of sea urchins and arthropods. Others such as the major histocompatibility complex (MHC) appear relatively recently and interestingly, only in animals that also possess a jaw. The natural history of CD1 is thus part of the wider story of immune system evolution and should be considered in this context. Most evidence indicates that CD1 probably evolved from a classical MHC class I (MHC I) gene at some point during vertebrate evolution. This chapter reviews the evidence for this phylogenetic relationship and attempts to connect CD1 to existing models of MHC evolution. This endeavor is facilitated today by the recent availability of whole genome sequence data from a variety of species. Investigators have used these data to trace the ultimate origin of the MHC to a series of whole genome duplications that occurred roughly 500 million years ago. Sequence data have also revealed homologs of the mammalian MHC I and MHC II gene families in virtually all jawed vertebrates including sharks, bony fishes, reptiles, and birds. In contrast, CD1 genes have thus far been found only in a subset of these animal groups. This pattern of CD1 occurrence in the genomes of living species suggests the emergence of CD1 in an early terrestrial vertebrate.

1
Introduction

The evolutionary history of CD1 is closely connected to the larger story of the evolution of the MHC. The MHC, in turn, has emerged as an important model for the more fundamental investigation of vertebrate genome evolution. Thus it is worth examining these broader topics to provide a conceptual framework for the evolution of CD1 [43]. Most of the theoretical models related to MHC evolution rely on known genetic mechanisms such as the expansion and contraction of gene families, duplication, deletion, neofunctionalization, chromosome translocation, and even whole genome duplication (polyploidization). These are processes that have played a fundamental role in the evolution of our own genetic history and that of all metazoan genomes. This history reaches hundreds of millions of years into the past and includes species that are long extinct but whose few descendants survive today, each carrying a genetic record that can illuminate both the present and the past. Piecing together this history can thus be likened to a form of paleo-molecular biology in which DNA sequences have replaced fossilized bone and rock-hammers have been traded in for computers. The recent flood of sequence data has ignited new interest in the study of genome evolution. Moreover, comparative immunology is a major driving force for many of the ongoing genome sequencing projects given that the evolution of the immune system is one of the major innovations that permitted the expansion of complex multicellular animals.

Given the structural similarities, it is often taken for granted that CD1 and the MHC share a common ancestry. This review examines the basis for this assumption and examines how CD1 fits into the established models of MHC evolution. To address this issue, we must piece together a phylogenetic history of CD1 using both protein sequences and the known ancestry of extant (living) animal species. By combining these data, together with relevant paleontological evidence, we can begin to formulate a model for the timing, origin, and evolution of CD1. Two essential theoretical principles underlie most evolutionary analysis. The first is the fundamental assumption of cladistics that two distinct species with a common characteristic likely shared a common ancestor from which that characteristic was derived. In the context of molecular evolution, this principle is typically applied to comparing aligned protein or DNA sequences. The second underlying assumption is that of maximum parsimony. In the context of creating a phylogenetic relationship between two characters, minimizing the total number of evolutionary steps required to explain a given set of data is probably the correct answer. These principles guide the evaluation of competing hypotheses within this chapter.

Instead of reiterating recent reviews on CD1 molecular biology and genetics in mammals, this review attempts to synthesize a number of broader topics in comparative immunology and genomic evolution with which CD1 intersects. An overview of the evolution of MHC and CD1 in the context of vertebrate evolution is presented first. This is followed by several new insights into CD1 evolution that have emerged from the recent discovery of CD1 homologs in birds. Lastly, a potential model for CD1 emergence is presented.

2
The MHC Paralogy Group

Most immunologists are familiar with the MHC locus present in the genomes of all mammals, at least in terms of the major regions devoted to the critical task of antigen presentation. It is a daunting stretch of DNA spanning over 3,600 kb of chromosome 6 in humans with 128 functional genes and 96 pseudogenes [1, 6]. Many of these genes are directly involved in various aspects of the adaptive immune system, but there are others involved in innate immunity and some that have functions completely unrelated to the immune system [40]. Interestingly, comparison of the genes in the human MHC locus to the rest of the genome has revealed the presence of duplicated or paralogous genes on multiple chromosomes [6, 21, 32, 35]. Paralogous genes arise from gene duplication *within* a given species at some point in its evolution. In humans, for example, the CD1A and CD1B genes are paralogs. In contrast, human CD1D and mouse CD1D are orthologs, as they derive from the same gene that was present in a common human–mouse ancestor and thus arose as the result of speciation and not gene duplication. Importantly, it is the presence and pattern of paralogous genes in a succession of animal species that has revealed a potentially key mechanism for the evolution of the MHC and perhaps all metazoan genomes.

The critical observation is that the concept of paralogy extends not just to single genes but also to large blocks of genes and even whole chromosomes. Paralogous segments of chromosomal DNA containing multiple genes (referred to as paralogons) can be found throughout the human genome [64].

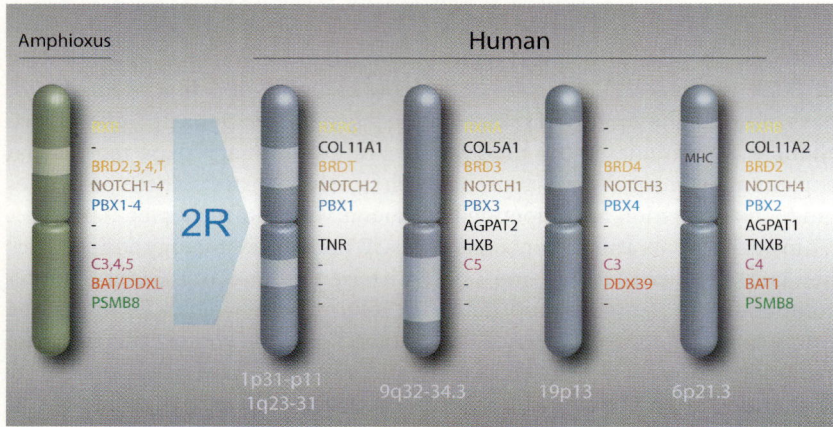

Fig. 1 Proto-MHC with anchor genes of the cephalochordate amphioxus and paralogous regions in the human genome. The proto-MHC is a syntenic array of anchor genes found on a single chromosome in invertebrates but do not include primordial MHC I or MHC II antigen presenting genes. The proto-MHC genes are shown in color with names to reflect the ancestry with the corresponding paralogous genes on human chromosome 1, 6, 9, and 19 [14]. Human genes not found in the amphioxus proto-MHC but still having paralogs within the human MHC paralogy group are in *black*. The proto-MHC genes are found on up to four separate chromosomes in jawed vertebrates but not necessarily in the same relative order or spacing. This shuffling is the result of chromosomal translocations and deletions that have accumulated over time. The quadruplication of the proto-MHC anchor genes in humans and other jawed vertebrates supports the 2R hypothesis in which two rounds whole genome duplication occurred during evolution of metazoans (see text for details). The MHC I and MHC II genes arose later in jawed vertebrates within one of the ancestral proto-MHC regions after the second vertebrate genome duplication event. Note that human chromosome 1 is thought to have undergone a pericentric inversion, which explains the separation of the paralogs onto both arms of the chromosome. The figure is a composite of data from several references [2, 12, 14, 21]. Genes are aligned across the figure for clarity; exact gene order or scale along the chromosomes is not implied

The MHC locus is itself part of linear array genes on chromosome 6 in humans that is at least partially duplicated on three other chromosomes in most jawed vertebrates [2, 15, 40]. These four paralogous regions located on chromosomes 1, 6, 9, and 19 in humans are collectively referred to as the MHC paralogy group, which is shown in Fig. 1. How did these paralogous segments arise and how is this related to the evolution of CD1? With these questions in mind, we can begin by exploring the evolutionary history of the MHC, and then later how this history relates to the emergence of CD1.

3
Genome Duplication and the Origin of the Proto-MHC

A certain debt is owed to the sea for the rapid progress in the CD1 field brought about by the discovery of alpha-galactosylceramide in a marine sponge [37, 54]. Similarly, to fully appreciate the evolutionary history of the MHC, we must once again return to the sea. Here, burrowed in the sandy bottom of many shallow tropical waters, it is possible to find the sea lancet or amphioxus (see photo in Fig. 2A). These modest invertebrates are cephalochordates that are thought to represent a critical transitional form that eventually led to the emergence of true vertebrates [25]. More importantly, for investigating the evolution of the immune system, amphioxus possess a locus of genes referred to as the proto-MHC. This nomenclature does *not* imply that amphioxus has genes encoding the peptide-binding MHC I and MHC II antigen-presenting molecules, but rather that these animals possess a linear array of anchor genes on a single chromosome that is conserved up to and including mammals [2, 12, 15]. Figure 1 illustrates some of the anchor genes (i.e., Notch, RXR, etc.) of the proto-MHC in amphioxus. It is the proto-MHC genes that are quadruplicated on four different chromosomes in jawed vertebrates, thus forming the core gene set of the MHC paralogy group (Fig. 1). The homologs of these proto-MHC genes are found within the present-day mammalian MHC locus, and it is this cluster of genes that is thought to be the primordial genomic scaffold on which MHC I, MHC II, and other members of the MHC-based adaptive immune system later evolved.

How did this proto-MHC go from a single copy in amphioxus to four in humans and other jawed vertebrates? A clue to the answer comes from the observation that it is not only the proto-MHC that exhibits this quadruplication phenomenon. Indeed, many other paralogous segments are found that exhibit a similar 1:4 ratio when comparing invertebrate to mammalian genomes [71]. Two non-mutually exclusive theories can account for the formation of these paralogous segments of DNA. One mechanism is simple en-bloc duplication in an ancestral species, possibly by copying a whole chromosome or a large segment of chromosome and incorporating this into a new germ line [2]. Although large- and small-scale chromosome duplication indeed occurs, in this stochastic model, a more random distribution from the observed 1:4 ratio might be expected [23]. A more sweeping model is thus required to explain the consistent ratio of paralogons.

A theory that accounts for the observed paralogy of genome segments is whole genome duplication or polyploidization; essentially a doubling of the number of chromosomes [64]. Genome duplication is a deceptively simple idea first proposed by Susumu Ohno in 1970 as a mechanism to provide the

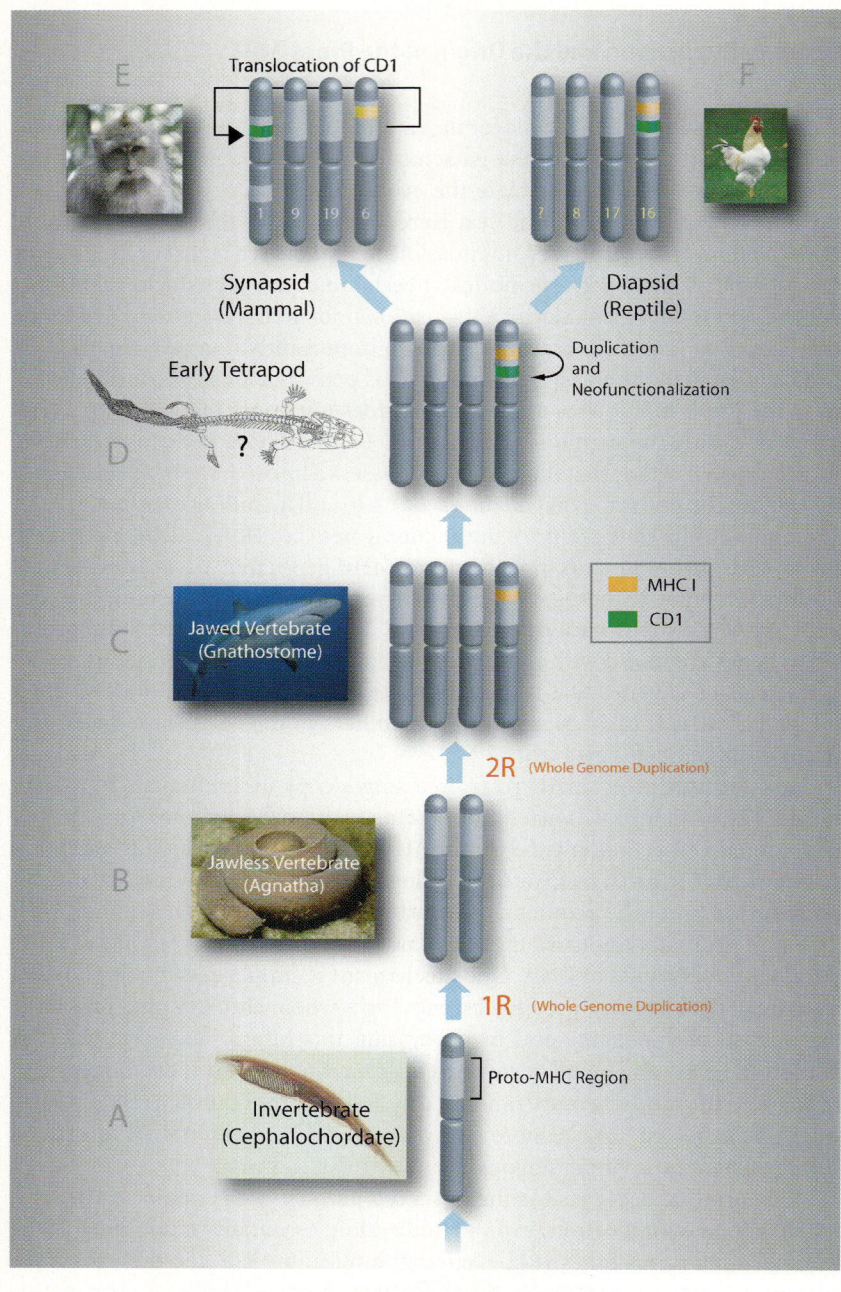

Translocation of CD1

Synapsid
(Mammal)

Diapsid
(Reptile)

Early Tetrapod

Duplication
and
Neofunctionalization

?

D

MHC I
CD1

Jawed Vertebrate
(Gnathostome)

C

2R (Whole Genome Duplication)

Jawless Vertebrate
(Agnatha)

B

1R (Whole Genome Duplication)

Proto-MHC Region

Invertebrate
(Cephalochordate)

A

◄──

Fig. 2A–F Genome duplication and CD1 locus translocation. The proto-MHC is an ancient array of genes present in invertebrates. Two successive rounds of genome duplication resulted in up to four chromosomal copies with these anchor genes (**A–C**). The MHC paralogy group for human chromosomes 1, 6, 9, and 19 are indicated (**E**). The assignment of specific chicken chromosomes to the MHC paralogy group (**F**) is preliminary (CCD, unpublished data). The MHC I and MHC II genes evolved within one of paralogons in an ancient ancestor of jawed vertebrates after the split from jawless fishes (**C**). The CD1 genes have not been identified in fish despite some efforts to find them. The CD1 genes have thus far been found only in mammals and birds, implying that CD1 was present in a common ancestor of birds and mammals but after the separation from fish; possibly in an early tetrapod (**D**). Furthermore, CD1 is linked to the MHC in birds (**F**), which supports the removal of CD1 from the MHC paralogy group despite its location on chromosome 1 in humans (**E**). The CD1 gene(s) likely translocated from a primordial MHC locus in an early mammalian ancestor after the bird–mammal split 310 million years ago (**D**). The CD1 and MHC have remained linked in birds, which is more likely to represent the ancestral state

genetic raw material for the evolution of increasingly complex life forms [57]. The theory has proven to be both popular and controversial, but compelling evidence for its essential predictions has been shown in plants, fungi, and more recently, vertebrate genomes [19, 63, 80, 81]. From a theoretical standpoint, duplicated genes or genomes provide a rapid mechanism for the evolution of novel gene functions (neofunctionalization) while still retaining an intact copy of the original (and potentially essential) gene [57]. Clearly, not every gene has corresponding paralogous segments on other chromosomes, and indeed only about 10% of the human genome shows clear evidence of this type of duplication [77]. This is no doubt a result of the dynamic nature of chromosome evolution, which has obfuscated the tell-tale signatures of genome duplication in the same way that tectonic and weathering forces obscure the geologic history of the earth's surface. Over hundreds of millions of years, duplicated chromosomes or chromosomal segments have become translocated, deleted, or otherwise rearranged, while, on a smaller scale, individual genes become neofunctionalized or silenced [20]. Thus, it is often challenging to piece together the original state of the ancestral genomic structure; hence the controversy.

The theory that two sequential rounds of genome duplication events occurred over the course of vertebrate evolution is commonly referred to as the 2R hypothesis [24, 57]. As described above, the prediction of this model is the 1:4 ratio rule of paralogous gene segments (X>2X>4X) when comparing early chordates prior to genome duplication and true jawed vertebrates after these duplication events (Fig. 1). Since not all genes follow this rule, there has been some disagreement about the validity of these segments as paralogs and of the 2R hypothesis in general [28, 29, 44]. Controversy not withstanding, analysis of whole genome sequence data increasingly supports the primary claim of the 2R hypothesis: that genome duplication has occurred at least once (and probably twice) during the early evolution of vertebrates from more primitive chordate ancestors [19, 21, 50, 64, 72]. Figure 2 illustrates the relevant steps in this model. Recent analysis of the amphioxus proto-MHC has provided strong evidence for an initial whole genome duplication [2, 63, 72]. These studies estimate that a duplication of the proto-MHC occurred approximately 600 million years ago (Mya) in an early jawless vertebrate ancestor *after* splitting off from the cephalochordate (amphioxus) lineage [2, 8, 79]. A second duplication is thought to have occurred in an early jawed vertebrate ancestor *after* splitting off from the jawless vertebrate lineage [19, 22]. This ancestral species subsequently gave rise to all jawed vertebrates, carrying with it the four paralogous copies of the proto-MHC found today in jawed vertebrates, one of which forms the core of the actual MHC locus found in all jawed vertebrates (Fig. 2). Whether two rounds of genome duplication took place, or a single round plus extensive localized segmental duplications, is still a matter of debate. However, the nature of these duplication events should become more apparent as additional whole genome sequences are analyzed.

4
Origin of the MHC Antigen-Presenting Molecules

Having set the stage for the emergence of the MHC I and MHC II antigen presentation genes found in all jawed vertebrates, it is now rather anticlimactic to reveal that the precise progenitor of these molecules remains a mystery. This is due to the absence of clear primordial MHC I or MHC II genes in any of the known extant jawed or jawless vertebrate species. Nevertheless, several theories have been put forward as to how these genes may have initially evolved [21]. One model suggests that the MHC II genes arose first by exon-shuffling that combined an immunoglobulin-like C domain with a peptide-binding region (PBR) whose origin is unclear [38]. The MHC I heavy chain was subsequently derived by the addition of another PBR exon to the MHC II β chain [38]. This relative order of MHC origin is supported by phylogenetic analysis of the relevant exons with the split between MHC I and MHC II estimated at approximately 500 Mya, just after the Cambrian explosion [27]. It is certainly plausible to speculate that the massive adaptive radiation of multicellular animals during that time period and the emergence of the MHC are somehow linked [27, 62]. Nevertheless, genes encoding a clear primordial

PBR that forms the critical antigen-binding domains of MHC I or MHC II genes have not been identified in any extant vertebrate or invertebrate species.

Despite the uncertainty of its origins, what is clear is the unambiguous presence of the MHC antigen-presenting genes in all jawed vertebrates (Gnathostomes). Therefore, the MHC I and MHC II genes likely evolved in an ancestral jawed vertebrate species very early *after* its split from the jawless vertebrate lineage. This timing for the emergence of the MHC-based adaptive immune system is inferred from two critical observations. The first is that virtually all jawed vertebrates share a conserved set of genes that have clear evolutionary homologs with the extensively characterized mammalian MHC-based adaptive immune system [14]. At a minimum, these include the genes that encode the αβ and γδ T cell receptors, MHC I and MHC II, and immunoglobulin molecules. Homologs of all of these components can be found in Chondrichthyes (cartilaginous fishes such as sharks, skates, and rays), teleosts (bony fishes), amphibians, reptiles, birds, and mammals [21]. The second is that no clear MHC I or MHC II homologs have been found in the more primitive jawless vertebrate species [49, 75]. Only hagfish and lampreys survive as the two living examples of the ancient lineage of jawless vertebrates and, despite some effort, no evidence of a primordial MHC gene has been found in either group. Thus, the precise origin of the MHC antigen-presenting genes remains an enigma.

5
Origin and Age of CD1

A working hypothesis of this discussion is that CD1 and MHC I share a common ancestry. This hypothesis is strongly supported by sequence alignments and structural data. However, the precise age of CD1 relative to MHC I has remained unresolved. This is due primarily to the lack of sequence data for the immune genes of lower vertebrates. Therefore, the most straightforward way to trace the origin of the CD1 genes is to identify clear orthologous sequences or transitional forms of CD1 in more phylogenetically distant species. It may then be possible to infer the age of CD1 by correlating the emergence of these genes with established vertebrate phylogenetic histories based on the paleontological record. Cartilaginous fish are the most primitive vertebrates that possess genes encoding MHC I [5, 31, 60, 65]. Thus, early efforts to determine the age of CD1 began by searching for primitive homologs in the spiny dogfish (*Squalus acanthias*), an abundant species of shark found in many oceans. However, clear CD1 homologs were not detected by degenerate PCR [78] or by data-mining of the available *S. acanthias* EST database (unpublished data).

Initial attempts to establish the timing for the origin of CD1 were also frustrated by the apparent absence of CD1 homologs in teleosts (bony fishes). Extensive searches of the public databases have thus far failed to reveal clear CD1 homologs in any of the five completed teleost genome sequences (*Danio rerio, Fugu rubripes, Tetraodon nigroviridis, Gasterosteus aculeatus, Oryzias latipes*) or other teleost EST libraries [51]. Despite the apparent absence of CD1 in both teleosts and sharks, these groups do possess highly divergent nonclassical MHC I genes [39, 70, 78]. Bearing in mind that the collection of genomic sequence data from lower vertebrates is still ongoing, the data examined thus far suggests that CD1 may not be as old as MHC I, but is rather a more recent innovation.

It is difficult to build a strong case for the emergence of CD1 based solely on the absence of these genes in lower aquatic jawed vertebrates, but that all retain MCH I genes. Nevertheless, if these observations are supported by future genomic sequence data from additional species, then it strengthens the probability that CD1 emerged after MHC I. However, there are two important qualifications that may explain the apparent absence of CD1 in teleosts and sharks. One is that extant teleosts exhibit a highly fragmented MHC that effectively unlinks MHC I, MHC II, and distributes other MHC-locus genes to virtually every chromosome in zebrafish [67, 68]. Thus, it is possible that the chaotic structure of the teleost genome may have contributed to the loss of CD1 and other genes. This fragmentation occurred after the separation of teleosts from sharks and other cartilaginous fishes. The second caveat is simply that whole genome sequence data is currently unavailable for sharks (although the available shark EST database is negative for CD1) and other ancient cartilaginous fishes. Sharks, unlike bony fish, retain the linkage of the MHC I and MHC II in a single locus and also have an overall slower rate of evolution compared to mammals [46, 58]. Therefore, these animals may have retained more primitive features of the primordial MHC locus. Further whole genome sequence data from cartilaginous fishes, teleosts, and also from a lobe-finned fish such as the Coelacanth will be required to support the findings of these initial surveys.

The failure to find CD1 homologs in sharks or bony fishes prompted the search for CD1 genes in other nonmammalian vertebrates. The chicken genome was used for this purpose since birds represent an evolutionary intermediate between mammals and fish. Three independent groups have recently characterized two clear evolutionary homologs of CD1 in the chicken *Gallus gallus* [48, 51, 66]. As described above, phylogenetic analysis assumes that a characteristic shared between two organisms implies the existence of a common ancestor from which the characteristic was derived. Therefore, evidence of CD1 homologs in both birds and mammals implies that a primordial CD1 gene was present in the common ancestor of both groups (Fig. 2). What was this common ancestor and when did it live?

The separation of birds and mammals from a common reptilian ancestor into two distinct lineages is one of the major milestones in vertebrate evolution: the Synapsid-Diapsid (S-D) split. Mammals emerged from the Synapsid lineage while birds derive from the Diapsid [41]. For the curious, these terms refer to the presence of one or two large openings in the skulls of the Synapsid and Diapsid lineages, respectively, which permit muscle attachment to the jaw. It is generally accepted that modern Aves arose from within the Archosauria group of Diapsid reptiles, more specifically the Theropod lineage of bipedal predatory dinosaurs [69]. Importantly, it is generally accepted from fossil evidence that the divergence of the Synapsid and Diapsid lineages occurred approximately 310 Mya [41, 42]. Thus, for the first time, the age of the CD1 gene family can be pushed back to before the existence of true mammals.

The timing of the S-D split from fossil evidence is well established in paleontology and therefore serves as a robust time calibration point for molecular clock analyses [41]. The molecular clock model uses the divergence time of two lineages derived from the geologic fossil record to calibrate an absolute time-scale for the branch lengths of a phylogenetic tree generated from sequence data. Based on the survey of the teleost genomes described above, our analysis assumes that CD1 genes evolved *after* the split of an ancestral tetrapod from a purely aquatic fish lineage. Figure 3 shows the resulting phylogenetic analysis with chicken CD1 representing the reptilian (Diapsid) branch and a broad array of mammal CD1 protein sequences representing the Synapsid branch. The node of these two branches represents the common ancestral CD1 protein at the time of the S-D split and is set to 310 Mya, thus allowing the remaining branch lengths to be interpreted as time. Using the zebrafish MHC I as the outgroup to root this tree, the split between teleost classical MHC I and CD1 is calculated to be 384 Mya (Fig. 3). Interestingly, this timing corresponds closely with the appearance of the first tetrapods in the Devonian fossil record roughly 365–385 Mya [3]. Briefly, this is the period in which primitive sarcopterygian fish made the initial transition from the aquatic to terrestrial environments; a point in evolution recently highlighted by the discovery of a Devonian fish with tetrapod-like limbs [3, 13]. In addition, the *Xenopus* amphibian MHC locus has recently been sequenced but lacks CD1 genes in the region examined [59]. These data suggest that the emergence of CD1 in the vertebrate genome occurred in the reptiliform lineage after the amphibian–reptile split. The early evolutionary history of frogs and other amphibians remains unclear, so a more precise timing of this split is not yet possible. However, the cumulative data thus far supports a model in which CD1 emerged in an early terrestrial vertebrate close to the

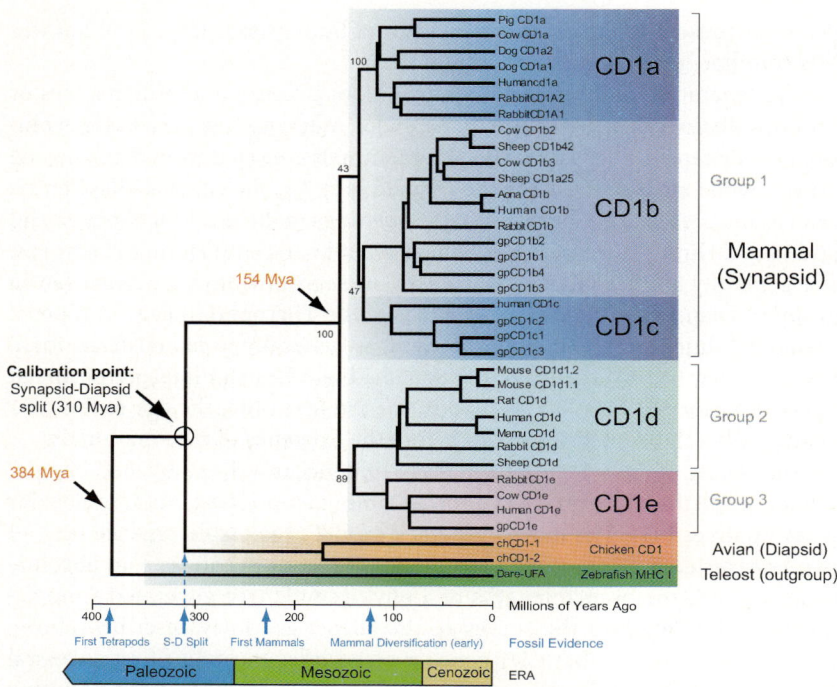

Fig. 3 Molecular clock analysis of the CD1 protein family. A rooted tree of aligned CD1 α1–3 protein sequences from various mammal species and the two chicken CD1 homologs was generated. Zebra fish classical MHC I was also aligned and used as the outgroup based on the assumption that MHC I and CD1 share a common ancestor. The phylogenetic tree was generated using the Neighbor-Joining method and calibrated using the bird–mammal split at 310 Mya [41, 42]. The separation of MHC I and CD1 is calculated at 384 Mya, which correlates with the approximate time (365–385 Mya) when tetrapods first appear in the fossil record. The molecular clock also indicates the separation of most mammal isoforms occurred at approximately 154 Mya. This value is consistent with a period in the Mesozoic fossil record when there were only a few mammal species. Note the transorder conservation of CD1 isoforms among diverse mammal orders, which further supports the divergence of CD1 into a multigene family in an early mammal ancestor. Bootstrap values for the nodes leading to mammal CD1 isoform divergence are indicated. A list of the taxa used for this analysis is available upon request from the author

transition from water to land (Figs. 2 and 3). More comprehensive genome sequence data from additional extant amphibian, reptile, and fish species will be required to support this model and to further define the origin and timing of CD1 evolution.

6
CD1 and the MHC Paralogy Group

The clear homology between MHC I and CD1 using both the amino acid sequence alignment and crystal structure data suggests that CD1 arose by gene duplication of a primordial MHC I. What is the genomic evidence for this model? As described above, the anchor genes that make up the MHC paralogy group in humans are present in two, three, or four copies on chromosomes 1, 6, 9, and 19. The human CD1 locus is located on chromosome 1 and is therefore unlinked to the MHC locus on chromosome 6 [4]. Mapping of the MHC paralogy group genes to parts of chromosome 1 quite reasonably suggested that CD1 was also part of this paralogy group, with the HLA genes being the paralogous partner [34]. However, the broader implications of this model are disconcerting. For example, this paralogy-based model of CD1 evolution necessarily forces the origin of the MHC I genes into an ancestral jawless vertebrate after the first round of genome duplication (Fig. 2B), despite the paradoxical observation that no primordial MHC I (or CD1) has been found in extant jawless vertebrates [49, 75]. It also implies that CD1 genes would have been present in the earliest jawed vertebrates, despite the apparent absence of CD1 in extant fish species. Preliminary analysis at the time of the original isolation of the CD1 genes suggested that CD1 and MHC I emerged at the same time, although later phylogenetic analysis raised some questions as to the extreme age of the CD1 genes [26, 47]. However, all of these models were based solely on the analysis of mammalian CD1 homologs. A resolution of these conflicting data requires the examination of CD1 genes from nonmammalian species that retain more primitive characteristics.

Comparative analysis with the chicken CD1 has been useful in developing a model that explains the extant chromosomal organization of the MHC and CD1 genes. The most striking feature of the chicken CD1 genes is that they map to within 50 kb of the chicken MHC I genes [48, 51, 66]. Therefore, the chicken genome data supports a model of CD1 evolution by gene duplication and neofunctionalization of an MHC I gene while *still linked* to the MHC locus rather than by genome duplication, as suggested by the paralogy hypothesis. Thus, the close linkage of CD1 with the MHC locus in the chicken probably reflects the ancestral state of CD1 originally found in the reptilian ancestor of both birds and mammals (Fig. 2D). This CD1-MHC linkage was maintained in the Diapsids (birds), while the nascent CD1 locus was translocated to a different chromosome in the Synapsid (mammal) lineage (Fig. 2E, F). The alternative model would be that the MHC and CD1 loci were originally separated (as the result of genome duplication) but that the CD1 locus rejoined the MHC locus in birds *after* the bird–mammal split. This scenario seems highly unlikely given the close proximity (~50 kb) of CD1 to MHC I in the chicken [48, 51, 66]. It is more parsimonious to hypothesize that the CD1 locus translocated to a different chromosome in the mammal lineage *after* the bird–mammal split (Fig. 2B). However, this does raise the question of why the CD1 locus in mammals paradoxically ended up on human chromosome 1 in proximity to other MHC paralogs. Despite this new question, the removal of CD1 as an MHC I paralog in the context of the 2R hypothesis eliminates a potential constraint on the timing of both MHC I and CD1 emergence. A more recent emergence of CD1 in an early terrestrial vertebrate is therefore more plausible since it reconciles predictions made by all of the existing data.

What factors could account for the difference in CD1–MHC linkage between birds and mammals? The separation of CD1 and the MHC to different chromosomes appears to be a consistent feature of mammalian genomes and thus probably happened relatively early in mammal evolution. This separation has been proposed as a hypothetical mechanism to preserve the unique features in divergent orthologous genes that may emerge during evolution [33]. For example, allowing a newly diversified nonclassical MHC I to remain within the highly plastic MHC locus increases the chances of gene conversion and potential loss of newly acquired functions. If this is true, then the theory must explain why it did not occur in chickens as well. However, the entire chicken MHC locus is only 2% the size of the total human MHC (~90 kb), making the rate of recombination within the avian MHC locus significantly lower and thus more stable over time. Therefore, there may be less selective pressure to separate the CD1 genes from the MHC in birds.

7
Mammalian CD1 Isoform Diversification

The human CD1 gene family is composed of five nonpolymorphic genes (CD1A, -B, -C, -D, and -E). The relatively close phylogenetic relationship between mammalian species has allowed easy identification of these prototypical CD1 isoforms in other mammal species by comparative sequence analysis [11, 17]. In fact, the homology between specific CD1 isoforms (orthologs) is typically higher between two mammalian species than among the multiple CD1 isoforms (paralogs) within a given species (Fig. 3). While there are differences in the total number of CD1 genes and specific CD1 isoform types that are present between mammal species, examples of each CD1 isoform (CD1A– E) have been found in at least two or more divergent mammalian orders [17]. This transorder conservation of isoform types suggests that the CD1 family of genes arose in an early mammalian ancestor, prior to the initial diversification of mammals around 125 Mya in the Cretaceous period [10, 30, 56]. Since the first mammal-like forms appear in the fossil record in the late Triassic about 220 Mya, the time range for mammal CD1 isoform divergence would be approximately 125–220 Mya [56]. Interestingly, the molecular clock analysis shown in Fig. 3 independently confirms this estimate. Examination of the clock analysis indicates that all of mammal CD1 isoforms diverged between 130 and 154 Mya, which is within the 125–220 Mya time framederived from the paleontological data (Fig. 3). This timing corresponds to a period when there were only a limited number of mouse-sized mammal species that lived in the shadows of the Mesozoic dinosaurs but that eventually radiated into the approximately 4,000 species known today [56]. Taken together, these data provide a cross-validation that supports the diversification of the CD1 multigene family in an early Mesozoic mammalian ancestor common to virtually all extant mammal species.

8
Microevolution of Primordial CD1

The discussion thus far has considered CD1 in the larger context of vertebrate genome and MHC evolution. In this last section, specific structural adaptations to the CD1 molecule are examined. In considering potential models for the structural evolution of CD1, it is logical to incorporate known experimental data on both CD1-mediated lipid antigen presentation and CD1 endosomal trafficking. For example, the MHC I requires a complex network of accessory molecules for effective presentation of peptides [14]. Similarly, the potential dependence of CD1 function on the coevolution or co-option of accessory molecules might also be hypothesized. However, if CD1 evolved from MHC I then it is likely that it went through a series on structural intermediates that would have reflected the switch from peptide to lipid binding. Thus, an early or transitional form of CD1 would likely have possessed a relatively shallow and charged antigen-binding pocket comparable to MHC I, which then expanded in size and became increasingly hydrophobic over time. It might then be postulated that the earliest evolutionary forms of CD1 would be restricted to binding small hydrophobic molecules or lipids with relatively short acyl chains. It is now clear that at least a subset of CD1 lipid antigens do not require internalization or processing to bind CD1 for subsequent recognition by T cells. These short-chain lipid and glycolipid antigens can be loaded directly onto fixed APC for recognition by T cells [45, 52, 53, 73]. Therefore, an early CD1 isoform would not *necessarily* require specialized molecules for antigen acquisition, internalization, processing, loading, or even the need for deep intracellular trafficking [52]. The initial evolutionary divergence of CD1 would therefore not be constrained by the need for specialized accessory proteins. A counter-argument to this model would be that none of the accessory molecules found for CD1 thus far appear to be strictly CD1-specific but rather have alternative physiological roles such as lipid binding and transport that CD1 has co-opted. Examples of these include molecules such as ApoE or saposins among others [76, 82]. Thus it is possible that the existence of any or all CD1 accessory molecules preceded the emergence of CD1.

The transition from a single CD1 gene to an extended gene family probably occurred by duplication and neofunctionalization in a manner similar to other multigene families, including MHC I itself. Each of the CD1 isoforms has evolved a slightly different intracellular pattern of traffic and it has been postulated that this allows the CD1 proteins as a group to broadly survey the intracellular environment of an APC for potential lipid antigens [17, 53, 74]. We have previously proposed a model in which the structural diversification of the CD1 antigen-binding pocket is driven by initial changes to the intracellular localization of the CD1 protein [17]. It is well known that some CD1 isoforms traffic from the cell surface in a manner that is dependent upon short endosomal sorting motifs located in the cytoplasmic tail of the CD1 heavy chain that serve as adaptor protein-binding sites [9]. Single nucleotide mutations resulting in changes to tyrosine and other critical amino acids in these sorting motifs are sufficient to completely alter the steady-state localization of CD1 [16]. Moreover, some lipids are preferentially sorted to different intracellular compartments based on the length of the acyl chains and independent of CD1 localization [55]. For example, short-chain lipids were shown to sort to recycling endosomes, whereas long-chain lipids sorted to late endosomes. The effect of acyl chain length on intracellular sorting of bacterial lipid antigens presented by CD1 has also been demonstrated [52]. Thus, mutations in the cytoplasmic tail resulting in trafficking changes could redirect a CD1 protein to previously inaccessible intracellular compartments, thereby exposing it to novel types of lipid antigens. Selective pressure would then act on mutations to the antigen-binding pocket in order to optimize the interaction of a new class of lipids found in that particular intracellular compartment. In general, the primary feature being altered would likely be the capacity of the CD1 pocket to accept lipids with different length acyl chains. Direct tests of this hypothesis are not possible, but evidence of this diversification process may be reflected in the unique structural differences and volumes that are observed between the various CD1 lipid-binding pockets. The cycle of gene duplication and diversification could be repeated in order to fine-tune the capacity of the cellular immune system to recognize lipid antigens acquired by CD1 from various intracellular locations.

The sequential diversification model of CD1 evolution outlined above raises the inevitable question of which extant CD1 isoform (if any) most closely resembles the primordial CD1 that we postulate must have existed at the time of the Synapsid-Diapsid split. It is clear from Fig. 3 that the relatively rapid diversification of the mammalian CD1 isoforms within a span of 24 million years (130–154 Mya) precludes assigning one of the mammal isoforms as being primordial with any statistical certainty. Instead of considering the global sequence alignment, specific structural features should be examined using a more cladistic approach. If we consider shared structural features between the avian chCD1–2 and the mammal CD1 isoforms, then the ancestral CD1 would appear to point more toward CD1a [51, 66]. For example, the human CD1a structure has the smallest antigen-binding pocket relative to the other known isoforms, consistent with the structural transition from MHC I to CD1 described above. In addition, although the human CD1a cytoplasmic tail has no known protein binding motifs, nonprimate CD1a orthologs contain a di-leucine-based adaptor protein binding motif in the cytoplasmic tail. Additional structural features linking chCD1–2 to CD1a have also been noted [51]. However, all of these correlations between chicken CD1 and mammal CD1a remain highly speculative without a wider sample of nonmammalian CD1 proteins for comparison.

9
Conclusion

It is now a straightforward task to obtain DNA sequence from virtually any living organism and to then perform comparative analysis between species. Ideally, the comparison of orthologous proteins between widely divergent species should include functional information as well. However, functional data is significantly harder to obtain from uncommon nonlaboratory species. For example, the role of CD1 in host defense has been shown for a variety of infectious diseases in the mouse, including parasite, bacterial, and viral disease models [18]. The conservation of CD1 homologs in birds suggests that it may have an important role in the avian immune system as well [51]. Was host-defense the primary function of CD1, at least in the early stages of its evolution? The chicken MHC locus is extremely compact, with only 19 genes spread over 90 kb [36]. Functional analysis of CD1 in this simpler chicken system, if it were possible, might provide useful insights into primitive functions of CD1 that are masked by the redundant layers of the more complex mammalian immune system.

Certainly many questions about the origin and evolution of CD1 remain to be answered. One question that stands out is the tentative correlation of the age of CD1, determined by molecular clock analysis, with the early colonization of land by vertebrates (Fig. 4). If this timing is supported by future data then the implications are certainly intriguing. Was CD1 simply a chance innovation that was retained as part of an overall expansion of the MHC I genes in early tetrapods? More interestingly, were there unique selective pressures found in the terrestrial environment that were absent in the purely aquatic setting? If so, then what were they? In considering these two distinct environments, the

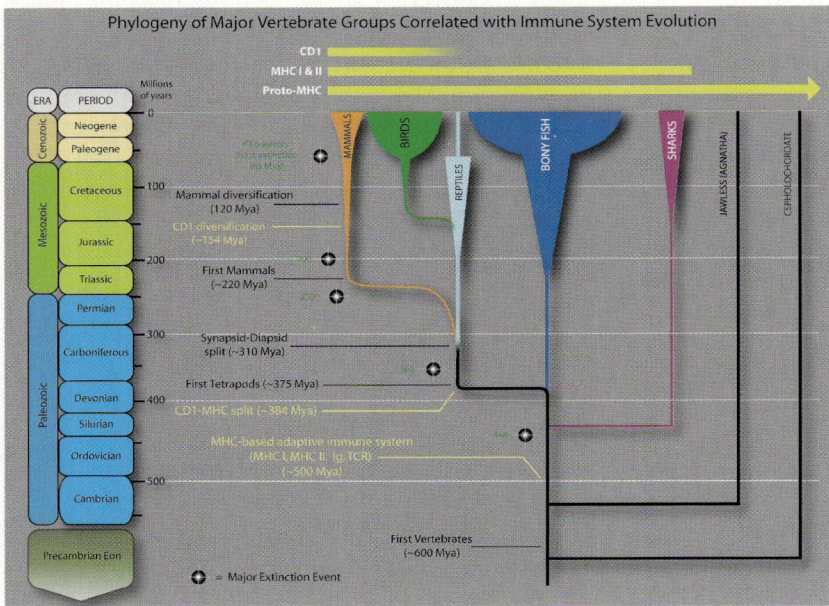

Fig. 4 Consensus phylogeny of major animal groups with milestones in immune system evolution. The tree represents a composite of available vertebrate evolution data and is derived from Benton [7]. The horizontal width is proportional to the number of species at any given time period based on the fossil record. The base of the tree starts at cephalochordates (amphioxus), although the proto-MHC has been found in even more primitive organisms. Jawless vertebrates possess a form of anticipatory immunity that is unrelated to the MHC or Ig genes [61]. The MHC-based adaptive immune genes emerged in an ancestral jawed vertebrate. Relevant time points in vertebrate immune system evolution are indicated in *yellow* and are discussed in the text. The current time points proposed for the origin and diversification of CD1 are based on the data calculated in Fig. 3. Thus far, CD1 has not been identified in fish or shark species, but their discovery in the future is still possible

most obvious difference might be the radical changes in anatomy (e.g., skin) and physiology that accompanied the evolutionary transition from water to land. In addition, strong selective pressures brought about by different microbial populations that exist in these two environments might also have played a role. Clearly, one of the major challenges to a broader understanding of the evolution of the immune system as a true system will be to develop and test models that encompass these broader concepts.

Lastly, there is the compelling mystery of the precise origins of the classical MHC I genes themselves from which we postulate CD1 later evolved. Based on its prevalence in living species, we assume that MHC I genes must have evolved in an early ancestral jawed vertebrate or perhaps even in a jawless fish that is now extinct. With only the genomes of two kinds of jawless fish left to examine, we may never find the immunological missing link to the MHC and CD1 antigen presenting molecules. In fact, we can only speculate that such an animal even existed since this was likely a cartilaginous species and these typically leave little trace in the fossil record. Any such animal is likely to be long extinct and with it, the evidence of the primitive form of the genes we wish to study. But there is still a chance that we will find the answer, locked away in the genome of that most elusive animal: those unknown to science. Perhaps somewhere in the dark crushing depths of the ocean where we humans, or our surrogate machines, have only just begun to explore, some small, blind eel-like creature lies curled in a rocky crevice waiting.

Acknowledgements The author would like to thank Annemieke deJong, Catherine Valentine, and Masanori Kasahara for reviewing the manuscript and Martin Flajnik for useful discussions on MHC evolution. The author also thanks Farish Jenkins for discussions of tetrapod evolution. Jenny Clack and Mike Coates kindly provided the early tetrapod drawing in Fig. 2.

References

1. The MHC sequencing consortium (1999) Complete sequence and gene map of a human major histocompatibility complex. Nature 401:921–923
2. Abi-Rached L, Gilles A, Shiina T, Pontarotti P, Inoko H (2002) Evidence of en bloc duplication in vertebrate genomes. Nat Genet 31:100–105
3. Ahlberg PE, Clack JA (2006) Palaeontology: a firm step from water to land. Nature 440:747–749
4. Albertson DG, Fishpool R, Sherrington P, Nacheva E, Milstein C (1988) Sensitive and high resolution in situ hybridization to human chromosomes using biotin labelled probes: assignment of the human thymocyte CD1 antigen genes to chromosome 1. EMBO J 7:2801–2805

5. Bartl S, Baish MA, Flajnik MF, Ohta Y (1997) Identification of class I genes in cartilaginous fish, the most ancient group of vertebrates displaying an adaptive immune response. J Immunol 159:6097–6104

6. Beck S, Trowsdale J (2000) The human major histocompatability complex: lessons from the DNA sequence. Annu Rev Genomics Hum Genet 1:117–137

7. Benton MJ (1997) Vertebrate palaeontology, 2nd edn. Chapman & Hall, New York

8. Blomme T, Vandepoele K, De Bodt S, Simillion C, Maere S, Van de Peer Y (2006) The gain and loss of genes during 600 million years of vertebrate evolution. Genome Biol 7:R43

9. Bonifacino JS, Traub LM (2003) Signals for sorting of transmembrane proteins to endosomes and lysosomes. Annu Rev Biochem 72:395–447

10. Calabi F, Jarvis JM, Martin L, Milstein C (1989) Two classes of CD1 genes. Eur J Immunol 19:285–292

11. Calabi F, Milstein C (2000) The molecular biology of CD1. Semin Immunol 12:503–509

12. Castro LF, Furlong RF, Holland PW (2004) An antecedent of the MHC-linked genomic region in amphioxus. Immunogenetics 55:782–784

13. Daeschler EB, Shubin NH, Jenkins FA Jr (2006) A Devonian tetrapod-like fish and the evolution of the tetrapod body plan. Nature 440:757–763

14. Danchin E, Vitiello V, Vienne A, Richard O, Gouret P, McDermott MF, Pontarotti P (2004) The major histocompatibility complex origin. Immunol Rev 198:216–232

15. Danchin EG, Pontarotti P (2004) Towards the reconstruction of the bilaterian ancestral pre-MHC region. Trends Genet 20:587–591

16. Dascher CC, Hiromatsu K, Xiong X, Sugita M, Buhlmann JE, Dodge IL, Lee SY, Roura-Mir C, Watts GF, Roy CJ, Behar SM, Clemens DL, Porcelli SA, Brenner MB (2002) Conservation of CD1 intracellular trafficking patterns between mammalian species. J Immunol 169:6951–6958

17. Dascher CC, Brenner MB (2003) Evolutionary constraints on CD1 structure: insights from comaparative genomic analysis. Trends Imm 24:412–418

18. Dascher CC, Brenner MB (2003) CD1 Antigen presentation and infectious disease. In: Herwald H (ed) Host response mechanisms in infectious disease. Basel Contributions to Microbiology, vol 10. Karger, pp 164–182

19. Dehal P, Boore JL (2005) Two rounds of whole genome duplication in the ancestral vertebrate. PLoS Biol 3:e314

20. Durand D, Hoberman R (2006) Diagnosing duplications – can it be done? Trends Genet 22:156–164

21. Flajnik MF, Kasahara M (2001) Comparative genomics of the MHC: glimpses into the evolution of the adaptive immune system. Immunity 15:351–162

22. Force A, Amores A, Postlethwait JH (2002) Hox cluster organization in the jawless vertebrate *Petromyzon marinus*. J Exp Zool 294:30–46

23. Gu X, Wang Y, Gu J (2002) Age distribution of human gene families shows significant roles of both large- and small-scale duplications in vertebrate evolution. Nat Genet 31:205–259

24. Hokamp K, McLysaght A, Wolfe KH (2003) The 2R hypothesis and the human genome sequence. J Struct Funct Genomics 3:95–110

25. Holland LZ, Laudet V, Schubert M (2004) The chordate amphioxus: an emerging model organism for developmental biology. Cell Mol Life Sci 61:2290–2308

26. Hughes AL (1991) Evolutionary origin and diversification of the mammalian CD1 antigen genes. Mol Biol Evol 8:185–201

27. Hughes AL, Nei M (1993) Evolutionary relationships of the classes of major histocompatibility complex genes. Immunogenetics 37:337–346

28. Hughes AL, da Silva J, Friedman R (2001) Ancient genome duplications did not structure the human Hox-bearing chromosomes. Genome Res 11:771–780

29. Hughes AL, Friedman R (2003) 2R or not 2R: testing hypotheses of genome duplication in early vertebrates. J Struct Funct Genomics 3:85–93

30. Ji Q, Luo ZX, Yuan CX, Wible JR, Zhang JP, Georgi JA (2002) The earliest known eutherian mammal. Nature 416:816–822

31. Kasahara M, Vazquez M, Sato K, McKinney EC, Flajnik MF (1992) Evolution of the major histocompatibility complex: isolation of class II A cDNA clones from the cartilaginous fish. Proc Natl Acad Sci U S A 89:6688–6692

32. Kasahara M, Hayashi M, Tanaka K, Inoko H, Sugaya K, Ikemura T, Ishibashi T (1996) Chromosomal localization of the proteasome Z subunit gene reveals an ancient chromosomal duplication involving the major histocompatibility complex. Proc Natl Acad Sci U S A 93:9096–9101

33. Kasahara M, Kandil E, Salter-Cid L, Flajnik MF (1996) Origin and evolution of the class I gene family: why are some of the mammalian class I genes encoded outside the major histocompatibility complex? Res Immunol 147:278–284; discussion 284–285

34. Kasahara M, Nakaya J, Satta Y, Takahata N (1997) Chromosomal duplication and the emergence of the adaptive immune system. Trends Genet 13:90–92

35. Katsanis N, Fitzgibbon J, Fisher EM (1996) Paralogy mapping: identification of a region in the human MHC triplicated onto human chromosomes 1 and 9 allows the prediction and isolation of novel PBX and NOTCH loci. Genomics 35:101–108

36. Kaufman J, Milne S, Gobel TW, Walker BA, Jacob JP, Auffray C, Zoorob R, Beck S (1999) The chicken B locus is a minimal essential major histocompatibility complex. Nature 401:923–925

37. Kawano T, Cui J, Koezuka Y, Toura I, Kaneko Y, Motoki K, Ueno H, Nakagawa R, Sato H, Kondo E, Koseki H, Taniguchi M (1997) CD1d-restricted and TCR-mediated activation of valpha14 NKT cells by glycosylceramides. Science 278:1626–1629

38. Klein J, O'HUigin C (1993) Composite origin of major histocompatibility complex genes. Curr Opin Genet Dev 3:923–930

39. Kruiswijk CP, Hermsen TT, Westphal AH, Savelkoul HF, Stet RJ (2002) A novel functional class I lineage in zebrafish (*Danio rerio*), carp (*Cyprinus carpio*), and large barbus (*Barbus intermedius*) showing an unusual conservation of the peptide binding domains. J Immunol 169:1936–1947

40. Kumanovics A, Takada T, Lindahl KF (2003) Genomic organization of the mammalian MHC. Annu Rev Immunol 21:629–657

41. Kumar S, Hedges SB (1998) A molecular timescale for vertebrate evolution. Nature 392:917–920

42. Lee MS (1999) Molecular clock calibrations and metazoan divergence dates. J Mol Evol 49:385–391

43. Litman GW, Cannon JP, Dishaw LJ (2005) Reconstructing immune phylogeny: new perspectives. Nat Rev Immunol 5:866–879

44. Lundin LG (1993) Evolution of the vertebrate genome as reflected in paralogous chromosomal regions in man and the house mouse. Genomics 16:1–19

45. Manolova V, Kistowska M, Paoletti S, Baltariu GM, Bausinger H, Hanau D, Mori L, De Libero G (2006) Functional CD1a is stabilized by exogenous lipids. Eur J Immunol 36:1083–1092

46. Martin AP, Naylor GJ, Palumbi SR (1992) Rates of mitochondrial DNA evolution in sharks are slow compared with mammals. Nature 357:153–155

47. Martin LH, Calabi F, Milstein C (1986) Isolation of CD1 genes: a family of major histocompatibility complex-related differentiation antigens. Proc Natl Acad Sci U S A 83:9154–9158

48. Maruoka T, Tanabe H, Chiba M, Kasahara M (2005) Chicken CD1 genes are located in the MHC: CD1 and endothelial protein C receptor genes constitute a distinct subfamily of class-I-like genes that predates the emergence of mammals. Immunogenetics 57:590–600

49. Mayer WE, Uinuk-Ool T, Tichy H, Gartland LA, Klein J, Cooper MD (2002) Isolation and characterization of lymphocyte-like cells from a lamprey. Proc Natl Acad Sci U S A 99:14350–14355

50. McLysaght A, Hokamp K, Wolfe KH (2002) Extensive genomic duplication during early chordate evolution. Nat Genet 31:200–204

51. Miller MM, Wang C, Parisini E, Coletta RD, Goto RM, Lee SY, Barral DC, Townes M, Roura-Mir C, Ford HL, Brenner MB, Dascher CC (2005) Characterization of two avian MHC-like genes reveals an ancient origin of the CD1 family. Proc Natl Acad Sci U S A 102:8674–8679

52. Moody DB, Briken V, Cheng TY, Roura-Mir C, Guy MR, Geho DH, Tykocinski ML, Besra GS, Porcelli SA (2002) Lipid length controls antigen entry into endosomal and nonendosomal pathways for CD1b presentation. Nat Immunol 3:435–442

53. Moody DB, Porcelli SA (2003) Intracellular pathways of CD1 antigen presentation. Nat Rev Immunol 3:11–22

54. Morita M, Motoki K, Akimoto K, Natori T, Sakai T, Sawa E, Yamaji K, Koezuka Y, Kobayashi E, Fukushima H (1995) Structure-activity relationship of alpha-galactosylceramides against B16-bearing mice. J Med Chem 38:2176–2187

55. Mukherjee S, Soe TT, Maxfield FR (1999) Endocytic sorting of lipid analogues differing solely in the chemistry of their hydrophobic tails. J Cell Biol 144:1271–1284

56. Novacek MJ (1997) Mammalian evolution: an early record bristling with evidence. Curr Biol 7: R489–R491

57. Ohno S (1970) Evolution by genome duplication. Springer-Verlag, New York Berlin Heidelberg

58. Ohta Y, Okamura K, McKinney EC, Bartl S, Hashimoto K, Flajnik MF (2000) Primitive synteny of vertebrate major histocompatibility complex class I and class II genes. Proc Natl Acad Sci U S A 97:4712–4717

59. Ohta Y, Goetz W, Hossain MZ, Nonaka M, Flajnik MF (2006) Ancestral organization of the MHC revealed in the amphibian Xenopus. J Immunol 176:3674–3685

60. Okamura K, Ototake M, Nakanishi T, Kurosawa Y, Hashimoto K (1997) The most primitive vertebrates with jaws possess highly polymorphic MHC class I genes comparable to those of humans. Immunity 7:777–790

61. Pancer Z, Amemiya CT, Ehrhardt GR, Ceitlin J, Gartland GL, Cooper MD (2004) Somatic diversification of variable lymphocyte receptors in the agnathan sea lamprey. Nature 430:174–180
62. Pancer Z, Cooper MD (2006) The evolution of adaptive immunity. Annu Rev Immunol 24:497–518
63. Panopoulou G, Hennig S, Groth D, Krause A, Poustka AJ, Herwig R, Vingron M, Lehrach H (2003) New evidence for genome-wide duplications at the origin of vertebrates using an amphioxus gene set and completed animal genomes. Genome Res 13:1056–1066
64. Panopoulou G, Poustka AJ (2005) Timing and mechanism of ancient vertebrate genome duplications – the adventure of a hypothesis. Trends Genet 21:559–567
65. Rast JP, Anderson MK, Strong SJ, Luer C, Litman RT, Litman GW (1997) alpha, beta, gamma, and delta T cell antigen receptor genes arose early in vertebrate phylogeny. Immunity 6:1–11
66. Salomonsen J, Sorensen MR, Marston DA, Rogers SL, Collen T, van Hateren A, Smith AL, Beal RK, Skjodt K, Kaufman J (2005) Two CD1 genes map to the chicken MHC, indicating that CD1 genes are ancient and likely to have been present in the primordial MHC. Proc Natl Acad Sci U S A 102:8668–8673
67. Sambrook JG, Figueroa F, Beck S (2005) A genome-wide survey of major histocompatibility complex (MHC) genes and their paralogues in zebrafish. BMC Genomics 6:152
68. Sato A, Figueroa F, Murray BW, Malaga-Trillo E, Zaleska-Rutczynska Z, Sultmann H, Toyosawa S, Wedekind C, Steck N, Klein J (2000) Nonlinkage of major histocompatibility complex class I and class II loci in bony fishes. Immunogenetics 51:108–116
69. Sereno PC (1999) The evolution of dinosaurs. Science 284:2137–2147
70. Shum BP, Rajalingam R, Magor KE, Azumi K, Carr WH, Dixon B, Stet RJ, Adkison MA, Hedrick RP, Parham P (1999) A divergent non-classical class I gene conserved in salmonids. Immunogenetics 49:479–490
71. Spring J (1997) Vertebrate evolution by interspecific hybridisation – are we polyploid? FEBS Lett 400:2–8
72. Spring J (2002) Genome duplication strikes back. Nat Genet 31:128–129
73. Sugita M, Grant EP, van Donselaar E, Hsu VW, Rogers RA, Peters PJ, Brenner MB (1999) Separate pathways for antigen presentation by CD1 molecules. Immunity 11:743–752
74. Sugita M, Peters PJ, Brenner MB (2000) Pathways for lipid antigen presentation by CD1 molecules: nowhere for intracellular pathogens to hide. Traffic 1:295–300
75. Suzuki T, Shin IT, Kohara Y, Kasahara M (2004) Transcriptome analysis of hagfish leukocytes: a framework for understanding the immune system of jawless fishes. Dev Comp Immunol 28:993–1003
76. Van den Elzen P, Garg S, Leon L, Brigl M, Leadbetter EA, Gumperz JE, Dascher CC, Cheng TY, Sacks FM, Illarionov PA, Besra GS, Kent SC, Moody DB, Brenner MB (2005) Apolipoprotein-mediated pathways of lipid antigen presentation. Nature 437:906–910
77. Venter JC, Adams MD, Myers EW, Li PW, Mural RJ, Sutton GG, Smith HO, Yandell M, Evans CA, Holt RA et al (2001) The sequence of the human genome. Science 291:1304–1351

78. Wang C, Perera TV, Ford HL, Dascher CC (2003) Characterization of a divergent non-classical MHC class I gene in sharks. Immunogenetics 55:57–61
79. Wang Y, Gu X (2000) Evolutionary patterns of gene families generated in the early stage of vertebrates. J Mol Evol 51:88–96
80. Wessler SR, Carrington JC (2005) The consequences of gene and genome duplication in plants. Curr Opin Plant Biol 8:119–121
81. Wolfe KH, Shields DC (1997) Molecular evidence for an ancient duplication of the entire yeast genome. Nature 387:708–713
82. Zhou D, Cantu C 3rd, Sagiv Y, Schrantz N, Kulkarni AB, Qi X, Mahuran DJ, Morales CR, Grabowski GA, Benlagha K, Savage P, Bendelac A, Teyton L (2004) Editing of CD1d-bound lipid antigens by endosomal lipid transfer proteins. Science 303:523–527

CTMI (2007) 314:27–50

Architecture of CD1 Proteins

D. M. Zajonc · I. A. Wilson (✉)

Department of Molecular Biology and Skaggs Institute of Chemical Biology, The Scripps Research Institute, 10550 North Torrey Pines Road, La Jolla, CA 92037, USA
wilson@scripps.edu

Abstract The CD1 family of glycosylated cell surface receptors binds and presents lipid antigens for T cell recognition and activation. Crystal structures of CD1-lipid complexes reveal differences in the mode of presentation of lipids by CD1 group 1 (CD1a, CD1b, and CD1c) and group 2 isoforms (CD1d). For group 1, especially CD1a and CD1b, the lipid backbone is anchored inside the hydrophobic binding grooves (lipid anchoring), whereas, for group 2 CD1d, a precise hydrogen-bonding network positions the polar ligand headgroups in well-defined orientation at the T cell recognition surface (headgroup positioning). In addition, small, but important, structural changes occur on the surface of CD1d upon binding of the potent invariant NKT cell agonist α-galactosylceramide due to increased polar interaction with the α1 and α2 helices. No such ligand-induced, conformational changes have yet been reported for any group 1 CD1 complexes, even upon binding of chemically diverse antigens, such as dual alkyl chain sphingolipids vs single alkyl chain lipopeptides. These structural data have already been successfully translated into the design of enhanced lipid activators of NKT cells and will likely continue for design of other chemotherapeutic agents or immunostimulatory compounds for a variety of immune-mediated diseases.

1
Introduction

CD1 is a family of nonpolymorphic, glycosylated cell-surface receptors that presents a growing number of structurally-diverse lipids, including mycobacterial mycolates (Beckman et al. 1994; Moody et al. 1997), lipoglycans (Sieling et al. 1995; Ernst et al. 1998; Fischer et al. 2004), diacylated sulfoglycolipids (Gilleron et al. 2004), lipopeptides (Moody et al. 2004; Van Rhijn et al. 2005), polyisoprenoids and phosphomycoketides (Moody et al. 2000; Matsunaga et al. 2004), small nonlipidic hydrophobic molecules (Van Rhijn et al. 2004), self and foreign glycosphingolipids (Kawano et al. 1997; Shamshiev et al. 1999; Miyamoto et al. 2001; Shamshiev et al. 2002; Schmieg et al. 2003; Wu et al. 2003; Goff et al. 2004; Jahng et al. 2004; Zhou et al. 2004b; Kinjo et al. 2005; Mattner et al. 2005; Wu et al. 2005; Yu et al. 2005), and phosphoglycerolipids (Joyce et al. 1998; Gumperz et al. 2000; Rauch et al. 2003; Agea et al. 2005), to specialized $\alpha\beta$ and $\gamma\delta$ T cells (Gumperz and Brenner 2001; Brigl and Brenner 2004; Das et al. 2004). The CD1 ligands that have been investigated as crystal structures of CD1–lipid complexes are represented in Fig. 1, and details about the structures are summarized in Table 1. Depending on the nature of the ligand, the corresponding CD1-restricted $\alpha\beta$ T cell or NKT cell can either contribute

Fig. 1A–E CD1 structure and crystallized ligands. **A** A representative CD1 molecule (α1, α2, and α3 domain of mCD1d) associated with β_2-microglobulin (β_2M) is shown with a semi-transparent surface and a ribbon diagram of the protein backbone. The sulfatide ligand (*yellow*) binds with the lipid backbone inserted into the binding groove, while the headgroup is exposed at the CD1d surface for T cell recognition. Asparagine-linked carbohydrate post-translational modifications of CD1 are shown in *grey*. **B** Overview of the key elements of the CD1 groove. A slice of the transparent CD1b binding groove is shown with the individual binding pockets, portals, and other structural elements depicted. **C** Crystallized CD1a ligands include natural sulfatide (Zajonc et al. 2003) and synthetic lipopeptides (Zajonc et al. 2005b), similar in structure to mycobacterial didehydroxymycobactins (Moody et al. 2004). **D** CD1b ligands include sphingolipids (ganglioside GM$_2$) (Gadola et al. 2002), phosphoglycerolipids (phosphatidylinositol) (Gadola et al. 2002), and mycobacterial mycolates (glucose monomycolate) (Batuwangala et al. 2004). Only the first of the four sugars was ordered in the crystal structure of CD1b-bound ganglioside GM$_2$. Phosphatidylinositol has been shown to activate CD1d-restricted T cells and has been eluted from and co-crystallized with CD1b. **E** Most crystallized CD1d antigens to date are galactose-containing sphingolipids, such as α-galactosylceramide (α-GalCer) (Koch et al. 2005; Zajonc et al. 2005a), α-galacturonosylceramide (Wu et al. 2006), and sulfatide (Zajonc et al. 2005c). Phosphatidylcholine was identified as an endogenously bound self-lipid (Giabbai et al. 2005)

to the killing of the microbe, initiate production of antibodies by activating B cells, or modulate various immune responses in mouse models of autoimmune diseases, allergic reactions, and tumor growth (Kronenberg 2005).

In addition to humans and mice, CD1 is found in all mammalian species studied to date, including guinea pig, sheep, cow, rhesus macaque, and chicken, as a representative of birds (Dascher et al. 1999; Brigl and Brenner 2004; Maruoka et al. 2005; Miller et al. 2005; Van Rhijn et al. 2006). However, this review will focus only on human and mouse CD1 for which crystal struc-

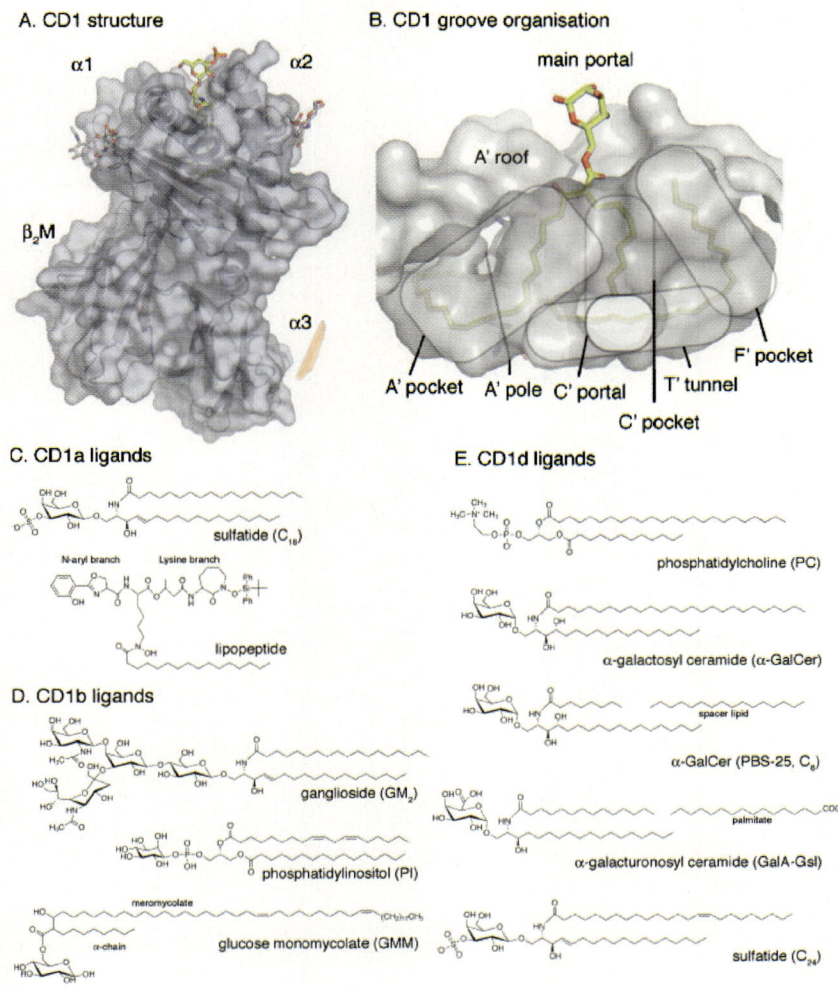

A. CD1 structure

α1   α2

β₂M

α3

B. CD1 groove organisation

main portal

A' roof

F' pocket

A' pocket   A' pole   C' portal   T' tunnel

C' pocket

C. CD1a ligands

sulfatide (C₁₈)

N-aryl branch   Lysine branch

lipopeptide

D. CD1b ligands

ganglioside (GM₂)

phosphatidylinositol (PI)

meromycolate

α-chain

glucose monomycolate (GMM)

E. CD1d ligands

phosphatidylcholine (PC)

α-galactosyl ceramide (α-GalCer)

spacer lipid

α-GalCer (PBS-25, C₈)

palmitate

α-galacturonosyl ceramide (GalA-Gsl)

sulfatide (C₂₄)

Table 1 CD1 lipid structures

Isotype (PDB code)	Ligand	Resolution (Å)	H bonds	T cell epitope	T cell antigen content	A' pocket content	F' pocket content	T' pocket content	C' pocket content	Reference
CD1a (1ONQ)	Bovine brain sulfatide extract	2.15	4	Sulfated-galactose + fatty acid tail	Yes	Sphingo-sine (C_{18})	Acyl (C_{18})	–	–	Zajonc et al. 2003
CD1a (1XZ0)	Lipopeptide (synthetic)	2.8	3	Terminal peptide (salicylic acid and cyclized lysine)	Model for DDM	Acyl (C_{16})	6 Amino acid peptide	–	–	Zajonc et al. 2005b
CD1b (1GZQ)	Phosphatidyl-inositol + detergent	2.25	1	Inositol	No	Acyl (C_{18})	C_{12}-detergent	C_{22}-detergent	Acyl (C_{16})	Gadola et al. 2002
CD1b (1GZP)	Ganglioside (GM$_2$) + detergent	2.8	1	Complex carbohydrate	Yes	Acyl (C_{18})	C_{12}-detergent	C_{22}-detergent	Sphingo-sine (C_{18})	Gadola et al. 2002
CD1b (1UQS)	Glucose monomycolate	3.0	1	Glucose	Yes	Meromy-colate (C_{50})	Meromy-colate (C_{50})	Meromy-colate (C_{50})	C_8-α-chain	Batuwangala et al. 2004
mCD1d (1CD1)	Uncharacterized endogenous lipid	2.67	-	N/A	No	Endoge-nous lipid	Endoge-nous lipid	–	–	Zeng et al. 1997
mCD1d (1ZHN)	Endogenous phosphatidyl-choline	2.8	3	Phosphoryl choline	No	Acyl (C_{24})	Acyl (C_{12})	–	–	Giabbai et al. 2005

Table 1 (continued)

Isotype (PDB code)	Ligand	Resolution (Å)	H bonds	T cell epitope	T cell antigen	A' pocket content	F' pocket content	T' pocket content	C' pocket content	Reference
hCD1d (1ZT4)	α-Galactosyl-ceramide (C_{26})	3.0	5	Galactose	Yes	Acyl (C_{26})	Phytosphingosine (C_{18})	–	–	Koch et al. 2005
mCD1d (1Z5L)	α-Galactosyl-ceramide (C_8) + palmitic acid	2.2	7	Galactose	Yes	Acyl (C_8) + Fatty acid (C_{16})	Phytosphingosine (C_{18})	–	–	Zajonc et al. 2005a
mCD1d (2FIK)	α-Galacturonosyl-ceramide + palmitic acid	1.8	5	Galacturonic acid	Yes	Acyl (C_{14}) + Fatty acid (C_{16})	Dihydro-sphingosine (C_{18})	–	–	Wu et al. 2006
mCD1d (2AKR)	cis-tetracosenoyl sulfatide	1.9	9	Sulfated galactose	Yes	Acyl ($C_{24:1}$)	Sphingosine (C_{18})	–	–	Zajonc et al. 2005c

Ten distinct CD1-lipid antigen structures have been crystallized to date. The T cell epitope represents the solvent accessible part of the bound ligand, but is not necessarily antigenic. All structural representations were prepared from the PDB coordinates listed below the CD1 isotype

tures are publicly available. The human family of CD1 antigen-presenting molecules were originally described as belonging either to group 1 (CD1a, CD1b, and CD1c) or group 2 (CD1d), while mice only express CD1d (Calabi et al. 1989). CD1e is not likely to present lipids to T cells because it is not detectable on the cell surface, but recently it has been shown to participate in intracellular lipid processing and subsequent loading onto other CD1 family members within endosomes. Therefore, CD1e constitutes a third group of CD1 molecules (Angenieux et al. 2000, 2005; de la Salle et al. 2005).

CD1 molecules are expressed as glycosylated proteins on many immune cells, including myeloid dendritic cells, thymocytes, B cells, and Langerhans cells, and they are structurally similar to their peptide-presenting, MHC class I analogs. CD1 forms a stable, noncovalently associated heterodimer with β_2-microglobulin (β_2M) of approximately 49 kDa molecular weight, including N-linked carbohydrates. Like MHC class I, the ectodomain, or CD1 heavy chain, is also organized into three domains, $\alpha1$, $\alpha2$, and $\alpha3$, and is anchored in the cell membrane by a transmembrane domain. The $\alpha1$ and $\alpha2$ domains combine to form the central binding groove of each CD1 isotype and differ significantly from one another in primary amino acid sequence and three-dimensional structure, whereas the $\alpha3$-domain is highly conserved among all isotypes and associates with β_2M (Fig. 1A). A tyrosine-based sorting motif, composed of tyrosine, two spacer amino acids, and a hydrophobic amino acid (YXXZ), is encoded on the short cytoplasmic tail of CD1b, CD1c, and CD1d to which various adaptor proteins (AP-1, AP-2, and AP-3) bind, but is absent in human CD1a (Sugita et al. 2004). As a result, CD1b–CD1d are sorted into late endosomal compartments (Jackman et al. 1998; Sugita et al. 1999, 2004; Moody and Porcelli 2003) that can load very long chain ($>C_{80}$) mycobacterial lipids, such as mycolates and acylated sulfotrehaloses onto CD1b or endogenous lipids onto CD1d (Chiu et al. 1999), whereas CD1a is mainly expressed on the cell surface, where it can capture lipids (Manolova et al. 2006), as it recycles via reinternalization into early sorting endosomes (Salamero et al. 2001).

A detailed discussion of CD1 trafficking is outlined in the chapter by M. Sugita et al., this volume, and these extensive studies of CD1 recycling lead to the general conclusion that differential sampling of the various intracellular compartments allows CD1 to effectively monitor the lipid content throughout most subcellular compartments of antigen-presenting cells. These isoform-specific differences in trafficking influence the chemical milieu and the sub-cellular co-localization of certain lipids in ways that affect antigen loading, which is required to understand the isoform-specific structural adaptations of the individual CD1 antigen binding grooves, as discussed in the following sections.

Over the past 5 years, a tremendous amount of structural data has clarified not only the architecture of the different CD1 isotypes themselves, but also their interaction with various lipid ligands (Table 1). These analyses have allowed definition of structural elements that are shared among the CD1 members, as well as isotype-specific adaptations, which have evolved to enable each CD1 isotype to differentially interact with the vast pools of endogenously synthesized and exogenously acquired lipids.

2
CD1 Binding Grooves

The CD1 binding grooves are composed of two main pockets, named A′ and F′, and are found in CD1a, CD1b, and CD1d (Zeng et al. 1997). An additional C′ pocket and T′ tunnel are unique to CD1b (Gadola et al. 2002). The central binding groove is formed by two anti-parallel α-helices (α1, α2), which sit on top of a six-stranded β-sheet platform. In comparison to their MHC counterparts, the CD1 helices are closer together and more elevated, and result in a configuration that gives rise to a deep and narrow groove, rather than the typical shallow cleft observed for binding peptides in classical MHC class I or II (Moody et al. 2005). This CD1 pocket nomenclature, first introduced for the mouse CD1d structure, originated from the terminal MHC class I pockets, which are called A and F (Zeng et al. 1997), at either end of the groove. The A′ and F′ pockets in CD1 are located in approximately equivalent locations to the A and F pockets in MHC class I, which bind the N and C-termini of peptide antigens (Zeng et al. 1997) Although the overall three-dimensional structures of individual members of the CD1 family are similar to one another, amino acid substitutions in the α1-α2 superdomain are responsible for shaping the individual grooves and for the formation of isotype-specific pockets. These pockets or tunnels are hydrophobic and reach deep inside the protein. As a result, the lipid backbone of all CD1 antigens is usually buried inside CD1 and shielded from the surrounding aqueous solvent (Fig. 1A). The different carbohydrate or peptide headgroups are exposed at the cell surface and serve as the major T cell epitopes.

2.1
CD1a

CD1a has the smallest of the binding groove with a volume of ~1,350 $Å^3$, which allows about 36 carbon atoms to fit into the groove (Zajonc et al. 2003). Compared to other isoforms, CD1a has an unusual A′ and F′ pocket structure. The general CD1 groove organization is illustrated in Fig. 1B) The A′ pocket is not directly connected to the CD1 surface and is only accessible through the more exposed F′ pocket. The CD1a-specific Arg73 points toward the α2-helix, where it forms a hydrogen bond with Thr158, thereby forming a large roof above the A′ pocket. In CD1b and mouse and human CD1d, a roof is also present, but the corresponding Tyr73 points down into the groove, so that the canopies of these isoforms are smaller and provide some direct access to the A′ pocket.

The center of the A′ pocket is defined by the A′ pole, which is formed by Val12 and Phe70 in CD1a. A similar pole is also formed by homologous residues in CD1b and CD1d, and it likely exists in CD1c, based on sequence comparisons. The two crystallized CD1a ligands, sulfatide sphingolipid (Zajonc et al. 2003) and a lipopeptide (Moody et al. 2004; Van Rhijn et al. 2005; Zajonc et al. 2005b), have to circle around this pole in order to bind optimally to the protein. This curved route leads to the observed S shape conformation of the lipid backbone in the CD1a binding groove (Fig. 2A, B). However, the A′ pole can only be partially encircled, as the A′ pocket is closed by Val28 in CD1a. Thus, the CD1a groove can be thought of as a long tube that terminates at the end of the A′ pocket and has its only entrance through the F′ pocket. Thus, the length of any alkyl chain that can be inserted into the A′ pocket is restricted by this unique, blunt-ended pocket and is predicted to correspond to approximately C_{16}. This pocket was, therefore, proposed to act as a molecular ruler to select ligands with at least one alkyl chain of a particular length (Zajonc et al. 2003). This limit presumably applies both to ligands with dual alkyl chains, such as common glycolipids, where the second alkyl chain must insert into the F′ pocket, and to lipopeptides with only one alkyl chain and a more complex peptidic headgroup, which binds in the F′ pocket in lieu of the second alkyl chain (Moody et al. 2004; Van Rhijn et al. 2005; Zajonc et al. 2005b).

Fig. 2A–J Overview of ligand binding to CD1. Ten crystal structures of CD1a, CD1b, and mouse and human CD1d in complex with different ligands have been published so far (Table 1). The CD1a and CD1b ligands are mainly bound by nonpolar van der Waals interactions between the ligand backbone and nonpolar amino acids that line the interior or the CD1 groove. These ligands are of different size and structure (**A–E**). In contrast, all of the CD1d ligands (**F–J**) are bound such that the conserved lipid antigen core structures with their polar moieties at the junction of the carbohydrate headgroup occupy a similar location with respect to the binding groove and are tightly anchored by a precise hydrogen-bonding network with hydrophilic CD1d residues. The lipid tail of CD1a-bound sulfatide (**A**) and CD1b-bound glucose monomycolate (**E**) reaches the CD1 surface for possible TCR contact, whereas all of the alkyl chains of the CD1d ligands are deeply buried inside the binding groove (**F–J**)

The crystal structure of CD1a in complex with a naturally derived sulfatide (Zajonc et al. 2003) revealed that the fatty acid tail, as well as the 3′-sulfated galactose moiety, are exposed on the CD1 surface and can both serve as antigenic T cell epitopes. The sulfated galactose headgroup is nestled between the α1-α2 helices and stabilized by four hydrogen-bond interactions with CD1a Arg73, Arg76, Ser77, and Glu154 for interaction with the TCR (Fig. 2A). Although previous studies demonstrated that the carbohydrate headgroup of sulfatides is the major TCR epitope of CD1a-restricted T cells (Shamshiev et al.

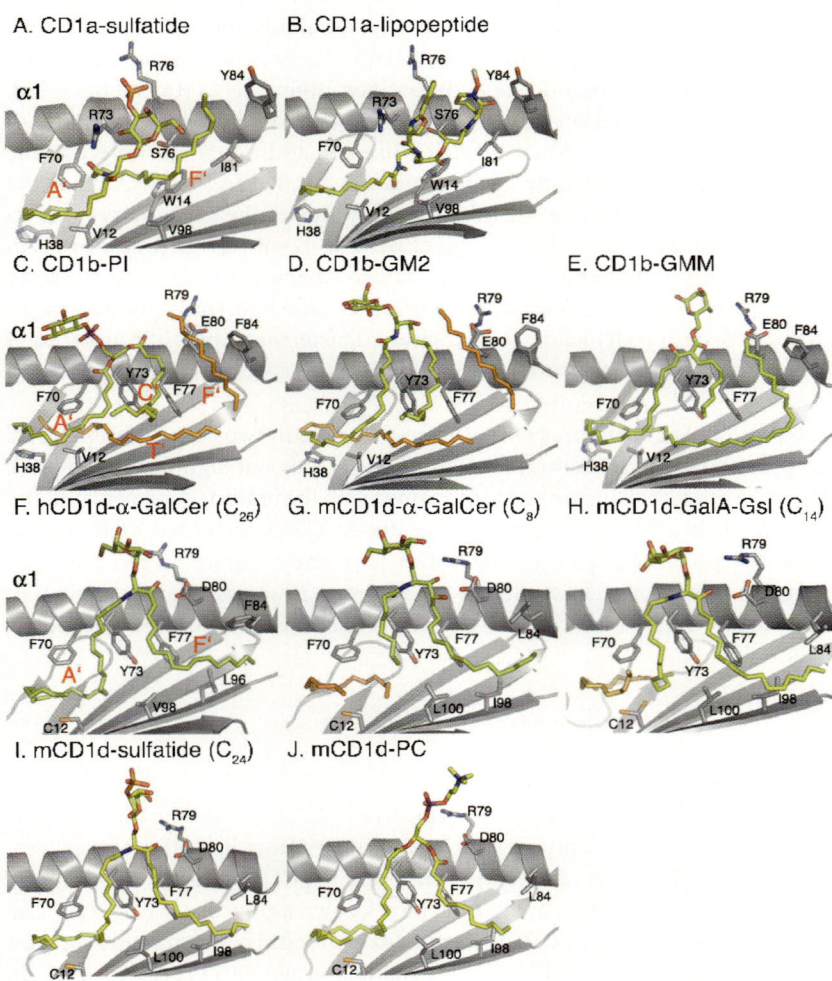

A. CD1a-sulfatide
B. CD1a-lipopeptide
C. CD1b-PI
D. CD1b-GM2
E. CD1b-GMM
F. hCD1d-α-GalCer (C_{26})
G. mCD1d-α-GalCer (C_8)
H. mCD1d-GalA-Gsl (C_{14})
I. mCD1d-sulfatide (C_{24})
J. mCD1d-PC

2002), it was later found that, in addition to the carbohydrate, the length and saturation state of the exposed fatty acid can directly affect T cell stimulation (Compostella et al. 2002), likely by direct contact with the complementarity determining regions (CDR) of their cognate TCRs. In this context, it should be noted, however, how little of the sulfatide ligand is exposed, in contrast to MHC class I or class II ligands, and that protein–protein interaction between CD1a and the TCR will likely contribute the majority of specific contacts in the CD1a–sulfatide–TCR ternary complex.

In addition to sphingolipids, didehydroxymycobactin lipopeptides have been identified as CD1a ligands (Moody et al. 2004). These lipopeptides belong to the family of iron-chelating mycobacterial mycobactins that scavenge iron with high affinity from host cells. Recently, the crystal structure of a structurally related, synthetic mycobactin antigen bound to CD1a (Zajonc et al. 2005b) illustrated that the lipopeptide is also anchored through insertion of its C_{16} alkyl chain into the A′ pocket, while the additional C_5-moiety of the N-amide linker to the lysine in the peptide is located in the junction of the A′ and F′ pockets. The N-aryl and lysine branches of the peptidic headgroup now fully occupy the F′ pocket (Fig. 2B). The N-aryl branch is located in a location that is similar to that of the sulfated galactose in the CD1a-sulfatide structure, whereas the cyclized lysine branch of the lipopeptide closely mimics the path of the fatty acid of the sulfatide. The terminal peptidic moieties of both peptide branches protrude slightly from the groove for presentation to T cells.

Overall, these structures of CD1a complexed with two very different kinds of lipids show that the overall structure of CD1a is not significantly altered, suggesting that each ligand has to maneuver into the binding groove to find the optimal fit. In addition to glycolipid epitopes, CD1a-restricted TCRs (Rosat et al. 1999; Shamshiev et al. 2002) also have the capacity to recognize, to a certain extent, peptide sequences, a feature that was previously attributed solely to MHC class I- and class II-restricted T cells (Garcia et al. 1999; Rudolph et al. 2006).

2.2
CD1b

Human CD1b has the largest binding groove ($\sim$2,200 Å^3) among the CD1 proteins described to date, and it is strikingly different from its CD1a counterpart. Not surprisingly, CD1b can bind the largest of the CD1 antigens, namely long chain ($\sim C_{80}$) fatty acids from mycobacteria known as mycolates (Fig. 1C). The first crystal structures of CD1b in complex with either phosphatidylinositol (PI) or GM$_2$ ganglioside (Fig. 2C, D) (Gadola et al. 2002) revealed that the binding groove was composed of four interconnected pockets, A′, C′, F′, and T′. The T′ tunnel was created by small, CD1b-specific glycine residues 98 and 116 on the β-sheet that cause a depression on the floor of the binding groove. The homologous residues Val98 and Leu116 in CD1a raise the β-sheet floor and occupy the space which would otherwise be the T′ tunnel in CD1a.

The alkyl chains of PI and GM2 ganglioside only occupy the A′ and C′ pockets, which corresponds to about half of the binding groove (~1,100 $Å^3$), so the F′ pocket and the T′ tunnel were occupied and stabilized by detergent molecules that were incorporated during refolding of the protein. These pocket factors are absent when other natural antigens, such as larger glucose monomycolates (GMMs) bind to CD1b (Batuwangala et al. 2004) and occupy most of the volume of the groove (Fig. 2E) (Batuwangala et al. 2004). Although these pocket factors were likely introduced during in vitro manipulation of CD1 proteins, this interesting result gave rise to the hypothesis that naturally occurring "spacer lipids" might normally bind at the bottom of the groove, beneath lipid antigens, to fill CD1 grooves or regulate antigen loading. Supporting this notion, studies carried out under physiological conditions, during the folding of the nascent polypeptide chain in the endoplasmic reticulum (ER) suggest that other spacer lipids can stabilize lipid complexes with human and mouse CD1d proteins, as subsequently seen in mouse CD1d (Zajonc et al. 2005a; Wu et al. 2006).

A second unique characteristic of CD1b is its open-ended C′ pocket. This pocket originates near the junction of the A′ and F′ pockets and descends into the groove and connects directly to the outer surface of CD1b via a structure known as the C′ portal, which is located distal to the TCR interaction surface (Fig. 1B). This second connection between the interior of the groove and the outer surface of CD1 might allow egress of alkyl chains that exceed the capacity of the C′ pocket, which corresponds approximately to C_{16}. For example, even the shorter of the two alkyl chains in glucose monomycolate can be up to C_{26}, and a recent study shows that such lipids are loaded into CD1b in an intact form, implying that they exit via the C′ portal with subsequent exposure to solvent (Cheng et al. 2006).

The individual headgroups of the CD1b-bound ligands, such as inositol phosphate of PI, the glucose of glucose monomycolate or the complex tetrasaccharide of GM_2, are exposed at the center of the binding groove and form a single hydrogen bond with CD1b. Not surprisingly, the headgroups of all crystallized CD1b antigens are not as well ordered as their respective lipid components, and for GM_2, only electron density for the first of the four sugars could be interpreted. As a result of the paucity of interaction between CD1b residues and the carbohydrate moieties of the bound ligands, these individual carbohydrate T cell epitopes project in different directions away from the binding groove and, hence, are likely recognized by the respective TCRs in a different context.

Whereas antigens with short lipid chains can readily be bound and exchanged to CD1a and CD1b proteins located at the cell surface, mycolic acids and acyl sulfotrehaloses with long alkyl chains have to be loaded onto CD1b in late endosomal or lysosomal compartments (Moody et al. 2002). The necessity for transport of antigens and CD1 proteins to late endosomal compartments for antigen loading has raised issues about how intracellular factors promote antigen insertion into CD1 grooves. The acidic pH of late endosomes relaxes both α-helices and facilitates the loading of long chain antigens onto CD1b (Moody et al. 2005). In addition, several lipid transfer proteins, such as GM_2 activator protein (Zhou et al. 2004a), saposins (Kang and Cresswell 2004; Winau et al. 2004; Zhou et al. 2004a), apolipoprotein E (van den Elzen et al. 2005), and microsomal triglyceride transfer protein (MTP) (Brozovic et al. 2004; Dougan et al. 2005) have been shown to be involved in the efficient presentation of various lipid antigens not only by CD1b, but also by CD1d.

2.3
CD1c

As no crystal structure of CD1c has yet been determined, information about its structure is inferred from amino acid sequence similarities with other CD1 proteins and the chemical structures of the antigens it presents. The known CD1c antigens are single alkyl chain phosphoisoprenoids (Moody 2001) and phosphomycoketides (Matsunaga et al. 2004), which are similar in structure, but synthesized by different enzyme systems. Whereas polyisoprenoid lipids contain repetitive isopentenyl pyrophosphate (C_5) units, the structurally similar mycoketide building block (C_5) is assembled from acetyl (C_2) and propionyl (C_3) units. As a result, every fourth carbon atom of the lipid backbone carries a methyl group. The multiple methyl branches on these antigens contrast with the unsubstituted alkyl chains that dominate the lipid anchors of antigens presented by other isoforms, implying that the individual pockets of the CD1c binding groove are unlikely to be as narrow as, for example, the A' pocket of CD1a, but instead will have a slightly greater diameter or multiple side pockets to accommodate the methyl substituents (Moody et al. 2005). As the CD1c ligands are single-chain ligands of intermediate size (C_{30-35}), the overall architecture of the CD1c binding groove may be a continuous pocket or channel, which is larger and wider than that of CD1a, but smaller and less complex than that of CD1b.

Based on sequence alignments with other CD1 isotypes, certain predictions regarding structural features of CD1c can be made based on the conservation of certain key residues. Firstly, CD1c is likely to have an A′ pocket based on the conservation of residues that form the key aspects of this structure in CD1b, CD1a, and CD1d (Phe10, His38, Trp40, Val98, Ile162, Phe169). Likewise, residues that form the central pole in the A′ pocket are conserved (Val12, Phe70), and human CD1c has a small glycine at position 28, suggesting that its A′ pocket is open-ended and can, therefore, be fully encircled by the ligand, similar to CD1b. Gly26, which is adjacent to Gly28, represents another small residue that is positioned such that it could potentially establish an alternate exit portal, similar to the C′ portal of CD1b. In all other CD1 structures, the bulkier side-chains of Asn26 or Thr26 exclude formation of this portal. In CD1c, it is predicted that the A′ pocket might be directly accessed from the solvent because it contains a phenylalanine residue at position 73, similar to mCD1d, which is unlikely to form an interdomain contact that could contribute to the A′ roof structure, in contrast to CD1a. However, no T′ tunnel is predicted for CD1c, as valine residues at positions 98 and 116 likely elevate the β-sheet floor, similar to CD1a and unlike the situation in CD1b. Also, CD1c is predicted to lack a C′ pocket as this potential space is likely occupied by Phe126 and Trp133. The F′ pocket varies in structure among the CD1 family members, and this likely holds true for CD1c, as fewer residues that line the F′ pocket in other isoforms are conserved in CD1c

2.4
CD1d

In 1997, the first crystal structure of mouse CD1d revealed the CD1 binding groove to be narrow, hydrophobic, and deep, unlike classical MHC molecules, which form a shallow and wider groove that is composed of multiple pockets (A–F) for anchoring peptide side chains (Zeng et al. 1997). Only two major pockets A′ and F′ were identified in CD1d in which additional electron density for an endogenous ligand was apparent, but not fully interpretable at that time. In 2005, this ligand was finally identified as phosphatidylcholine (PC), which was acquired during folding of the protein in the ER of insect cells (Giabbai et al. 2005). Empty binding grooves have not been observed for mouse CD1d that comes from natively folded protein, so it seems plausible that a pocket-stabilizing factor is bound until it is replaced with another antigen during the course of its trafficking through various intracellular compartments. This scenario is in part reminiscent of the binding of the invariant chain to MHC class II molecules, which is later cleaved and replaced by other, higher-affinity peptides in the MHC class II endosomal compartments.

Recently, various crystal structures have been determined for human and mouse CD1d bound to either α-galactosylceramide (α-GalCer) (Koch et al.

2005; Zajonc et al. 2005a), α-galacturonosylceramide (Wu et al. 2006), phosphatidylcholine (Giabbai et al. 2005), and sulfatide (Zajonc et al. 2005c) (Table 1 and Fig. 2F–J). Human and mouse CD1d crystal structures have also been determined with either the highly stimulatory antigen for Vα14+ NKT cells, α-galactosylceramide (Fig. 2F), or a potent variant with a truncated fatty acyl unit, PBS-25 (Fig. 2G). These structures revealed an intricate hydrogen-bonding network that is formed between the polar moieties of the sphingolipid backbone and the galactose headgroup (Fig. 3) with the hydrophilic residues of mouse CD1d (Arg79, Asp80, Asp153, and Thr156) and the corresponding residues in human CD1d. The complexity of this hydrogen-bonding network has not been observed for the group 1 CD1a and CD1b isoforms, so it appears unique to CD1d and seems to account for these antigens binding with unusually high affinity. Thus, in contrast to group 1 CD1, where the ligand binding is dominated by extensive hydrophobic and van der Waals interactions, CD1d ligands appear to be oriented initially in the binding groove by this hydrogen bond network, rather than the initial encounter being dictated primarily by insertion of the alkyl chains until they optimally fill the groove, as observed for the A′ pocket of CD1a. We suggest that these two separate binding processes could be defined as lipid-anchoring and headgroup-anchoring, respectively. Consistent with these observations, the electron density for the headgroup of all CD1d bound ligands is much better defined than those of the group 1 CD1 bound ligands.

Consistent with this headgroup anchoring hypothesis, mutational studies (Kamada et al. 2001) have suggested that the crucial residues in CD1d that are necessary for NKT cell activation either participate in this hydrogen-bond network with the ligand and thereby stabilize the antigenic headgroup for proper TCR engagement (Arg79, Asp80, Asp153, and Thr156) or are predicted to directly interact with the TCR (Glu83, Arg79) to facilitate CD1–lipid antigen–TCR ternary complex formation (Kamada et al. 2001). Comparison of the hydrogen-bond networks that CD1d establishes with a variety of ligands has led to identification of several CD1 residues that are conserved in interactions with the ligand and can, therefore, be thought of as core residues (Fig. 3). Aspartate at position 80 in the α1-helix interacts with the 3′-OH group of the various sphingosine species, whereas aspartate at position 153 in mouse CD1d or position 151 in human CD1d consistently stabilizes the various headgroups through interaction with either the 2′- and 3′-OH groups of galactose or the 2′-OH of 3′-sulfated galactose. Threonine at position 156 in mouse CD1d or the homologous threonine at position 154 in human CD1d interacts with the oxygen of the O-glycosidic linkage and with the sphingosine backbone nitrogen. Similar polar interactions are formed between CD1d and phosphatidylcholine (Fig. 3E). Additional residues, such as arginine at

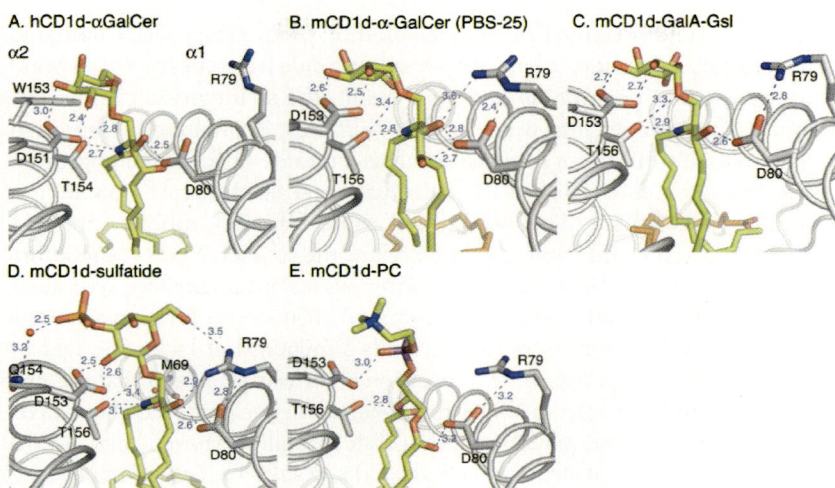

Fig. 3A–E CD1d hydrogen-bonding network. CD1d ligands (*yellow sticks*) are stabilized by hydrogen bonds (*blue dashed lines*) between the α1 and α2-helices of either human CD1d (**A**) or mouse CD1d (**B–E**). The invariant NKT cell ligands α-galactosylceramide (**A** and **B**) and α-galacturonosylceramide (**C**) are shown in the *top row* and reveal a slightly different lateral position of the galactose, due to differences in the corresponding hydrogen-bond interactions with CD1d residues or to different protein side chains that interact with the galactose of α-galactosylceramide (Trp153 in human CD1d and Gly155 in mouse CD1d). The sulfatide ligand (**D**) is presented differently, due to its β-glycosidic linkage and the concomitant alteration in hydrogen-bond interactions. However, the same core set of CD1d residues is involved in interacting with the ligand in all five structures (Asp80, Asp153, and Thr156 for mouse and Asp80, Asp151, and Thr154 for human CD1d)

position 79 in mouse CD1d, can provide additional specificity for the ligand, but are also in a suitable location for interacting with the incoming TCR.

Interestingly, mouse and human CD1d are very similar in structure and in their binding of α-galactosylceramide. The only difference between human and mouse CD1d occurs around tryptophan at position 153 in the human isoform, which raises and tilts the galactose headgroup slightly, whereas the corresponding mouse residue is a much smaller glycine (Gly155), which does not influence ligand binding (Fig. 3A, B). Both α-galactosylceramide and α-galacturonosylceramide activate NKT cells, but α-galactosylceramide is a much more potent antigen. Most of the polar interactions between the two ligands and CD1d residues are conserved; however, slight structural differences, such as the lack of the 4′-OH group in α-galacturonosylceramide, affect the fine positioning of the ligand in the binding groove (Fig. 2H). Compared to α-galactosylceramide, α-galacturonosylceramide lacks the hydrogen bond with aspartate at position 80 and, as a result, the sphingosine chain is inserted slightly deeper into the F′ pocket (Fig. 3C). This altered interaction results in an overall tilt of α-galacturonosylceramide in the binding groove, which leads to lateral shift of the galacturonosyl headgroup by about 1 Å along the CD1 surface. This tilt in turn could lead to a different interaction with the TCR and, hence, could explain the weaker T cell stimulation. Interestingly, α-galactosylceramide induces slight, but important, structural changes in the α1-helix, which causes more intimate association with the ligand. As α-galacturonosylceramide binds similarly, but lacks one hydrogen bond with the key aspartate at position 80, it was proposed that the two hydrogen bonds between the 3′-OH and 4′-OH of the ceramide backbone of α-galactosylceramide and Asp80 are responsible for pulling the α1-helix toward the ligand. The induced structural changes also result in a formation of a roof above the F′ pocket, which increases the T cell recognition surface and could provide additional specificity for ligand discrimination. Overall, these extensive interactions between the ligand headgroup and the α1-α2 superdomain show how headgroup anchoring results in an induced fit with CD1d.

In contrast to these two α-linked glycosphingolipids, sulfatide has a β-linkage between the galactose and the sphingosine backbone. Therefore, the presentation and exposure of its sulfogalactosyl headgroup is completely different. The headgroup projects away from the binding groove (Fig. 3D), whereas the above-described α-linked ligands form more extensive contacts with aspartate at position 153 of the α2-helix of CD1d (Fig. 3A–C). Not surprisingly, sulfatide is not an antigen recognized by the canonical TCR of invariant NKT cells, but rather activates another subset of noninvariant NKT cells (Jahng et al. 2004) in the mouse model of experimental autoimmune encephalomyelitis (EAE) as well as human CD1a-restricted T cells from human MS patients (Shamshiev et al. 1999, 2002). Understanding the molecular details of the underlying interactions among CD1a or CD1d and sulfatide-reactive T cells might provide a rationale for the design of chemotherapeutic agents that could control the initiation of T cell-mediated autoimmune diseases.

A second interesting feature was the observation of an electron density in the A′ pocket of the short-chain α-galactosylceramide-CD1d structure (Zajonc et al. 2005a), which did not correspond to α-galactosylceramide. This second ligand density was later determined to be an endogenously acquired palmitic acid (Wu et al. 2006) and demonstrates that relatively short CD1 ligands can be complemented by pocket stabilizing factors in order to fully fill the groove. These endogenously bound factors might then give rise to different fine positioning of the ligand and thereby have an indirect effect on antigen presentation and recognition by T cells. Furthermore, several variants of α-galactosylceramide that express truncated alkyl chains, such as OCH (Miyamoto et al. 2001), PBS-25 (Goff et al. 2004), and a di-unsaturated fatty acid ($C_{20:2}$) α-galactosylceramide (Yu et al. 2005) do indeed modulate the initial T_H0 response toward an accentuated T_H2-like phenotype. However, the mechanism of presentation of these four ligands is likely to be very similar, as all of the key structural elements that would maintain the hydrogen-bond network with CD1d are preserved. Therefore, it is likely that the altered cytokine production in response to these antigens could be a result of the different loading properties or different cellular distribution, which can lead to different signaling strengths of these α-galactosylceramide variants (Oki et al. 2004), rather than structural changes in the ligand presentation or TCR interaction.

2.5
CD1e

The molecular structure of CD1e has not yet been determined, but great progress has been achieved in characterizing the intracellular function of this molecule. CD1e is expressed as several alternatively spliced proteins in dendritic cells (Angenieux et al. 2000). The intracellular trafficking of CD1e was extensively studied in mature and immature dendritic cells (Angenieux et al. 2005) and, finally, its involvement in the lysosomal processing of complex phosphatidylinositol mannosides (PIMs), necessary for T cell presentation of PIMs by CD1b, was established (de la Salle et al. 2005).

CD1e is cleaved into a soluble, active form in CD1b$^+$ lysosomes of mature DCs, where it is proposed to act as a lipid chaperone. A recent model suggests that CD1e binds glycolipids, such as phosphatidylinositol hexamannosides (PIM-6), in a central cavity, similar to the binding of other CD1 members. Unlike the presentation of these lipids at the cell surface, as in other CD1 isotypes, CD1e activates α-mannosidases that further process hexamannosylated PIM-6 to di-mannosylated PIM-2, which can then subsequently be presented by CD1b (de la Salle et al. 2005).

Therefore, CD1e does not itself display lipids at the cell surface, but instead its function is to facilitate glycolipid processing and presentation by other CD1 members similar to lipid transfer proteins.

3
T Cell Receptors

The crystal structures of invariant human Vα24 iNKT cell TCRs, paired with Vβ11 (Gadola et al. 2006; Kjer-Nielsen et al. 2006) and other α-galactosylceramide reactive, non-Vα24$^+$ TCRs (Gadola et al. 2006) have been reported. Although ternary CD1-lipid-TCR crystal structures are not available, docking models based on available MHC–peptide–TCR structures have adapted the canonical diagonal TCR orientation to predict how NKT cell TCRs bind to CD1d. In these models, CDR3α, CDR3β and CDR1β contact the ligand, while CDR2β binds to the α1-helix (Gadola et al. 2006). One of the two crystallized Vα24 TCRs displayed a positively charged, preformed binding pocket composed of residues from CDR1α and CDR3α from the α-chain and CD1β CDR3β from the β-chain, which could accommodate and interact with the galactose headgroup of α-galactosylceramide (Kjer-Nielsen et al. 2006). In addition, the positive charge of the TCR binding pocket would be well suited to neutralize the additional negative charge of the galacturonosyl headgroup. Although these structures give important structural insights into the NKT cell recognition of CD1d-presented glycolipids, the current lack of a CD1α-galactosylceramide–TCR ternary complex makes it difficult to formulate detailed predictions about glycolipid recognition, especially to explain the observed differences in biological response to α-galactosylceramide and α-galacturonosylceramide.

4
Conclusion

CD1 members bind a wide variety of lipids, glycolipids, and lipopeptides within their hydrophobic binding pockets and present the polar headgroups of the ligands for T cell recognition (De Libero and Mori 2005; Moody et al. 2005). Some lipids can be presented by all CD1 isotypes, including sulfatide (Shamshiev et al. 2002), whereas other glycolipids, such as glucose monomycolate, can only be presented by one isotype, CD1b, due to their size. However, through determination of the structures of various CD1d–glycolipid complexes, differences in the binding and presentation of ligands between group1 CD1 and group2 CD1 is now being elucidated. For group 1 CD1, most of the binding energy and specificity appears to be derived from extensive, nonpolar, van der Waals contacts between hydrophobic CD1 residues and the alkyl chain of the bound ligand. While this scenario is in part true for ligands that are presented by CD1d, additional binding energy and specificity is conferred by an extensive hydrogen-bonding network between the headgroup of the ligand and several highly conserved CD1d residues. As a result, most of the T cell epitopes are presented in a predetermined orientation, which gives rise to exceptionally ordered electron density that is not observed with CD1a or CD1b bound ligands. This positioning of the T cell epitope can facilitate T cell recognition, which could explain the high potency of the NKT cell ligands that perhaps influences the time course of NKT cell activation, which leads to the rapid production of IL-4 and IFN-γ within 4 h after TCR ligation.

With the identification of a pocket-stabilizing factor, many interesting questions arise. Firstly, is there also a spacer lipid for the F′ pocket and how do these factors compare with the identification of phosphatidylcholine as an endogenously bound ligand in a similar expression system? How are these factors removed from the groove upon ligand binding? Are lipid transfer proteins involved and, if so, what exact role do these proteins have in lipid loading and unloading? Is there, for example, a transient CD1–saposin complex that can be captured and examined structurally to gain insight into the lipid loading mechanism?

One of the most intriguing questions regarding T cell recognition deals with the differences between invariant and variant TCRs. How is it possible that some TCRs are so specific for their presented T cell epitope, such as the CD1b-restricted T cell line LDN5 that recognizes glucose monomycolate, but not if the carbohydrate epitope is changed from glucose to either mannose or galactose (Moody et al. 1997)? On the other hand, several antigens with differing chemical structures have recently been identified, which all have the capacity to stimulate the same invariant Vα14 expressing T cells. It is not yet clear how the model antigen α-galactosylceramide (Kawano et al. 1997), microbial α-glycuronosylceramides from *Sphingomonas* (Kinjo et al. 2005; Mattner et al. 2005; Sriram et al. 2005), the self-antigen isoglobotrihexosylceramide (iGB3) (Zhou et al. 2004b), and possibly mycobacterial phosphatidylinositol-tetramannoside (PIM-4) (Fischer et al. 2004) can use their markedly differing glycans to activate the same types of TCRs. Therefore, the structural determination of the CD1–glycolipid complexes bound to their respective TCRs is the next major step in elucidating the immunological properties of lipid-recognizing T cells in human diseases.

References

Agea E, Russano A, Bistoni O, Mannucci R, Nicoletti I, Corazzi L, Postle AD, De Libero G, Porcelli SA, Spinozzi F (2005) Human CD1-restricted T cell recognition of lipids from pollens. J Exp Med 202:295–308

Angenieux C, Salamero J, Fricker D, Cazenave JP, Goud B, Hanau D, de La Salle H (2000) Characterization of CD1e, a third type of CD1 molecule expressed in dendritic cells. J Biol Chem 275:37757–37764

Angenieux C, Fraisier V, Maitre B, Racine V, van der Wel N, Fricker D, Proamer F, Sachse M, Cazenave JP, Peters P, Goud B, Hanau D, Sibarita JB, Salamero J, de la Salle H (2005) The cellular pathway of CD1e in immature and maturing dendritic cells. Traffic 6:286–302

Batuwangala T, Shepherd D, Gadola SD, Gibson KJ, Zaccai NR, Fersht AR, Besra GS, Cerundolo V, Jones EY (2004) The crystal structure of human CD1b with a bound bacterial glycolipid. J Immunol 172:2382–2388

Beckman EM, Porcelli SA, Morita CT, Behar SM, Furlong ST, Brenner MB (1994) Recognition of a lipid antigen by CD1-restricted $\alpha\beta+$ T cells. Nature 372:691–694

Brigl M, Brenner MB (2004) CD1: Antigen presentation and T cell function. Annu Rev Immunol 22:817–890

Brozovic S, Nagaishi T, Yoshida M, Betz S, Salas A, Chen D, Kaser A, Glickman J, Kuo T, Little A, Morrison J, Corazza N, Kim JY, Colgan SP, Young SG, Exley M, Blumberg RS (2004) CD1d function is regulated by microsomal triglyceride transfer protein. Nat Med 10:535–539

Calabi F, Jarvis JM, Martin L, Milstein C (1989) Two classes of CD1 genes. Eur J Immunol 19:285–292

Cheng TY, Relloso M, Van Rhijn I, Young DC, Besra GS, Briken V, Zajonc DM, Wilson IA, Porcelli S, Moody DB (2006) Role of lipid trimming and CD1 groove size in cellular antigen presentation. EMBO J 25:2989–2999

Chiu YH, Jayawardena J, Weiss A, Lee D, Park SH, Dautry-Varsat A, Bendelac A (1999) Distinct subsets of CD1d-restricted T cells recognize self-antigens loaded in different cellular compartments. J Exp Med 189:103–110

Compostella F, Franchini L, De Libero G, Palmisano G, Ronchetti F, Panza L (2002) CD1a-binding glycosphingolipids stimulating human autoreactive T-cells: synthesis of a family of sulfatides differing in the acyl chain moiety. Tetrahedron 58:8703–8708

Das H, Sugita M, Brenner MB (2004) Mechanisms of $V\delta1$ $\gamma\delta$ T cell activation by microbial components. J Immunol 172:6578–6586

Dascher CC, Hiromatsu K, Naylor JW, Brauer PP, Brown KA, Storey JR, Behar SM, Kawasaki ES, Porcelli SA, Brenner MB, LeClair KP (1999) Conservation of a CD1 multigene family in the guinea pig. J Immunol 163:5478–5488

De la Salle H, Mariotti S, Angenieux C, Gilleron M, Garcia-Alles LF, Malm D, Berg T, Paoletti S, Maitre B, Mourey L, Salamero J, Cazenave JP, Hanau D, Mori L, Puzo G, De Libero G (2005) Assistance of microbial glycolipid antigen processing by CD1e. Science 310:1321–1324

De Libero G, Mori L (2005) Recognition of lipid antigens by T cells. Nat Rev Immunol 5:485–496

Dougan SK, Salas A, Rava P, Agyemang A, Kaser A, Morrison J, Khurana A, Kronenberg M, Johnson C, Exley M, Hussain MM, Blumberg RS (2005) Microsomal triglyceride transfer protein lipidation and control of CD1d on antigen-presenting cells. J Exp Med 202:529–539

Ernst WA, Maher J, Cho S, Niazi KR, Chatterjee D, Moody DB, Besra GS, Watanabe Y, Jensen PE, Porcelli SA, Kronenberg M, Modlin RL (1998) Molecular interaction of CD1b with lipoglycan antigens. Immunity 8:331–340

Fischer K, Scotet E, Niemeyer M, Koebernick H, Zerrahn J, Maillet S, Hurwitz R, Kursar M, Bonneville M, Kaufmann SH, Schaible UE (2004) Mycobacterial phosphatidylinositol mannoside is a natural antigen for CD1d-restricted T cells. Proc Natl Acad Sci U S A 101:10685–10690

Gadola SD, Zaccai NR, Harlos K, Shepherd D, Castro-Palomino JC, Ritter G, Schmidt RR, Jones EY, Cerundolo V (2002) Structure of human CD1b with bound ligands at 2.3 Å, a maze for alkyl chains. Nat Immunol 3:721–726

Gadola SD, Koch M, Marles-Wright J, Lissin NM, Shepherd D, Matulis G, Harlos K, Villiger PM, Stuart DI, Jakobsen BK, Cerundolo V, Jones EY (2006) Structure and binding kinetics of three different human CD1d-α-galactosylceramide-specific T cell receptors. J Exp Med 203:699–710

Garcia KC, Teyton L, Wilson IA (1999) Structural basis of T cell recognition. Annu Rev Immunol 17:369–397

Giabbai B, Sidobre S, Crispin MD, Sanchez-Ruiz Y, Bachi A, Kronenberg M, Wilson IA, Degano M (2005) Crystal structure of mouse CD1d bound to the self ligand phosphatidylcholine: a molecular basis for NKT cell activation. J Immunol 175:977–984

Gilleron M, Stenger S, Mazorra Z, Wittke F, Mariotti S, Bohmer G, Prandi J, Mori L, Puzo G, De Libero G (2004) Diacylated sulfoglycolipids are novel mycobacterial antigens stimulating CD1-restricted T cells during infection with *Mycobacterium tuberculosis*. J Exp Med 199:649–659

Goff RD, Gao Y, Mattner J, Zhou D, Yin N, Cantu C 3rd, Teyton L, Bendelac A, Savage PB (2004) Effects of lipid chain lengths in α-galactosylceramides on cytokine release by natural killer T cells. J Am Chem Soc 126:13602–13603

Gumperz JE, Brenner MB (2001) CD1-specific T cells in microbial immunity. Curr Opin Immunol 13:471–478

Gumperz JE, Roy C, Makowska A, Lum D, Sugita M, Podrebarac T, Koezuka Y, Porcelli SA, Cardell S, Brenner MB, Behar SM (2000) Murine CD1d-restricted T cell recognition of cellular lipids. Immunity 12:211–221

Jackman RM, Stenger S, Lee A, Moody DB, Rogers RA, Niazi KR, Sugita M, Modlin RL, Peters PJ, Porcelli SA (1998) The tyrosine-containing cytoplasmic tail of CD1b is essential for its efficient presentation of bacterial lipid antigens. Immunity 8:341–351

Jahng A, Maricic I, Aguilera C, Cardell S, Halder RC, Kumar V (2004) Prevention of autoimmunity by targeting a distinct, noninvariant CD1d-reactive T cell population reactive to sulfatide. J Exp Med 199:947–957

Joyce S, Woods AS, Yewdell JW, Bennink JR, De Silva AD, Boesteanu A, Balk SP, Cotter RJ, Brutkiewicz RR (1998) Natural ligand of mouse CD1d1: cellular glyco-sylphosphatidylinositol. Science 279:1541–1544

Kamada N, Iijima H, Kimura K, Harada M, Shimizu E, Motohashi S, Kawano T, Shinkai H, Nakayama T, Sakai T, Brossay L, Kronenberg M, Taniguchi M (2001) Crucial amino acid residues of mouse CD1d for glycolipid ligand presentation to Vα14 NKT cells. Int Immunol 13:853–861

Kang SJ, Cresswell P (2004) Saposins facilitate CD1d-restricted presentation of an exogenous lipid antigen to T cells. Nat Immunol 5:175–181

Kawano T, Cui J, Koezuka Y, Toura I, Kaneko Y, Motoki K, Ueno H, Nakagawa R, Sato H, Kondo E, Koseki H, Taniguchi M (1997) CD1d-restricted and TCR-mediated activation of Vα14 NKT cells by glycosylceramides. Science 278:1626–1629

Kinjo Y, Wu D, Kim G, Xing GW, Poles MA, Ho DD, Tsuji M, Kawahara K, Wong CH, Kronenberg M (2005) Recognition of bacterial glycosphingolipids by natural killer T cells. Nature 434:520–525

Kjer-Nielsen L, Borg NA, Pellicci DG, Beddoe T, Kostenko L, Clements CS, Williamson NA, Smyth MJ, Besra GS, Reid HH, Bharadwaj M, Godfrey DI, Rossjohn J, McCluskey J (2006) A structural basis for selection and cross-species reactivity of the semi-invariant NKT cell receptor in CD1d/glycolipid recognition. J Exp Med 203:661–673

Koch M, Stronge VS, Shepherd D, Gadola SD, Mathew B, Ritter G, Fersht AR, Besra GS, Schmidt RR, Jones EY, Cerundolo V (2005) The crystal structure of human CD1d with and without α-galactosylceramide. Nat Immunol 8:819–826

Kronenberg M (2005) Toward an understanding of NKT cell biology: progress and paradoxes. Annu Rev Immunol 23:877–900

Manolova V, Kistowska M, Paoletti S, Baltariu GM, Bausinger H, Hanau D, Mori L, De Libero G (2006) Functional CD1a is stabilized by exogenous lipids. Eur J Immunol 36:1083–1092

Maruoka T, Tanabe H, Chiba M, Kasahara M (2005) Chicken CD1 genes are located in the MHC: CD1 and endothelial protein C receptor genes constitute a distinct subfamily of class-I-like genes that predates the emergence of mammals. Immunogenetics 57:590–600

Matsunaga I, Bhatt A, Young DC, Cheng TY, Eyles SJ, Besra GS, Briken V, Porcelli SA, Costello CE, Jacobs WR Jr, Moody DB (2004) *Mycobacterium tuberculosis* pks12 produces a novel polyketide presented by CD1c to T cells. J Exp Med 200:1559–1569

Mattner J, Debord KL, Ismail N, Goff RD, Cantu C 3rd, Zhou D, Saint-Mezard P, Wang V, Gao Y, Yin N, Hoebe K, Schneewind O, Walker D, Beutler B, Teyton L, Savage PB, Bendelac A (2005) Exogenous and endogenous glycolipid antigens activate NKT cells during microbial infections. Nature 434:525–529

Miller MM, Wang C, Parisini E, Coletta RD, Goto RM, Lee SY, Barral DC, Townes M, Roura-Mir C, Ford HL, Brenner MB, Dascher CC (2005) Characterization of two avian MHC-like genes reveals an ancient origin of the CD1 family. Proc Natl Acad Sci U S A 102:8674–8679

Miyamoto K, Miyake S, Yamamura T (2001) A synthetic glycolipid prevents autoimmune encephalomyelitis by inducing T_H2 bias of natural killer T cells. Nature 413:531–534

Moody DB (2001) Polyisoprenyl glycolipids as targets of CD1-mediated T cell responses. Cell Mol Life Sci 58:1461–1474

Moody DB, Porcelli SA (2003) Intracellular pathways of CD1 antigen presentation. Nat Rev Immunol 3:11–22

Moody DB, Reinhold BB, Guy MR, Beckman EM, Frederique DE, Furlong ST, Ye S, Reinhold VN, Sieling PA, Modlin RL, Besra GS, Porcelli SA (1997) Structural requirements for glycolipid antigen recognition by CD1b-restricted T cells. Science 278:283–286

Moody DB, Ulrichs T, Muhlecker W, Young DC, Gurcha SS, Grant E, Rosat JP, Brenner MB, Costello CE, Besra GS, Porcelli SA (2000) CD1c-mediated T-cell recognition of isoprenoid glycolipids in *Mycobacterium tuberculosis* infection. Nature 404:884–888

Moody DB, Briken V, Cheng TY, Roura-Mir C, Guy MR, Geho DH, Tykocinski ML, Besra GS, Porcelli SA (2002) Lipid length controls antigen entry into endosomal and nonendosomal pathways for CD1b presentation. Nat Immunol 3:435–442

Moody DB, Young DC, Cheng TY, Rosat JP, Roura-Mir C, O'Connor PB, Zajonc DM, Walz A, Miller MJ, Levery SB, Wilson IA, Costello CE, Brenner MB (2004) T cell activation by lipopeptide antigens. Science 303:527–531

Moody DB, Zajonc DM, Wilson IA (2005) Anatomy of CD1-lipid antigen complexes. Nat Rev Immunol 5:387–399

Oki S, Chiba A, Yamamura T, Miyake S (2004) The clinical implication and molecular mechanism of preferential IL-4 production by modified glycolipid-stimulated NKT cells. J Clin Invest 113:1631–1640

Rauch J, Gumperz J, Robinson C, Skold M, Roy C, Young DC, Lafleur M, Moody DB, Brenner MB, Costello CE, Behar SM (2003) Structural features of the acyl chain determine self-phospholipid antigen recognition by a CD1d-restricted invariant NKT (iNKT) cell. J Biol Chem 278:47508–47515

Rosat JP, Grant EP, Beckman EM, Dascher CC, Sieling PA, Frederique D, Modlin RL, Porcelli SA, Furlong ST, Brenner MB (1999) CD1-restricted microbial lipid antigen-specific recognition found in the CD8+ αβ-T cell pool. J Immunol 162:366–371

Rudolph MG, Stanfield RL, Wilson IA (2006) How TCRs bind MHCs, peptides, and coreceptors. Annu Rev Immunol 24:419–466

Salamero J, Bausinger H, Mommaas AM, Lipsker D, Proamer F, Cazenave JP, Goud B, de la Salle H, Hanau D (2001) CD1a molecules traffic through the early recycling endosomal pathway in human Langerhans cells. J Invest Dermatol 116:401–408

Schmieg J, Yang G, Franck RW, Tsuji M (2003) Superior protection against malaria and melanoma metastases by a C-glycoside analogue of the natural killer T cell ligand α-galactosylceramide. J Exp Med 198:1631–1641

Shamshiev A, Donda A, Carena I, Mori L, Kappos L, De Libero G (1999) Self glycolipids as T-cell autoantigens. Eur J Immunol 29:1667–1675

Shamshiev A, Gober HJ, Donda A, Mazorra Z, Mori L, De Libero G (2002) Presentation of the same glycolipid by different CD1 molecules. J Exp Med 195:1013–1021

Sieling PA, Chatterjee D, Porcelli SA, Prigozy TI, Mazzaccaro RJ, Soriano T, Bloom BR, Brenner MB, Kronenberg M, Brennan PJ et al (1995) CD1-restricted T cell recognition of microbial lipoglycan antigens. Science 269:227–230

Sriram V, Du W, Gervay-Hague J, Brutkiewicz RR (2005) Cell wall glycosphingolipids of Sphingomonas paucimobilis are CD1d-specific ligands for NKT cells. Eur J Immunol 35:1692–1701

Sugita M, Grant EP, van Donselaar E, Hsu VW, Rogers RA, Peters PJ, Brenner MB (1999) Separate pathways for antigen presentation by CD1 molecules. Immunity 11:743–752

Sugita M, Cernadas M, Brenner MB (2004) New insights into pathways for CD1-mediated antigen presentation. Curr Opin Immunol 16:90–95

Van den Elzen P, Garg S, Leon L, Brigl M, Leadbetter EA, Gumperz JE, Dascher CC, Cheng TY, Sacks FM, Illarionov PA, Besra GS, Kent SC, Moody DB, Brenner MB (2005) Apolipoprotein-mediated pathways of lipid antigen presentation. Nature 437:906–910

Van Rhijn I, Young DC, Im JS, Levery SB, Illarionov PA, Besra GS, Porcelli SA, Gumperz J, Cheng TY, Moody DB (2004) CD1d-restricted T cell activation by nonlipidic small molecules. Proc Natl Acad Sci U S A 101:13578–13583

Van Rhijn I, Zajonc DM, Wilson IA, Moody DB (2005) T-cell activation by lipopeptide antigens. Curr Opin Immunol 17:222–229

Van Rhijn I, Koets AP, Im JS, Piebes D, Reddington F, Besra GS, Porcelli SA, van Eden W, Rutten VP (2006) The bovine CD1 family contains group 1 CD1 proteins, but no functional CD1d. J Immunol 176:4888–4893

Winau F, Schwierzeck V, Hurwitz R, Remmel N, Sieling PA, Modlin RL, Porcelli SA, Brinkmann V, Sugita M, Sandhoff K, Kaufmann SH, Schaible UE (2004) Saposin C is required for lipid presentation by human CD1b. Nat Immunol 5:169–174

Wu DY, Segal NH, Sidobre S, Kronenberg M, Chapman PB (2003) Cross-presentation of disialoganglioside GD3 to natural killer T cells. J Exp Med 198:173–181

Wu D, Xing GW, Poles MA, Horowitz A, Kinjo Y, Sullivan B, Bodmer-Narkevitch V, Plettenburg O, Kronenberg M, Tsuji M, Ho DD, Wong CH (2005) Bacterial glycolipids and analogs as antigens for CD1d-restricted NKT cells. Proc Natl Acad Sci U S A 102:1351–1356

Wu D, Zajonc DM, Fujio M, Sullivan BA, Kinjo Y, Kronenberg M, Wilson IA, Wong CH (2006) Design of NKT-cell activators: structure and function of a microbial glycosphingolipid bound to mouse CD1d. PNAS 103:3972–3977

Yu KO, Im JS, Molano A, Dutronc Y, Illarionov PA, Forestier C, Fujiwara N, Arias I, Miyake S, Yamamura T, Chang YT, Besra GS, Porcelli SA (2005) Modulation of CD1d-restricted NKT cell responses by using N-acyl variants of α-galactosylceramides. Proc Natl Acad Sci U S A 102:3383–3388

Zajonc DM, Elsliger MA, Teyton L, Wilson IA (2003) Crystal structure of CD1a in complex with a sulfatide self antigen at a resolution of 2.15 A. Nat Immunol 4:808–815

Zajonc DM, Cantu C, Mattner J, Zhou D, Savage PB, Bendelac A, Wilson IA, Teyton L (2005a) Structure and function of a potent agonist for the semi-invariant natural killer T cell receptor. Nat Immunol 8:810–818

Zajonc DM, Crispin MD, Bowden TA, Young DC, Cheng TY, Hu J, Costello CE, Rudd PM, Dwek RA, Miller MJ, Brenner MB, Moody DB, Wilson IA (2005b) Molecular mechanism of lipopeptide presentation by CD1a. Immunity 22:209–219

Zajonc DM, Maricic I, Wu D, Halder R, Roy K, Wong CH, Kumar V, Wilson IA (2005c) Structural basis for CD1d presentation of a sulfatide derived from myelin and its implications for autoimmunity. J Exp Med 202:1517–1526

Zeng Z, Castano AR, Segelke BW, Stura EA, Peterson PA, Wilson IA (1997) Crystal structure of mouse CD1: an MHC-like fold with a large hydrophobic binding groove. Science 277:339–345

Zhou D, Cantu C 3rd, Sagiv Y, Schrantz N, Kulkarni AB, Qi X, Mahuran DJ, Morales CR, Grabowski GA, Benlagha K, Savage P, Bendelac A, Teyton L (2004a) Editing of CD1d-bound lipid antigens by endosomal lipid transfer proteins. Science 303:523–527

Zhou D, Mattner J, Cantu C 3rd, Schrantz N, Yin N, Gao Y, Sagiv Y, Hudspeth K, Wu YP, Yamashita T, Teneberg S, Wang D, Proia RL, Levery SB, Savage PB, Teyton L, Bendelac A (2004b) Lysosomal glycosphingolipid recognition by NKT cells. Science 306:1786–1789

CTMI (2007) 314:51–72

Structure and Biology of Self Lipid Antigens

G. De Libero (✉) · L. Mori

Department of Research, University Hospital, Basel, Switzerland
gennaro.delibero@unibas.ch

Abstract Self lipid antigens induce selection and expansion of autoreactive T cells which have a role in immunoregulation and disease pathogenesis. Here we review the important biological rules which determine lipid immunogenicity. The impact of lipid structure, synthesis, traffic, membrane distribution and CD1 loading are discussed.

1
Introduction

T cells recognize glycolipids associated with CD1 antigen-presenting molecules. The CD1–glycolipid complexes are structurally related to MHC–peptide complexes and this may explain the capacity of the TCR αβ to interact with both types of complexes. Although important immunological properties of lipid-specific T cells remain to be disclosed, it is clear that certain aspects of their biology resemble those of peptide-specific T cells. This is the case for thymic selection, upregulation of chemokine receptors necessary for thymus exit, acquisition of phenotype typical of naïve cells in the periphery and of memory or effector cells after antigen encounter and challenge.

T cells recognizing self glycolipids can be operationally divided into two groups. T cells restricted by CD1d which express a semi-invariant TCR, composed of the invariant Vα24-Jα18 and variable Vβ11 chains in humans (Vα14-Jα18 paired with Vβ8.2, Vβ7 or Vβ2 chains in mice) are included in the first group. Because of the conserved TCR structure, these cells are known as invariant NK T cells. NKT cells are activated by the neutral self glycosphingolipid isogloboside 3 (iGb3) (Zhou et al. 2004b) and by a variety of bacterial glycolipids such as α-glucuronosylceramide and α-galacturonosylceramide (Kinjo et al. 2005; Mattner et al. 2005). Both bacterial glycolipids are produced by *Sphingomonas*, bacteria which do not synthesize lipopolysaccharide (Kawahara et al. 1999) and which rarely cause disease in humans. NKT cells are also stimulated during infection with *Ehrlichia muris* (Mattner et al. 2005), another Gram-negative bacterium which does not produce LPS. It has been suggested that the immune system has evolved this type of recognition to promptly react to LPS-deficient bacteria. NKT cells also react to the sponge-derived glycolipid, α-galactosylceramide (α-GalCer), which behaves as a superagonist for this cell population. α-GalCer has been instrumental in studying responsiveness of NKT cells and their involvement in immunoregulation, as well as protection from infections and pathogenesis of autoimmune diseases (Godfrey and Kronenberg 2004).

T cells belonging to the second group express a variety of TCR heterodimers, apparently without bias for unique V or J genes, and they are restricted by CD1a, CD1b, CD1c and CD1d molecules. Among these diverse CD1-restricted T cells, evidence to date has not yet revealed a strong bias for CD4 and CD8 co-receptors in identifying subpopulations preferentially restricted to CD1 molecules, in contrast with T cells that recognize MHC molecules. Human CD1-restricted T cells may express CD4 or CD8 and, in some cases, are CD4 and CD8 double-negative.

A major question is whether lipid-specific T cells are a minor population of T cells or whether instead they present at high frequencies such that they could represent an effector arm of the immune response. A limited number of studies have addressed this important issue. In an initial report, it was found that human T cells reacting to self-glycosphingolipids are present in the circulating blood at the same frequency as classically MHC-restricted and peptide-specific T cells (Shamshiev et al. 1999). These initial studies have been confirmed by ongoing studies showing that T cells specific for sulfatides are present at frequencies of 1 in 2,000–10,000 T cells. These frequencies are very similar to those detected for myelin protein-specific and MHC class II-restricted T cells. Other studies have investigated the frequency of T cells recognizing microbial lipid antigens (Kawashima et al. 2003; Ulrichs et al. 2003) and have also shown that T cells with these specificities can be easily detected and isolated. Thus, lipid-specific T cells do not represent a unique and rare population of lymphocytes and are activated in immune responses against infectious microorganisms, tumour cells and are also involved in autoimmunity.

2
Nature of Self Lipids Stimulating T Cells

The two most prominent families of self lipids which stimulate T cells are sphingolipids and phospholipids. The structure of some immunogenic self lipids are shown in Figs. 1, 2 and 3. The sphingolipids gangliosides, sphingomyelin and sulfatides (Shamshiev et al. 1999, 2000) and the phospholipids phosphatidylcholine (PC), phosphytidylethanolamine (PE) and phosphatidylglycerol (PG) have been found to stimulate specific human T cells (Agea et al. 2005). Also, the ganglioside GD3, which is enriched in human tumours of neuroectodermal origin, stimulates specific T cells after immunization (Wu et al. 2003). Mouse T cells reacting to phosphatidylinositol (PI),

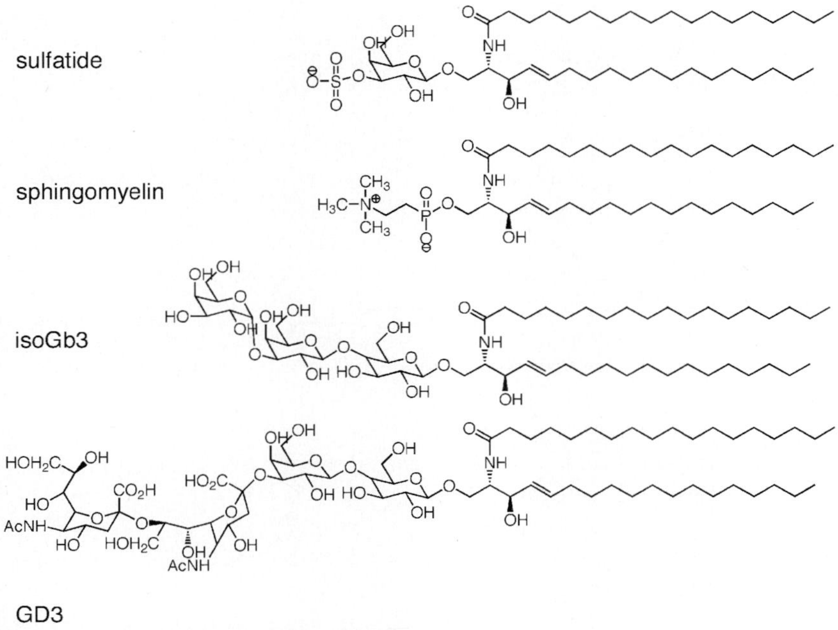

Fig. 1 Structures of immunogenic sphingolipids

PE and PG have also been described (Gumperz et al. 2000). NKT cells are reactive against the self iGb3 (Zhou et al. 2004b), which is generated during the lysosomal degradation of isogloboside 4. Importantly, the structure of the sphingoid base and of the associated fatty acids determine the half-life of the lipid, its distribution in the membranes and association with membrane proteins (Pomorski et al. 2001), thus also influencing the immunogenicity of the lipid (see below).

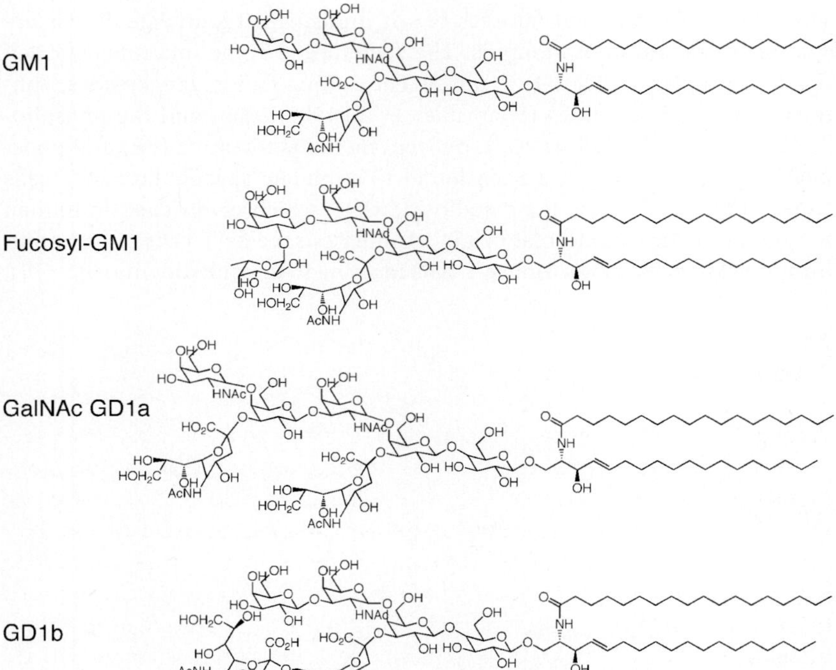

Fig. 2 Structures of immunogenic gangliosides

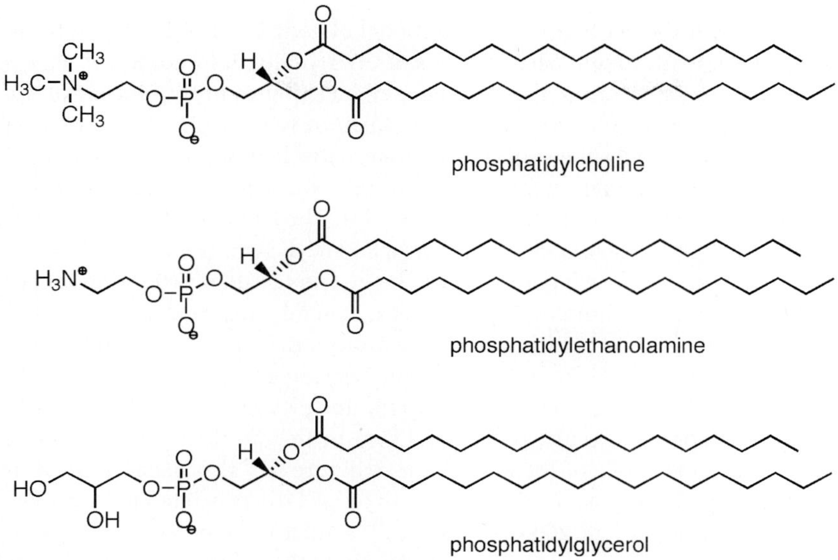

Fig. 3 Structures of immunogenic phospholipids

2.1
Structure of Self Lipids Stimulating T Cells

Sphingolipids have a backbone made of the basic alcohol sphingosine or a related long-chain base, which usually contains between 14 and 24 carbon atoms. Bases with up to two double bonds as well as one additional hydroxyl group may also be present. Sphingosine combines in amide linkage with a fatty acid to form a ceramide, which contains a free hydroxyl group combining with another component. When phosphate is added to ceramide, followed by choline, sphingomyelin is formed. This lipid is very abundant in all cell membranes. When glucose or galactose are added, glycosylceramides are generated. Synthases of mammalian cells link glucose or galactose monosaccharides to ceramide with a beta glycosidic bond, thus conferring a definable orientation to the polar head of the glycosphingolipid (GSL). This has important consequences with respect to antigen recognition by the TCR.

2.2
How the Structure of the Lipid Moiety Influences TCR Recognition

The hydrophobic part of GSL directly participates in the immunogenicity of GSLs through several discernible mechanisms. The importance of the acyl chain structure was described in the model of ganglioside GM1 recognition (Shamshiev et al. 2000). When a series of GM1 analogues were tested, it was clear that the structure of the ceramide tail contributes to the efficacy of the lipid when measured in vitro. The lyso form of GM1, which lacks the acyl chain and bears only the sphingosine base, as well as the sugar component devoid of ceramide, are not recognized by GM1-specific T cells, probably because these compounds do not bind to CD1. The length of the acyl chain is also important because GM1 containing a C18 acyl chain is more stimulatory than the analogue bearing a C24 acyl chain. The fact that GSLs with longer acyl chains are less immunogenic is not a general rule, because in another model of self lipid recognition, sulfatide molecules bearing a C24 acyl chain are more immunogenic than the analogue bearing a C18 acyl chain. As both GM1 and sulfatide are presented by CD1b, this difference is not ascribed to the presentation molecule, but more likely to the specificity of individual TCR. The importance of the acyl chain structure has also been outlined in another model antigen, i.e. PE recognition by a CD1d-restricted mouse T cell hybridoma (Rauch et al. 2003). These T cells are activated by PE containing at least one unsaturated acyl chain, with the cis configuration of double bonds being mandatory. These structural requirements were associated with a more efficient binding to CD1d. Similar constraints apply to the response of human T cells which specifically recognize phosphatidylcholine from pollens and discriminate the length and saturation of acyl chains (Agea et al. 2005).

In the GM1 recognition model, it was also found that modifications to the sphingosine base, namely the presence of a sphinganine, which unlike sphingosine does not bear unsaturated bonds, also decreases GM1 immunogenicity. This finding suggests that the rigidity of the base is also important, although the mechanism by which these lipid alterations influence T cell activation is not yet fully clear. Sphinganine is less polar than sphingosine and thus might also modify the critical micelle concentration (CMC), so that the capacity of GM1 to be solubilized and therefore to be delivered to CD1 might be affected. The CMC is an important biophysical property of lipids, which has two consequences of immunological relevance. If lipids are aggregated in a form that prevents their transfer to CD1 as monomers, this phenomenon may lead to overestimation of the lipid concentration which activates T cells. Also, differing solubilities and CMCs may render the comparison of immunogenicity between lipid analogues difficult.

The presence of a less rigid lipid base may also affect the orientation inside CD1 and the stability of binding. This latter mechanism has been found to play a role when an analogue of α-GalCer with a truncated sphingosine, called OCH, was tested (Miyamoto et al. 2001; Oki et al. 2004). This ligand induces a strong IL-4 release by NKT cells and a weak IFN-γ response. This effect likely depends on the fast off rate of OCH from CD1d and a reduced interaction with the TCR. As a consequence, activated T cells do not upregulate CD40 ligand, which is important for efficient IFN-γ secretion (Oki et al. 2005). Recent studies suggest that substitution of phytosphingosine with sphinganine in OCH also generates a compound which preferentially induces IL-4 secretion (Ndonye et al. 2005).

The importance of the lipid tail may have great relevance during immune responses against self lipids in vivo. Different tissues synthesize complex GSL using the most abundant fatty acids available inside their constitutive cells. This leads to the accumulation of GSL, which differ in their fatty acid composition and, therefore, may have immunologically different behaviours. Furthermore, the type of fatty acid used may change during ontogenesis and modifications of lipid metabolism occur after oncogenesis, viral transformation, cell activation and growth (Hakomori 1981). It is tempting to speculate that in these instances the immune system may be confronted with unusual GSL to which it is not tolerant and thus specific immunity is readily initiated.

The mechanisms of thymic selection and central tolerance of T cells recognizing self lipids have not yet been investigated. Mouse and human NKT cells are positively selected on double-positive thymocytes which express CD1d. Positive selection of NKT cells requires co-stimulation by a still unidentified member of the protein family called signalling lymphocytic activation molecule (SLAM). SLAM molecules are expressed by immature NKT cells and make homotypic interactions with other unidentified SLAM molecules expressed by CD4 and CD8 double-positive thymocytes. Upon this interaction, the SLAM protein expressed by NKT cells signals through a SLAM-associated protein (SAP) and contributes to further maturation of NKT cells (MacDonald and Schumann 2005). SAP is a key molecule, which probably facilitates recruitment of Fyn to the TCR. Indeed, in SAP-deficient patients and mice, either NKT cells or other non-MHC-restricted T cells do not develop (Borowski and Bendelac 2005). It is not clear whether T cells bearing a receptor interacting with self GSL undergo the same type of negative selection as peptide-specific T cells. Furthermore, it is not known how broad the repertoire of GSL in the thymus is, thus permitting induction of central tolerance to this type of antigenic lipids.

2.3
How the Structure of the Polar Part Influences TCR Recognition

The polar head of lipid antigens has two main functions. First, it makes direct interactions with residues of the alpha helices of CD1, thus assisting in forming stable CD1–lipid complexes, facilitating TCR interaction. Secondly, it participates directly in the cognate interaction with the TCR. The specificity of recognition is therefore dependent on the presence of the antigen residues making both types of interactions. The positioning of the polar residues is also dictated by the structure of the lipid moiety, as outlined in the section above, and thus the final shape of the lipid–CD1 complex is influenced by both the polar and apolar parts of the antigen.

Some complex glycolipid antigens require trimming of their terminal sugars, in order to generate immunogenic molecules. This has been shown with a synthetic di-galactosylceramide molecule, which stimulates NKT cells only after the terminal galactose is cleaved, thus generating the stimulatory α-GalCer (Prigozy et al. 2001). A second example is the presentation of the mycobacterial hexamannosylated phosphatidyl-myo-inositol (PIM_6) antigens (de la Salle et al. 2005). PIM_6s are characterized by the presence of six mannoses, which are trimmed into the dimannosylated molecules (PIM_2) by the lysosomal α-mannosidase. PIM_2s are then presented by CD1b to specific T cells. Recently, the important role of CD1e has been identified in processing of PIM_6. CD1e is able to bind PIM_6 and facilitates its processing to PIM_2 by the enzyme acidic α-mannosidase present in lysosomes (de la Salle et al. 2005).

T cells recognizing processed self GSL have not been isolated so far. In the GM1 model, this antigen, which contains an large glycan, is recognized as an intact molecule and does not require any processing, as shown by the ability of recombinant CD1 proteins to present the antigen in the absence of APCs. Also, gangliosides which lack individual sugars present in GM1 are not recognized. Furthermore, more complex gangliosides, such as GD1a, GD1b, GT1b, and GQ1b are also recognized by the same T cells without processing (Shamshiev et al. 2000). These more complex gangliosides have additional sialic acid units, which make them more negatively charged as compared to GM1. The TCR of these specific T cells makes cognate interaction with the α-helices of CD1b (Melian et al. 2000) and hence it is unlikely that it binds to the sugars only. Furthermore, the sequence of the TCR complementarity determining region 3 (CDR3) has a length comparable to that of MHC-restricted TCR and, therefore, it is also unlikely that this CDR3 region forms a cavity accommodating the additional sialic acid sugars. Another possibility is that more distal sialic acid residues assume a position that is lateral to the CD1–TCR interface so that they do not sterically hinder the contacts between CD1, TCR and the sugars common to GM1. This model resembles recognition of long peptides associated with MHC class II molecules (Stern et al. 1994). This latter possibility is suggested by the fact that fucosyl-GM1 is not recognized by these T cells (Fig. 4). In this ganglioside, the terminal fucose is linked with an alpha 1–2 glycosidic bond, thus assuming a disposition very different

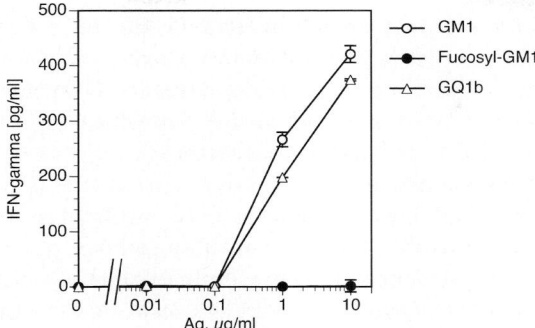

Fig. 4 Comparison of immunogenicity of gangliosides

from that of the sialic acid residues present in the other tested gangliosides. These results confirm the fine antigen specificity of the TCR and show that, like peptide-specific T cells, lipid-specific T cells also show a certain degree of cross-reactivity between different lipid antigens. Whether this cross-reactivity may lead to autoreactive responses remains to be investigated.

3
Where Glycolipids and Phospholipids Are Synthesized

The cellular localization of the enzymes which synthesize glycolipids and phospholipids influences the capacity of these lipids to bind to CD1 molecules.

The enzymes responsible for ceramide synthesis are located on the cytosolic membrane leaflet of the endoplasmic reticulum (ER) (Mandon et al. 1992). Then ceramide is transported to the trans-Golgi cisternae by a dedicated lipid transfer protein called CERT (Hanada et al. 2003) or is translocated inside the luminal membrane of ER in which it can be utilized to generate galactosylceramide in some cell types (van Meer and Holthuis 2000). Therefore, if ceramide binds to nascent CD1 molecules, a limiting step might be its translocation into the ER lumen. Ceramide is the common precursor of sphingomyelin and GSL. Sphingomyelin is predominantly synthesized in the luminal part of Golgi apparatus vesicles (Futerman et al. 1990) and is formed by the transfer of phosphorylcholine on the 1-hydroxyl group of ceramide. This requires the translocation of ceramide to the luminal leaflet of Golgi. After its synthesis, sphingomyelin traffics to the plasma membrane following the secretory pathway.

The Golgi apparatus is also the place where sugars are added to ceramide and GSL are synthesized. Glucosylceramide (GlcCer) is synthesized on the cytosolic leaflet of the Golgi apparatus (Jeckel et al. 1992). A major fraction of newly synthesized GlcCer is rapidly transported to the plasma membrane by a non-Golgi pathway and then rapidly degraded (Warnock et al. 1994). Alternatively, GlcCer is translocated in the luminal leaflet of Golgi vesicles and further modified by addition of other sugars.

Lactosylceramide (LacCer) is the GSL synthesized after GlcCer by the addition of a galactose moiety and is the common precursor for the GSL series. LacCer synthesis, as well as synthesis of more complex glycosylated lipids which contain sialic acid, occurs on the luminal leaflet of Golgi membranes (Lannert et al. 1998). GM3 and GD3 synthesis occurs in early Golgi compartments, whereas complex gangliosides are predominantly synthesized in the *trans* Golgi (Allende et al. 2000; Giraudo et al. 1999). These GSL then reach the plasma membrane following the secretory pathway. Because GSL and sphingomyelin are synthesized in the Golgi lumen and are not substrates for lipid translocators, they are localized exclusively in the noncytosolic leaflet of membranes.

Phospholipids are synthesized in the endoplasmic reticulum. The enzymes involved in phospholipid synthesis have their active sites facing the cytosol, in which the required metabolites are present. After their synthesis, phospholipids move to the luminal leaflet of ER. This movement is very fast and is facilitated by scramblases, which thus equilibrate the distribution of phospholipids across the ER membrane. The luminal localization of phospholipids may explain their association with nascent CD1d (Giabbai et al. 2005; Zajonc et al. 2005) and CD1b (Garcia-Alles et al. 2006) molecules. In the plasma membrane, phospholipid flippases specifically remove phospholipids containing free aminogroups (PS and PE) from the extracellular leaflet, generating an asymmetric phospholipids composition (Holthuis et al. 2003). How phospholipids are loaded on CD1 molecules in lysosomes is not clear.

4
Regulation of Antigenic Self Lipid Synthesis

Several mechanisms appear to participate in the regulation of antigenic self lipid synthesis. Ganglioside generation is influenced by intrinsic properties of the sugar transferases such as their enzymatic kinetics, localization within the Golgi compartments, and the contiguous presence of other transferases. For example, N-acetyl-galactosyl-transferase and galactosyltransferase II form a complex, which accepts GM3 and generates GM1, without releasing GM2 (Giraudo et al. 2001). This may explain why GM2, which is an intermediate of GM1 synthesis, is poorly represented in membranes.

Another mechanism of glycolipid regulation is based on the relative abundance and activity of glycosyltransferases which have common substrates (Ruan and Lloyd 1992; Yamashiro et al. 1993). The presence of increased amounts of GM3 synthase leads to accumulation of GSL of the ganglioside series (Dumonceaux and Carlsen 2001; Prinetti et al. 2003). This may result in important changes in cell behaviour, including the capacity to adhere to other cells in vitro, formation of metastasis in vivo and resistance to fenretinide.

The physicochemical characteristics of each GSL, the trafficking capacity through membranes of different organelles and the availability of required sugar substrates, may also contribute to their relative abundance.

Finally, gene regulation of sugar transferases influences GSL synthesis. Indeed, in transformed cells and during ontogenesis transcription of transferase genes undergo profound changes, thus influencing the type of accumulating GSL. Also, feedback regulation on gene transcription exerted by accumulated GSL or phosphorylation of glycosyl transferases and the pH of their environment may affect GSL synthesis.

5
Lipid Traffic in the Cell

The ER and Golgi are the two organelles in which immunogenic self lipids are synthesized. Therefore, the mechanisms regulating lipid traffic from these cellular compartments to the membranes of other compartments are important because they regulate membrane lipid composition as well as the possible loading of CD1 molecules.

The ER is a highly dynamic center of lipid distribution. The lipids synthesized in the ER or moving to the ER may be efficiently transferred to other organelles through the combined action of different lipid transfer proteins (LTP) (Holthuis and Levine 2005). These proteins are characterized by the capacity to bind and transport lipid monomers across aqueous phases. Most LTP bind lipid with some degree of specificity, with a 1:1 stoichiometry, and have the capacity to extract lipids from membranes. Several LTPs are composed of domains conferring the lipid-binding capacity and of domains, which may exert functions such as recognition of proteins associated with other organelles, gene regulation or GTPase regulation.

The specific transfer between two compartments is assured by the presence of additional LTP protein domains, some of which are specific for the donor membrane and others for the acceptor membrane. This unique structure allows precise transport and also explains why transfer of bound lipid is rapid. The presence of two domains increases the affinity of binding to the membranes and allows the formation of a bridge, thus avoiding random navigation in the cytoplasmic space. The effects of cytoplasmic LTP on lipid presentation to T cells have not been investigated and it is possible that LTP involved in trafficking of relevant self lipids may have important roles.

Another mechanism controlling lipid distribution in the membranes is provided by the biophysical characteristics of each lipid. For example, sphingolipids synthesized in the Golgi do not traffic to the ER and move only to the plasma membrane through anterograde transport vesicles. The reason why they are not incorporated in retrograde transport vesicles seems to be related to their capacity to form large numbers of hydrogen bonds, leading to formation of rigid lipid domains in the membrane of Golgi. Similar mechanisms may also occur in sorting lipids in the endosomal compartment. In early endosomes, lipids in more fluid microdomains more easily recycle to plasma membrane, whereas lipids in less fluid ones traffic to late endosomes. This may also explain why glycolipids with similar structures but differing in the length of the lipid tail traffic with different preferences: the ones with short lipid preferentially recycling in the early endosomal compartment, the ones with long lipids reaching the late endosomal compartment. An elegant example has been provided with analogues of the mycobacterial antigen glucose monomycolate which bears acyl chains of different length (Moody et al. 2002). Lipid differences in recycling may have important consequences for the loading of CD1 molecules. Indeed, phospholipids commonly recycling in early endosomes are efficiently presented by CD1a (Agea et al. 2005), which also recycles in this compartment (Moody and Porcelli 2003), whereas more complex GSL, such as gangliosides, reach late endosomes and are presented by CD1b (Shamshiev et al. 1999), recycling in this compartment.

Another important feature of late endosomes is the capacity to sort proteins and lipids into multivesicular bodies (MVB), small vesicles which bud towards the same endosomal lumen. Lipid composition of MVB is different from that of endosomal membranes, as they are enriched in cholesterol and the negatively charged lipids bis-(monoacylglycero)-phosphate and phosphatidylinositol-3-phosphate. Complex glycolipids which are degraded in lysosomes are sorted in the MVB membrane leaflet facing the endosomal lumen. This location allows their processing and might also aid in transfer to CD1 molecules, which recycle in the same compartment. Furthermore, in late endosomes LTP such as saposins and GM2-activator protein are present, which behave as liftases and facilitate GSL attack by hexohydrolases and GSL loading on CD1 molecules (Zhou et al. 2004a).

6
Where Self Lipids Are Loaded on CD1

The ER is the first compartment in which endogenous lipids may associate with CD1 molecules. During CD1d assembly, the microsomal triglyceride transfer protein (MTP) plays an important role in its stabilization (Brozovic et al. 2004), likely by promoting binding of phospholipids (Dougan et al. 2005) such as PC, which is associated with nascent CD1d (Giabbai et al. 2005). Whether MTP is also important in stabilization of other CD1 molecules is not clear.

During assembly, a subpopulation of CD1d molecules form complexes with the invariant chain (Ii) and MHC class II molecules (Jayawardena-Wolf et al. 2001; Kang and Cresswell 2002). This association drives this population of CD1d molecules to late endosomes and might have relevance during inflammation in which the cellular levels of Ii also change.

Recent data show that newly synthesized CD1d (Zajonc et al. 2005) and CD1b molecules (Garcia-Alles et al., submitted) may associate with spacer molecules, during their assembly inside ER. These spacers stabilize CD1d and CD1b during their traffic to the cell membrane and likely also prevent binding of lipids with long acyl chains. Therefore, it is unlikely that complex GSL, which are synthesized inside the luminal part of Golgi, associate with nascent CD1d and CD1b molecules. Upon reaching the cell surface, CD1 molecules recycle into late endosomal compartments in which the low pH facilitates their partial denaturation (Ernst et al. 1998) and loading with other lipid antigens.

An exception to this scenario is CD1a, which recycles in early endosomes. In this compartment, CD1a is proximal to lipid molecules that do not traffic further in deeper compartments because of the lack of tyrosine containing cytoplasmic tail motifs, which mediated internalization through binding to adaptor protein complexes. How self lipids might be extracted from early endosomal membranes is unclear, since no LTP such as saposins and GM2 activator are present in these organelles. One possibility is that lipoproteins present in serum, and which upon internalization are sorted in the recycling endosomes, may provide this function. This is supported by the finding that serum lipids control the maintenance of CD1a molecules with appropriate conformation on the cell surface (Manolova et al. 2006). In the absence of serum, CD1a molecules maintain their plasma membrane location, but are altered and lose the capacity to present lipid antigens. This behaviour does not depend on the recycling properties, since hybrid CD1a molecules expressing the CD1b cytoplasmic tail and recycling in late endosomes behave as wild type CD1a. Most likely the unique structure of CD1a accounts for

this dependence on exogenous lipid and lipoproteins. Indeed, the CD1a F'
pocket, which represents the portal through which lipids enter the groove, is
partially open towards the upper part of the molecule facing the extracellular
space (Zajonc et al. 2003). This may facilitate ready exchange of lipids when
appropriate acceptors such as membranes or lipoproteins come in contact
with the lipid-binding part of CD1a.

Complex glycolipids traffic in late endosomes where they are loaded
on CD1 molecules present in the same compartment. This is facilitated by
saposins and GM2 activator, which participate in glycolipid degradation as
well as their loading on CD1 molecules. The importance of saposins in CD1
loading is outlined by a series of findings with both mouse and human CD1-
restricted T cells. Mice lacking functional prosaposin gene do not develop
normal numbers of NKT cells (Zhou et al. 2004a). Furthermore, presentation
of α-GalCer is partially impaired when saposin-deficient APCs are used (Kang
and Cresswell 2004; Zhou et al. 2004a). When saposins were tested in a CD1d
loading assay in vitro with sulfatide, saposins A and C were more efficient than
saposin B, whereas saposin D was inactive (Zhou et al. 2004a). In a third study,
it was found that CD1b-restricted presentation by human saposin-deficient
dendritic cells of mycobacterial lipoarabinomannan, glucosylmonomycolate
and mycolic acid was inefficient. Loading of these antigens required the presence of saposin C and not of saposin B (Winau et al. 2004). These studies
suggest that each saposin may preferentially interact with individual CD1
proteins. However, this conclusion is not supported by the published data,
and another possibility can be considered. Saposins and GM2 activator preferentially bind different types of lipids and therefore it is the type of lipid
antigen to be loaded which selects the LTP involved in CD1 loading. For
example, when mouse CD1d is loaded with sulfatide, saposins A and C are
very efficient, whereas they are inactive in loading α-GalCer. Instead, GM2
activator, which binds α-GalCer, is very efficient in assisting the formation of
the CD1d-α–GalCer complex (Zhou et al. 2004a).

7
Role of Self Glycolipids in Diseases

The identification of the possible role of self lipid-specific T cells in human
diseases is a difficult task. First, there is a limited number of studies conducted
in human diseases and therefore it is still premature to make final conclusions.
Secondly, to investigate the role of these cells in vivo, it is important to
investigate disease models in animals which can be manipulated. As small
rodents do not express group I CD1 molecules, they have not been useful

for this purpose. However, mice have been instrumental in investigations into the role of NKT cells, which also recognize self lipids, and these studies have provided direct evidence of the important regulatory function of these cells. The function of NKT cells has already been appropriately reviewed (Bendelac et al. 1997; Godfrey and Kronenberg 2004; Kronenberg and Gapin 2002; Taniguchi et al. 2003; Van Kaer 2005) and this discussion focuses on how self lipid-reactive T cells restricted by group I CD1 molecules may have a role in human diseases.

7.1
Multiple Sclerosis

Multiple sclerosis (MS) is an autoimmune disease characterized by areas in the brain becoming demyelinated as result of autoimmune attack. Activated T cells accumulate at the borders of the lesions in the brain and in the perivascular spaces and are likely to contribute to persistence of inflammation. These T cells are mostly specific for myelin components such as myelin proteins and myelin lipids. In the circulating blood of MS patients, there is a high frequency of T cells recognizing gangliosides, sulfatide and sphingomyelin (Shamshiev et al. 1999). These self glycosphingolipids can be presented by all CD1 molecules expressed on the cell surface without apparent bias for any particular isoform (Shamshiev et al. 2002). The T cell response against self lipids appears to be more pronounced in patients with the primary progressive form of MS (Pender et al. 2003), which is also the more malignant form of this disease. Patients with primary progressive MS also develop high titers of anti-glycolipid antibodies in the CSF and serum (Acarin et al. 1996; Sadatipour et al. 1998). These findings support the hypothesis that myelin lipids are highly immunogenic in patients, and it is likely that the specific T and B cell immune responses are correlated with the progression of MS.

Another important finding is that mice with experimental allergic en-cephalomyelitis (EAE), a model of autoimmune disease which leads to brain lesions and paralysis and resembles MS in some respects, show increased numbers of CD1d-restricted and sulfatide-specific T cells. Interestingly, these T cells accumulate in the brain at the time of the disease peak, whereas in disease-free animals they are mostly present in the spleen (Jahng et al. 2004). If mice are immunized with sulfatide before EAE induction, a milder form of disease develops.

Additional data supporting the importance of self lipid-specific immunity is provided by the EAE model in guinea pigs, which, in contrast to mice, express group I CD1 molecules. EAE in guinea pigs is exacerbated (Kusunoki et al. 1988; Moore et al. 1984) or inhibited (Mullin et al. 1986) by injecting gangliosides present in myelin. Self lipids also induce generation of specific antibodies in MS patients (Arnon et al. 1980; Endo et al. 1984; Kanter et al. 2006), in mice (Kanter et al. 2006) and in guinea pigs (Schwerer et al. 1984) with EAE.

An open question remains: How are self lipid-reactive T cells activated? One possibility is that some T cells cross-react with microbial lipoglycans. However, this remains a hypothesis, as there is no experimental evidence for this possibility. An alternative mechanism is that during infection there is a modulation of self lipid metabolism, which facilitates their synthesis and presentation by CD1 molecules. Indeed, when dendritic or monocytic cells are infected with different types of bacteria or stimulated with different bacterial products, they increase the de novo synthesis of glycosphingolipids and acquire the capacity to stimulate CD1-restricted and glycolipid-specific T cells (De Libero et al. 2005). Thus, infection promotes recognition of induced self lipids, which might result in disease exacerbation. This mechanism is observed independently of the bacteria used for infection and is in accordance with the findings that MS attacks are more frequent after infection, although there is no evidence of association with a unique infectious agent.

7.2
Guillaume Barré Syndrome

Guillaume Barré syndrome (GBS) is a postinfectious autoimmune neuropathy caused by the presence of autoantibodies cross-reacting with gangliosides present in myelin and in the lipopolysaccharides (LPS) of some *Campylobacter jejuni* strains (Willison and Yuki 2002), which usually only causes enteritis. Chemical analyses of the core oligosaccharides of neuropathy-associated *C. jejuni* strains have revealed structural homology with human gangliosides (Moran and Prendergast 2001). Serum antibodies against gangliosides are found in one-third of GBS patients but are generally absent in enteritis cases. It is assumed that the antibodies are induced by antecedent infection with *C. jejuni*, and subsequently react with nerve tissue, causing damage. Although there is still no evidence for a direct role of self lipid-specific T cells in this disease, the observation that most GBS patients produce IgG antibodies specific for lipid structures supports the possibility that these T cells might be present and help glycolipid-specific B cells to switch to Ig isotypes. That these patients might also have a genetic predisposition to the development of this type of autoimmune response remains an open possibility.

8
Conclusions

The capacity of T cells to react against self lipids shows the high plasticity of T cell recognition and has important consequences for immune response. The apparent lack of functional polymorphism in CD1 molecules raises questions concerning the evolutionary mechanism that forced this type of antigen recognition. The hydrophobic structures of the self glycolipids responsible for anchoring to CD1 molecules may have provided an important evolutionary constraint. However, it not clear why CD1 molecules have not acquired polymorphic residues on the two alpha helices which make cognate interactions with the TCR. Lack of polymorphism might simplify the design of novel types of vaccines inducing the proliferation of self lipid-specific T cells with immunoregulatory or protective immune functions.

References

Acarin N, Rio J, Fernandez AL, Tintore M, Duran I, Galan I, Montalban X (1996) Different antiganglioside antibody patterns between relapsing-remitting and progressive multiple sclerosis. Acta Neurol Scand 93:99–103

Agea E, Russano A, Bistoni O, Mannucci R, Nicoletti I, Corazzi L, Postle AD, De Libero G, Porcelli SA, Spinozzi F (2005) Human CD1-restricted T cell recognition of lipids from pollens. J Exp Med 202:295–308

Allende ML, Li J, Darling DS, Worth CA, Young WW Jr (2000) Evidence supporting a late Golgi location for lactosylceramide to ganglioside GM3 conversion. Glycobiology 10:1025–1032

Arnon R, Crisp E, Kelley R, Ellison GW, Myers LW, Tourtellotte WW (1980) Antiganglioside antibodies in multiple sclerosis. J Neurol Sci 46:179–186

Bendelac A, Rivera MN, Park SH, Roark JH (1997) Mouse CD1-specific NK1. T cells: development, specificity, and function. Annu Rev Immunol 15:535–562

Borowski C, Bendelac A (2005) Signaling for NKT cell development: the SAP-FynT connection. J Exp Med 201:833–836

Brozovic S, Nagaishi T, Yoshida M, Betz S, Salas A, Chen D, Kaser A, Glickman J, Kuo T, Little A, Morrison J, Corazza N, Kim JY, Colgan SP, Young SG, Exley M, Blumberg RS (2004) CD1d function is regulated by microsomal triglyceride transfer protein. Nat Med 10:535–539

De la Salle H, Mariotti S, Angenieux C, Gilleron M, Garcia-Alles LF, Malm D, Berg T, Paoletti S, Maitre B, Mourey L, Salamero J, Cazenave JP, Hanau D, Mori L, Puzo G, De Libero G (2005) Assistance of microbial glycolipid antigen processing by CD1e. Science 310:1321–1324

De Libero G, Moran AP, Gober H-J, Rossy E, Shamshiev A, Chelnokova O, Mazorra Z, Vendetti S, Sacchi A, Prendergast MM, Sansano S, Tonevitsky A, Landmann R, Mori L (2005) Bacterial infections promote T cell recognition of self-glycolipids. Immunity 22:763–772

Dougan SK, Salas A, Rava P, Agyemang A, Kaser A, Morrison J, Khurana A, Kronenberg M, Johnson C, Exley M, Hussain MM, Blumberg RS (2005) Microsomal triglyceride transfer protein lipidation and control of CD1d on antigen-presenting cells. J Exp Med 202:529–539

Dumonceaux T, Carlsen SA (2001) Isogloboside biosynthesis in metastatic R3230AC cells results from a decreased GM3 synthase activity. Arch Biochem Biophys 389:187–194

Endo T, Scott DD, Stewart SS, Kundu SK, Marcus DM (1984) Antibodies to glycosphingolipids in patients with multiple sclerosis and SLE. J Immunol 132:1793–1797

Ernst WA, Maher J, Cho S, Niazi KR, Chatterjee D, Moody DB, Besra GS, Watanabe Y, Jensen PE, Porcelli SA, Kronenberg M, Modlin RL (1998) Molecular interaction of CD1b with lipoglycan antigens. Immunity 8:331–340

Futerman AH, Stieger B, Hubbard AL, Pagano RE (1990) Sphingomyelin synthesis in rat liver occurs predominantly at the cis and medial cisternae of the Golgi apparatus. J Biol Chem 265:8650–8657

Garcia-Alles LF, Versluis K, Maveyraud L, Vallina AT, Sansano S, Bello NF, Gober HJ, Guillet V, de la Salle H, Puzo G, Mori L, Heck AJ, De Libero G, Mourey L (2006) Endogenous phosphatidylcholine and a long spacer ligand stabilize the lipid-binding groove of CD1b. EMBO J 25:3684–3692

Giabbai B, Sidobre S, Crispin MD, Sanchez-Ruiz Y, Bachi A, Kronenberg M, Wilson IA, Degano M (2005) Crystal structure of mouse CD1d bound to the self ligand phosphatidylcholine: a molecular basis for NKT cell activation. J Immunol 175:977–984

Giraudo CG, Rosales Fritz VM, Maccioni HJ (1999) GA2/GM2/GD2 synthase localizes to the trans-Golgi network of CHO-K1 cells. Biochem J 342:633–640

Giraudo CG, Daniotti JL, Maccioni HJ (2001) Physical and functional association of glycolipid N-acetyl-galactosaminyl and galactosyl transferases in the Golgi apparatus. Proc Natl Acad Sci U S A 98:1625–1630

Godfrey DI, Kronenberg M (2004) Going both ways: immune regulation via CD1d-dependent NKT cells. J Clin Invest 114:1379–1388

Gumperz JE, Roy C, Makowska A, Lum D, Sugita M, Podrebarac T, Koezuka Y, Porcelli SA, Cardell S, Brenner MB, Behar SM (2000) Murine CD1d-restricted T cell recognition of cellular lipids. Immunity 12:211–221

Hakomori S (1981) Glycosphingolipids in cellular interaction, differentiation, and oncogenesis. Annu Rev Biochem 50:733–764

Hanada K, Kumagai K, Yasuda S, Miura Y, Kawano M, Fukasawa M, Nishijima M (2003) Molecular machinery for non-vesicular trafficking of ceramide. Nature 426:803–809

Holthuis JC, Levine TP (2005) Lipid traffic: floppy drives and a superhighway. Nat Rev Mol Cell Biol 6:209–220

Holthuis JC, van Meer G, Huitema K (2003) Lipid microdomains, lipid translocation and the organization of intracellular membrane transport. Mol Membr Biol 20:231–241

Jahng A, Maricic I, Aguilera C, Cardell S, Halder RC, Kumar V (2004) Prevention of autoimmunity by targeting a distinct, noninvariant CD1d-reactive T cell population reactive to sulfatide. J Exp Med 199:947–957

Jayawardena-Wolf J, Benlagha K, Chiu YH, Mehr R, Bendelac A (2001) CD1d endosomal trafficking is independently regulated by an intrinsic CD1d-encoded tyrosine motif and by the invariant chain. Immunity 15:897–908

Jeckel D, Karrenbauer A, Burger KN, van Meer G, Wieland F (1992) Glucosylceramide is synthesized at the cytosolic surface of various Golgi subfractions. J Cell Biol 117:259–267

Kang SJ, Cresswell P (2002) Regulation of intracellular trafficking of human CD1d by association with MHC class II molecules. EMBO J 21:1650–1660

Kang SJ, Cresswell P (2004) Saposins facilitate CD1d-restricted presentation of an exogenous lipid antigen to T cells. Nat Immunol 5:175–181

Kanter JL, Narayana S, Ho PP, Catz I, Warren KG, Sobel RA, Steinman L, Robinson WH (2006) Lipid microarrays identify key mediators of autoimmune brain inflammation. Nat Med 12:138–143

Kawahara K, Kuraishi H, Zahringer U (1999) Chemical structure and function of glycosphingolipids of *Sphingomonas* spp and their distribution among members of the alpha-4 subclass of Proteobacteria. J Ind Microbiol Biotechnol 23:408–413

Kawashima T, Norose Y, Watanabe Y, Enomoto Y, Narazaki H, Watari E, Tanaka S, Takahashi H, Yano I, Brenner MB, Sugita M (2003) Cutting edge: major CD8. T cell response to live bacillus Calmette-Guerin is mediated by CD1 molecules. J Immunol 170:5345–5348

Kinjo Y, Wu D, Kim G, Xing G-W, Poles MA, Ho DH, Tsuji M, Kawahara K, Wong C-H, Kronenberg M (2005) Recognition of bacterial glycosphingolipids by natural killer T cells. Nature 434:520–525

Kronenberg M, Gapin L (2002) The unconventional lifestyle of NKT cells. Nat Rev Immunol 2:557–568

Kusunoki S, Yu RK, Kim JH (1988) Induction of experimental autoimmune encephalomyelitis in guinea pigs using myelin basic protein and myelin glycolipids. J Neuroimmunol 18:303–314

Lannert H, Gorgas K, Meissner I, Wieland FT, Jeckel D (1998) Functional organization of the Golgi apparatus in glycosphingolipid biosynthesis. Lactosylceramide and subsequent glycosphingolipids are formed in the lumen of the late Golgi. J Biol Chem 273:2939–2946

MacDonald HR, Schumann J (2005) The need for natural killer T cells. Nat Med 11:256–257

Mandon EC, Ehses I, Rother J, van Echten G, Sandhoff K (1992) Subcellular localization and membrane topology of serine palmitoyltransferase, 3-dehydrosphinganine reductase, and sphinganine N-acyltransferase in mouse liver. J Biol Chem 267:11144–11148

Manolova V, Kistowska M, Paoletti S, Baltariu GM, Bausinger H, Hanau D, Mori L, De Libero G (2006) Functional CD1a is stabilized by exogenous lipids. Eur J Immunol 36:1083–1092

Mattner J, DeBord KL, Ismail N, Goff RD, Cantu C 3rd, Zhou D, Saint-Mezard P, Wang V, Gao Y, Yin N, Hoebe K, Schneewind O, Walker D, Beutler B, Teyton L, Savage PB, Bendelac A (2005) Both exogenous and endogenous glycolipid antigens activate NKT cells during microbial infections. Nature 434:525–529

Melian A, Watts GF, Shamshiev A, De Libero G, Clatworthy A, Vincent M, Brenner MB, Behar S, Niazi K, Modlin RL, Almo S, Ostrov D, Nathenson SG, Porcelli SA (2000) Molecular recognition of human CD1b antigen complexes: evidence for a common pattern of interaction with alpha beta TCRs. J Immunol 165:4494–4504

Miyamoto K, Miyake S, Yamamura T (2001) A synthetic glycolipid prevents autoimmune encephalomyelitis by inducing TH2 bias of natural killer T cells. Nature 413:531–534

Moody DB, Porcelli SA (2003) Intracellular pathways of CD1 antigen presentation. Nat Rev Immunol 3:11–22

Moody DB, Briken V, Cheng TY, Roura-Mir C, Guy MR, Geho DH, Tykocinski ML, Besra GS, Porcelli SA (2002) Lipid length controls antigen entry into endosomal and nonendosomal pathways for CD1b presentation. Nat Immunol 3:435–442

Moore GR, Traugott U, Farooq M, Norton WT, Raine CS (1984) Experimental autoimmune encephalomyelitis. Augmentation of demyelination by different myelin lipids. Lab Invest 51:416–424

Moran AP, Prendergast MM (2001) Molecular mimicry in *Campylobacter jejuni* and *Helicobacter pylori* lipopolysaccharides: contribution of gastrointestinal infections to autoimmunity. J Autoimmun 16:241–256

Mullin BR, Patrick DH, Poore CM, Rupp BH, Smith MT (1986) Prevention of experimental allergic encephalomyelitis by ganglioside GM4. A follow-up study. J Neurol Sci 73:55–60

Ndonye RM, Izmirian DP, Dunn MF, Yu KO, Porcelli SA, Khurana A, Kronenberg M, Richardson SK, Howell AR (2005) Synthesis and evaluation of sphinganine analogues of KRN7000 and OCH. J Org Chem 70:10260–10270

Oki S, Chiba A, Yamamura T, Miyake S (2004) The clinical implication and molecular mechanism of preferential IL-4 production by modified glycolipid-stimulated NKT cells. J Clin Invest 113:1631–1640

Oki S, Tomi C, Yamamura T, Miyake S (2005) Preferential T(h)2 polarization by OCH is supported by incompetent NKT cell induction of CD40L and following production of inflammatory cytokines by bystander cells in vivo. Int Immunol 17:1619–1629

Pender MP, Csurhes PA, Wolfe NP, Hooper KD, Good MF, McCombe PA, Greer JM (2003) Increased circulating T cell reactivity to GM3 and GQ1b gangliosides in primary progressive multiple sclerosis. J Clin Neurosci 10:63–66

Pomorski T, Hrafnsdottir S, Devaux PF, van Meer G (2001) Lipid distribution and transport across cellular membranes. Semin Cell Dev Biol 12:139–148

Prigozy TI, Naidenko O, Qasba P, Elewaut D, Brossay L, Khurana A, Natori T, Koezuka Y, Kulkarni A, Kronenberg M (2001) Glycolipid antigen processing for presentation by CD1d molecules. Science 291:664–667

Prinetti A, Basso L, Appierto V, Villani MG, Valsecchi M, Loberto N, Prioni S, Chigorno V, Cavadini E, Formelli F, Sonnino S (2003) Altered sphingolipid metabolism in N-(4-hydroxyphenyl)-retinamide-resistant A2780 human ovarian carcinoma cells. J Biol Chem 278:5574–5583

Rauch J, Gumperz J, Robinson C, Skold M, Roy C, Young DC, Lafleur M, Moody DB, Brenner MB, Costello CE, Behar SM (2003) Structural features of the acyl chain determine self-phospholipid antigen recognition by a CD1d-restricted invariant NKT (iNKT) cell. J Biol Chem 278:47508–47515

Ruan S, Lloyd KO (1992) Glycosylation pathways in the biosynthesis of gangliosides in melanoma and neuroblastoma cells: relative glycosyltransferase levels determine ganglioside patterns. Cancer Res 52:5725–5731

Sadatipour BT, Greer JM, Pender MP (1998) Increased circulating antiganglioside antibodies in primary and secondary progressive multiple sclerosis. Ann Neurol 44:980–983

Schwerer B, Kitz K, Lassmann H, Bernheimer H (1984) Serum antibodies against glycosphingolipids in chronic relapsing experimental allergic encephalomyelitis. Demonstration by ELISA and relation to serum in vivo demyelinating activity. J Neuroimmunol 7:107–119

Shamshiev A, Donda A, Carena I, Mori L, Kappos L, De Libero G (1999) Self glycolipids as T-cell autoantigens. Eur J Immunol 29:1667–1675

Shamshiev A, Donda A, Prigozy TI, Mori L, Chigorno V, Benedict CA, Kappos L, Sonnino S, Kronenberg M, De Libero G (2000) The alphabeta T cell response to self-glycolipids shows a novel mechanism of CD1b loading and a requirement for complex oligosaccharides. Immunity 13:255–264

Shamshiev A, Gober HJ, Donda A, Mazorra Z, Mori L, De Libero G (2002) Presentation of the same glycolipid by different CD1 molecules. J Exp Med 195:1013–1021

Stern LJ, Brown JH, Jardetzky TS, Gorga JC, Urban RG, Strominger JL, Wiley DC (1994) Crystal structure of the human class IIMHC protein HLA-DR1 complexed with an influenza virus peptide. Nature 368:215–221

Taniguchi M, Harada M, Kojo S, Nakayama T, Wakao H (2003) The regulatory role of Valpha14. NKT cells in innate and acquired immune response. Annu Rev Immunol 21:483–513

Ulrichs T, Moody DB, Grant E, Kaufmann SH, Porcelli SA (2003) T-cell responses to CD1-presented lipid antigens in humans with *Mycobacterium tuberculosis* infection. Infect Immun 71:3076–3087

Van Kaer L (2005) Alpha-galactosylceramide therapy for autoimmune diseases: prospects and obstacles. Nat Rev Immunol 5:31–42

Van Meer G, Holthuis JC (2000) Sphingolipid transport in eukaryotic cells. Biochim Biophys Acta 1486:145–170

Warnock DE, Lutz MS, Blackburn WA, Young WW Jr, Baenziger JU (1994) Transport of newly synthesized glucosylceramide to the plasma membrane by a non-Golgi pathway. Proc Natl Acad Sci U S A 91:2708–2712

Willison HJ, Yuki N (2002) Peripheral neuropathies and anti-glycolipid antibodies. Brain 125:2591–2625

Winau F, Schwierzeck V, Hurwitz R, Remmel N, Sieling PA, Modlin RL, Porcelli SA, Brinkmann V, Sugita M, Sandhoff K, Kaufmann SH, Schaible UE (2004) Saposin C is required for lipid presentation by human CD1b. Nat Immunol 5:169–174

Wu DY, Segal NH, Sidobre S, Kronenberg M, Chapman PB (2003) Cross-presentation of disialoganglioside GD3 to natural killer T cells. J Exp Med 198:173–181

Yamashiro S, Ruan S, Furukawa K, Tai T, Lloyd KO, Shiku H (1993) Genetic and enzymatic basis for the differential expression of GM2 and GD2 gangliosides in human cancer cell lines. Cancer Res 53:5395–5400

Zajonc DM, Elsliger MA, Teyton L, Wilson IA (2003) Crystal structure of CD1a in complex with a sulfatide self antigen at a resolution of 2.15 A. Nat Immunol 4:808–815

Zajonc DM, Cantu C 3rd, Mattner J, Zhou D, Savage PB, Bendelac A, Wilson IA, Teyton L (2005) Structure and function of a potent agonist for the semi-invariant natural killer T cell receptor. Nat Immunol 6:810–818

Zhou D, Cantu C, 3rd Sagiv Y, Schrantz N, Kulkarni AB, Qi X, Mahuran DJ, Morales CR, Grabowski GA, Benlagha K, Savage P, Bendelac A, Teyton L (2004a) Editing of CD1d-bound lipid antigens by endosomal lipid transfer proteins. Science 303:523–527

Zhou D, Mattner J, Cantu C 3rd, Schrantz N, Yin N, Gao Y, Sagiv Y, Hudspeth K, Wu YP, Yamashita T, Teneberg S, Wang D, Proia RL, Levery SB, Savage PB, Teyton L, Bendelac A (2004b) Lysosomal glycosphingolipid recognition by NKT cells. Science 306:1786–1789

CTMI (2007) 314:73–110
© Springer-Verlag Berlin Heidelberg 2007

Structures and Functions of Microbial Lipid Antigens Presented by CD1

B. E. Willcox[1] (✉) · C. R. Willcox[2] · L. G. Dover[3] · G. Besra[3]

[1]CRUK Institute for Cancer Studies, Edgbaston, B15 2TT Birmingham, United Kingdom
b.willcox@bham.ac.uk

[2]Institute for Biomedical Research, Edgbaston, B15 2TT Birmingham, United Kingdom

[3]School of Biosciences, Edgbaston, B15 2TT Birmingham, United Kingdom

Abstract The CD1 family of proteins has evolved to bind a range of endogenous and foreign lipids and present these at the cell surface for antigen-specific recognition by T cells. The distinct intracellular trafficking pathways of CD1 molecules indicate that collectively, they have the potential to survey the endocytic system widely for antigen, consistent with a role in the presentation of lipids derived from intracellular microbial pathogens. In keeping with this idea, CD1a, CD1b, CD1c and CD1d have now been shown to present foreign lipid antigens derived from mycobacteria, Gram-negative bacteria and also protozoan species to T cells. These antigens are extremely diverse chemically, and include naturally occurring lipopeptide, glycolipid and phospholipid structures that are distinct from mammalian lipids. CD1-restricted mycobacterial lipids defined to date derive from the highly complex microbial cell envelope. They play a variety of physiological roles for the microbe, including formation of the plasma membrane and protective cell wall and as metabolic intermediates in iron-scavenging pathways. In each case, alkyl chains of CD1-restricted lipid antigens are accommodated within a deep hydrophobic groove in the membrane-distal $\alpha 1$-$\alpha 2$ domains of the CD1 molecule, with hydrophilic elements solvent-exposed and accessible for recognition by the T cell receptor. Variation in the number, length and saturation of alkyl chains, and the precise chemistry and chirality of the lipid headgroup, clearly exert dominant influences on antigenicity, mediated by effects on CD1 binding and T cell receptor recognition. In the context of structural studies of CD1–lipid complexes, these data suggest that the CD1 isoforms have evolved binding specificities for different classes of foreign lipids, and strongly support a model for antigen recognition involving fine discrimination of lipid headgroup components by the $\alpha\beta$ T cell receptor. In this review, we summarise our current knowledge of foreign lipid antigens bound by CD1, focusing on the roles their distinct structural features play in presentation and T cell antigen recognition, and their likely function in antimicrobial T cell responses.

1
Introduction

The CD1 family of proteins present lipid antigens to T cells. Originally defined using monoclonal antibodies that stained human thymocytes (McMichael et al. 1979), the human family consists of four proteins – CD1a, CD1b, CD1c and CD1d – directly involved in lipid presentation at the cell surface. A fifth family member, CD1e, is expressed intracellularly and may facilitate lipid presentation by other CD1 molecules (de la Salle et al. 2005). Although encoded on chromosome 1 outside the major histocompatibility complex (MHC) by genes that exhibit extremely limited allelic polymorphism (Han et al. 1999), CD1 molecules are related to MHC class I molecules in terms of gene structure, homology and domain organisation, suggesting a common evolutionary origin. Like MHC class I, CD1 molecules are type I transmembrane proteins that contain $\alpha 1$, $\alpha 2$ and $\alpha 3$ domains and associate noncovalently with $\beta 2$-microglobulin. Based on sequence similarities in the $\alpha 1$ and $\alpha 2$ domains, the CD1 family was split into two subsets, with the relatively closely related CD1a, CD1b and CD1c isoforms assigned to group 1, and the more distantly related

CD1d to group 2 (Calabi et al. 1989). Whereas the human genome contains single copies of CD1a, CD1b, CD1c, CD1d and CD1e genes, these isoforms are expanded or deleted in other species of mammals (Brigl and Brenner 2004; Van Rhijn et al. 2006).

2
T Cell Recognition of Microbial Antigens Restricted by CD1 Molecules

Similarities to MHC class I molecules and expression on antigen-presenting cells suggested a role for CD1 molecules in T cell recognition. This idea was first confirmed by studies that used antibodies specific for CD1 isoforms to establish that CD1a and CD1c molecules were targets for recognition by $\alpha\beta$ and $\gamma\delta$ cytotoxic T lymphocyte lines, respectively (Porcelli et al. 1989). This work left the question of whether CD1 proteins could present antigen unresolved. However, studies of the proliferative and cytotoxic responses of an $\alpha\beta$ TCR $^+$ CD4$^-$CD8$^-$ T cell line specific for *Mycobacterium tuberculosis* antigen indicated recognition was absolutely dependent on the presence of CD1b on the presenting cell, but unaffected by the presence of MHC class I molecules. This study provided the first direct evidence for CD1-mediated antigen presentation and suggested a role for CD1 molecules in antimicrobial immunity (Porcelli et al. 1992).

2.1
A Specialised Role for CD1 in Microbial Lipid Presentation

The first evidence that the antigens presented by CD1 molecules were bio-chemically distinct from those presented by MHC molecules came from stud-ies on CD1b-restricted $\alpha\beta$ TCR$^+$ T cell lines specific for *M. tuberculosis* (Beck-man et al. 1994). In contrast to class II MHC-restricted recognition by an *M. tuberculosis*-specific T cell clone, CD1b-restricted recognition was insensitive to prior protease treatment of *M. tuberculosis* antigen. Organic extractions of mycobacterial sonicates indicated the stimulating activity was highly hy-drophobic, and fractionation steps revealed that the CD1b-restricted antigen was mycolic acid, a prevalent lipid of the cell wall of mycobacteria and related genera of bacteria (Fig. 1). As outlined below, subsequent studies have defined other microbial lipids as antigens presented by the group 1 molecules CD1b (Gilleron et al. 2004; Moody et al. 1997; Sieling et al. 1995), CD1c (Moody et al. 2000b), and CD1a (Moody et al. 2004), and more recently by the group 2 molecule CD1d (Amprey et al. 2004; Fischer et al. 2004; Kinjo et al. 2005; Mattner et al. 2005; Sriram et al. 2005; Wu et al. 2005), and support the idea that CD1 molecules predominantly present lipid antigens.

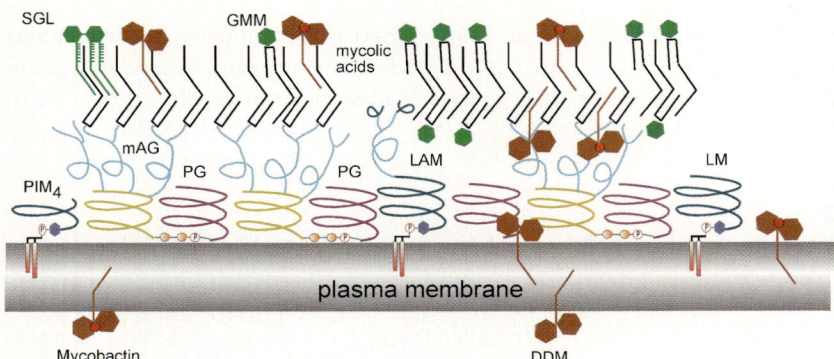

Fig. 1 Schematic representation of the cell envelope of *Mycobacterium tuberculosis (M. tb)*, with relevant antigenic lipids highlighted. Like most bacteria, the *M. tb* envelope consists of a plasma membrane with an associated peptidoglycan layer (*PG*). However, a distinguishing feature of mycobacteria is the presence of an additional thick cell wall layer containing mycolic acids esterified to arabinogalactan (mycolyl arabinogalactan, *mAG*). The antigenic lipids of *M. tb* are located throughout the envelope. A subset, including phosphatidyl inositol mannosides (*PIMs*), Lipomannan (*LM*) and Lipoarabinomannan (*LAM*), are anchored via their phosphatidyl inositol core structure to the outer leaflet of the plasma membrane. Others are noncovalently associated with the cell wall, including nonesterified mycolic acid, glucose monomycolate (*GMM*), and sulfoglycolipids (*SGL*). The precise locations of the acylated siderophore mycobactin and the related lipid Didehydroxymycobactin (*DDM*) are unclear, but since they are involved in iron capture and delivery to the mycobacterium, it is conceivable they are present in both the cell wall and plasma membrane

Crystallographic studies on murine CD1d confirmed an overall structural similarity to MHC class I molecules, and provided the first insights into the distinct structural adaptations necessary for lipid presentation (Zeng et al. 1997). The α1, α2 and α3 domains of the CD1d heavy chain adopted a secondary and tertiary structure similar to MHC class I proteins and associated in an analogous fashion with β2-microglobulin. Despite these similarities, the key distinction was that the α1α2 domains of CD1d formed an antigen-binding groove that was substantially larger and deeper relative to that of MHC class I, and was lined with nonpolar residues, consistent with adaptation to binding lipids. Subsequent structures of CD1 proteins presenting individual lipid antigens have confirmed that the hydrophobic groove formed by the α1α2 platform directly binds the nonpolar alkyl chains of lipid antigens. These studies highlight the conserved structure of such alkyl chains relative to microbial antigenic peptides, a factor that may provide an explanation for the lack of allelic variation of individual CD1 isoforms compared to the highly polymorphic class I and class II MHC gene families. In particular, structures of group 1 CD1 molecules (Batuwangala et al. 2004; Gadola et al. 2002; Zajonc et al. 2005b) have provided a more detailed picture of microbial lipid presentation, and recently the structure of murine CD1d in complex with a bacterial glycolipid has been determined (Wu et al. 2006). While a comprehensive discussion of such CD1–lipid complex structures is outside the scope of this review, relevant details are discussed below in relation to specific antigens.

In addition to structural adaptation to presentation of lipid antigens, the expression patterns (reviewed by Blumberg et al., this volume) and intracellular trafficking pathways of CD1 molecules (reviewed by Brenner et al., this volume) exhibit functionally important differences from MHC class I molecules. Briefly, whereas MHC class I molecules are expressed on the surface of most types of nucleated cells, CD1 expression is mainly restricted to professional APCs. Also, whereas MHC class I molecules are specialised to present peptides derived from cytosolic antigens, CD1 trafficking pathways have evolved to acquire antigen in the endocytic pathway, and intersect those utilised by a diverse range of intracellular pathogens. These include bacterial genera such as *Mycobacterium*, *Legionella* and *Salmonella*, as well as protozoa such as *Leishmania*, which enter the cell by endocytosis, suggesting CD1 proteins are likely to have evolved to target such intracellular microbes. As outlined below, the chemical structures of lipids derived from such pathogens are highly distinct from mammalian lipids, and consequently immune surveillance of lipid antigens is likely to provide important contributions to antimicrobial immunity.

In summary, the picture emerging is that by presenting chemically distinct foreign lipid species to T cells, CD1 molecules are likely to play important roles in immune responses to microbial pathogens, including medically important bacterial species such as *M. tuberculosis*. Understanding the structures of CD1-restricted exogenous lipid antigens, and the molecular and immunological basis of their recognition, could promote the development of novel therapeutic strategies based on lipid-specific immunity. In this review, we summarise the current knowledge concerning microbial lipid antigens presented by group 1 and group 2 CD1 molecules, and discuss their potential significance in antimicrobial immune responses. The antigens defined to date illustrate the diversity of bacterial lipids, emphasise major differences in structure to endogenous host counterparts, and reflect the nature of the pathogen–host relationship.

3
Group 1 CD1-Restricted Lipid Antigens

3.1
CD1a Presentation of Didehydroxymycobactin

Recent studies have defined lipopeptides as a novel class of antigen presented by CD1 (Moody et al. 2004). Early experiments showed that a $CD8^+$ T cell line (CD8-2), previously generated from random donor peripheral blood in the presence of organic extracts of *M. tuberculosis*, was capable of lysing $CD1^+$ macrophages infected with *M. tuberculosis* and recognised an antigen present in the lipid fraction in a CD1a-restricted fashion (Rosat et al. 1999). Extractions from whole mycobacteria using a variety of solvents suggested the activating antigen was noncovalently associated with the cell wall and polar in nature. Ultimately, Fourier transform ion cyclotron resonance mass spectroscopy (FITCR-MS) methods led to the identification of the antigen as didehydroxymycobactin (DDM, Fig. 1, 2), a molecule closely related to mycobactin, a mycobacterial lipopeptide with iron-scavenging properties (Moody et al. 2004). DDM consists of a complex headgroup that is peptidic in nature but synthesised by nonribosomal mycobacterial enzymes, linked via acylation of a lysine moiety to a single alkyl chain of approximately 20 carbons (Fig. 2). This structure therefore differs radically from sulfatide self-antigens that bind to CD1a, which are sphingolipids with two alkyl chains and sulphated sugar headgroups. The structure of DDM differs from mycobactin in that it lacks two hydroxyl groups and bears an unusual α-methyl serine moiety (Fig. 1). DDM therefore may function as a direct metabolic precursor of mycocbactin that becomes modified at each lysine residue, hydroxylation of which is critical in enabling the mature siderophore to bind ferric iron with an extremely high (10^{-26} M) affinity (Snow 1970).

The identification of DDM has highlighted siderophores and their precursors as a novel group of bacterial antigens targeted by the CD1 pathway. In infection, bacteria require host iron to support a wide variety of metabolic functions. They scavenge host iron by producing cell-associated and secreted siderophores, which together enable them to bind host iron and deliver it to the bacterium (Wooldridge and Williams 1993). Mycobacteria make a number of siderophores, including mycobactin and related compounds. Siderophore function is thought to be important for mycobacterial growth and virulence, and this is underlined by the complex enzymatic machinery devoted to their synthesis: mycobactin synthesis in *M. tuberculosis* is controlled by a set of ten mycobactin synthase genes (MbtA to MbtJ) encoded in the mycobactin locus (Quadri et al. 1998) that direct the biosynthesis of the iron-binding

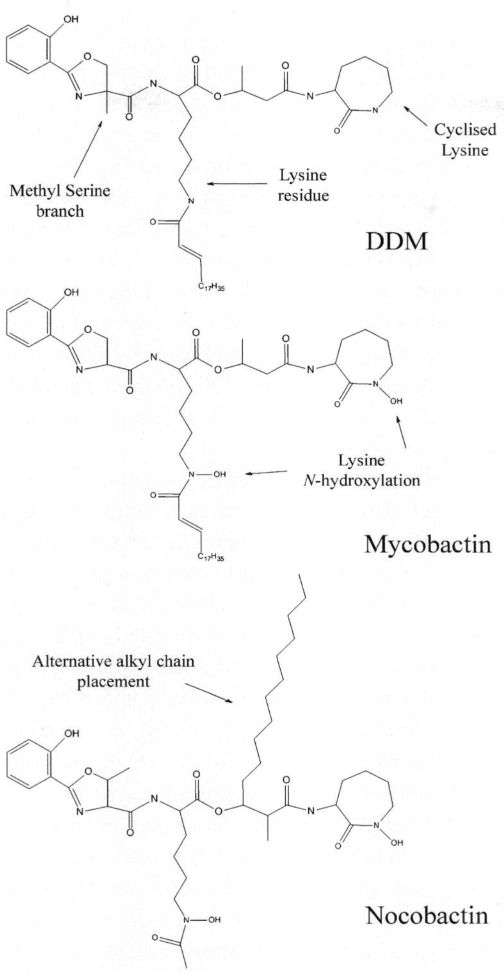

Fig. 2 CD1a-restricted presentation of Didehydroxymycobactin. Didehydroxymy-cobactin (*DDM, top*, derived from *M. tb*) consists of a peptidic headgroup containing methyl serine, lysine and cyclised lysine moieties connected by peptide bonds, acylated by the central lysine residue to a C17 hydrocarbon tail that facilitates binding to CD1a. The structure of the functional mycobactin siderophores (*middle*) differs from DDM in that there are hydroxyl substituents on the two lysine moieties, and they also lack a methyl group on the serine branch. However, such differences are still compatible with binding to CD1a (Zajonc 2005a). The nocobactins, produced by species of *Nocardia* bacteria (*bottom panel*, derived from *Nocardia asteroides*), are iron-binding siderophores structurally related to mycobactins that are also linked to hydrocarbon chains (albeit positioned differently to that of the mycobactins). The length of the alkyl chain present in different *Nocardia* species is currently unclear

core of the siderophores and a further four genes clustered in the *mbt2* locus whose products add the long acyl chain (Card et al. 2005; LaMarca et al. 2004). Not surprisingly, expression of such genes is regulated and becomes de-repressed only in low-iron conditions (Dussurget et al. 1999). However, this occurs normally during growth in host cells and is required for *M. tuberculosis* survival in human macrophages (De Voss et al. 2000). Consistent with this hypothesis, production of the DDM intermediate by *M. tuberculosis*-infected DCs was readily detected only when bacteria were grown under low-iron conditions (Moody et al. 2004). Since CD1a-restricted T cells are able to kill mycobacteria-infected cells in vitro (Stenger et al. 1997), it has been suggested that presentation of DDM and similar antigens may represent an early warning system highlighting intracellular pathogen infection, whereby bacterial metabolites that are important for adaptation to intracellular growth are targeted for immune recognition.

The precise role of the DDM lipopeptide structure in T cell recognition was analysed by comparing recognition of a range of naturally occurring variants of DDM purified from *M. tuberculosis* (Moody et al. 2004). These studies highlighted a number of concepts that had previously emerged from studies on CD1b- and CD1c-restricted recognition of foreign lipids. Firstly, a number of natural DDM variants were recognised, with the length and saturation of the alkyl chain an important factor in recognition, and DDM variants with shorter (C18 rather than C20) or saturated chains exhibiting decreased potencies. Secondly, changes to the lipid headgroup play a critical role in recognition. This was evident since natural mycobactins were not recognised, suggesting hydroxylation of the lysine residues, which is critical in permitting iron chelation by mycobactin, in some way abolishes recognition. Also, eliminating the butyric acid/cyclic lysine branch of the peptide headgroup significantly reduced recognition (Moody et al. 2004), as did modifications to the α-methylserine branch (Zajonc et al. 2005a), consistent with a key role for the lipid headgroup in recognition. Therefore, as for CD1b antigen recognition, the T cell response to DDM was specific for the structure of peptide headgroup, and the length and saturation of the lipid tail.

As with other CD1 isoforms, CD1a does not solely present one type of lipid antigen, as CD1a is known to mediate recognition of sulfatides and other self lipids (Brigl and Brenner 2004; Shamshiev et al. 2002) in addition to DDM. Recent crystallographic structures in complex with the foreign mycobactin lipopeptide (Zajonc et al. 2005a) and a self antigen sulfatide (Zajonc et al. 2003) now suggest molecular mechanisms of how the CD1a groove can present such structurally divergent classes of self and foreign lipids. The hydrophobic A' pocket, which protrudes deep into CD1a and is not directly accessible at the presumed TCR contact site, can accommodate the sphingosine chain of sulfatide, or the single alkyl chain of mycobactin. In contrast, the F' pocket, which is the most shallow and readily accessible compartment of the CD1 groove, can bind either the fatty acid chain from sulfatide or the peptidic moiety from mycobactin. This binding mode enables key portions of the sulfatide or mycobactin headgroups to protrude from the CD1 groove. Although TCR binding of CD1a with lipopeptide analogues has not yet been reported, this evidence strongly favours the hypothesis that fine discrimination of the precise structures of the DDM peptide headgroup moiety can be controlled by differential interactions of the peptide with the TCR (Zajonc et al. 2005a). Therefore, CD1-restricted TCRs, like MHC-restricted TCRs, can discriminate polypeptide sequences.

The extent to which lipopeptides other than DDM may be presented by CD1a molecules is unclear. Mammalian lipopeptides, generated by acylation of peptides produced by mammalian ribosomes to yield structures analogous to DDM and mycobactin, are candidate self ligands for CD1a molecules (Casey 1995). Furthermore, peptidases have been shown to regulate the recognition of certain CD1d-presented antigens, raising the possibility of lipopeptide presentation by other CD1 isoforms (Moody et al. 2004). Further studies are likely to clarify some of these issues. It is also somewhat unclear whether other bacterial siderophore-related molecules may be presented by CD1. The majority of siderophores produced by bacteria are soluble, secreted molecules lacking long acyl chains, and are therefore unlikely to bind to CD1 molecules in their unmodified forms. Production of cell-envelope-associated siderophores incorporating hydrocarbon chain linkages is unusual and appears to be restricted to mycobacteria (which produce the mycobactins) and the related genus *Nocardia* (which produce related siderophores known as nocobactins in which the hydrocarbon chain placement is different) (Fig. 2). The reason for this is probably the lipophilic cell envelope characteristic of these bacteria and the benefit provided by a short-term storage system for iron before it is passed into the cytoplasm of the bacterium (Ratledge and Dover 2000). Since mycobactins are widely produced by mycobacteria, it seems likely that DDM-related structures from species other than *M. tuberculosis* may be targets for CD1-restricted recognition. These include bacteria such as *M. avium*, which is a major cause of disease in immunocompromised patients. Although antigen recognition by the CD8-2 clone was restricted to variants of DDM, it is also possible that the mycobactin structure itself might be presented by CD1a (Zajonc et al. 2005a) and become a target for recognition by other CD1a-restricted T cells with subtly different specificity for the hydroxylated peptidic headgroup, although whether recognition could tolerate mycobactin-bound iron is unclear. Furthermore, it is also conceivable that either nocobactins or nocobactin-related molecules are presented for T cell recognition by CD1 in an analogous fashion to DDM. Nocobactins are produced by numerous *Nocardia* species (Ratledge and Snow 1974), including *Nocardia asteroides*, the species that is most commonly associated with human disease, typically in immunocompromised patients (Fig. 2).

3.2
CD1b Presentation of Mycobacterial Lipid Antigens

The earliest CD1b-restricted antigen to be reported was mycolic acid, a lipid derived from *M. tuberculosis* (Beckman et al. 1994). Since this discovery, a range of other CD1b-restricted foreign lipids have been identified, all of which derive from the mycobacterial cell envelope (Fig. 1) and have no close structural homologues in mammalian cells. These include lipoarabinomannan (LAM), lipomannan (LM) and phosphatidylinositol mannosides (PIMs) (Ernst et al. 1998; Sieling et al. 1995), glucose monomycolate (GMM) (Moody et al. 1997), and sulfoglycolipids (Gilleron et al. 2004). These studies highlight a potential role for CD1b in immunity to pathogenic mycobacteria.

3.2.1
Mycolic Acid and Glucose Monomycolate

Characterisation of mycolic acid as the CD1b-restricted *M. tuberculosis* antigen recognised by the αβ T cell line DN1, derived from a healthy donor by stimulation with *M. tuberculosis* lysate, provided the first evidence that CD1 can present foreign lipids to T cells. Mycolic acids are a family of characteristic α-branched, β-hydroxy fatty acids produced by *M. tuberculosis* and other species of actinomyces bacteria (Figs. 1, 3a). They are present either as free mycolic acids, or as esters of glycerol, a mannosylphospholipid, arabinogalactan and trehalose, key components of the cell walls of mycobacteria, corynebacteria and *Nocardia*. As such, they are extremely abundant, constituting about 40% of the cell wall skeleton (Brennan and Nikaido 1995). In addition, mycolic acids present in mycobacterial cell walls are distinguishable from those of other genera by certain structural features. They are the largest (C_{70} to C_{90}), with the longest α-branch (up to C_{26}), and extremely long meromycolate chains (typically C_{60}) that often contain additional functional groups such as methyl branches, cyclopropane rings, or double bonds (Brennan and Nikaido 1995) (Fig. 3a). The saturated α branches and long meromycolate chains of mycolic acids are thought to favour close packing of hydrocarbon chains in the mycobacterial cell wall, contributing to its rigidity and low permeability. Their importance for *M. tuberculosis* is emphasised by the mode of action of two antituberculosis drugs, isoniazid and ethionamide, which inhibit mycolic acid synthesis (Brennan and Nikaido 1995).

The molecular determinants of CD1b-restricted mycolate recognition have been addressed in relation to αβ T cell clones specific for free mycolic acid (Grant et al. 2002; Porcelli et al. 1992)and for glucose monomycolate (GMM) (Moody et al. 1997) (Fig. 3a), a glucose ester of mycolic acid. Studies on GMM recognition by the LDN5 T cell clone, derived from the skin lesion of a leprosy patient by stimulation with *M. leprae* and *M. phlei* sonicate, have addressed the role of both lipid and headgroup structure in recognition (Moody et al. 1997). Recognition was specific for the characteristic mycobacterial α-branched, β-hydroxy mycolic acid structure of GMM, because synthetic analogues lacking the α branch, or with the β-hydroxy group modified or removed, abolished recognition. Consistent with this, a variety of non-mycolyl glycolipids similar to GMM were not recognised (Moody et al. 1997). Recognition was tested against GMM from a range of mycobacterial species, including *M. tuberculosis*,

---

Fig. 3a–d CD1b-restricted lipid antigens. **a** Mycolic acids present in the cell wall of actinomyces bacteria. The antigens depicted share the characteristic α-branched, β-hydroxy structure of mycolic acid, but differ in chain length and headgroup derivitisation. Mycobacterial mycolic acids (*top three structures*) have longer hydrocarbon chains than mycolic acids derived from corynebacteria (corynomycolate) or *Nocardia* (α-mycolate), with the α branch C_{22-26}, and the meromycolate branch up to C_{90} in length. Mycobacterial mycolic acids can be separated into three classes (α, methoxy, keto) depending on the presence of different functional groups on the meromyolate chain. Glucose monomycolate (GMM) is a glucose ester of mycolic acid, recognised by the LDN5 T cell clone. **b** Highly specific recognition of glucose-6-monomycolate (GMM) by the LDN5 T cell clone. LDN5 recognition of GMM shows exquisite specificity for the carbohydrate headgroup. Recognition requires the carbohydrate moiety, since mycolic acid is not activatory. Recognition is specific for the type of carbohydrate, since neither naturally occurring mycolate esters of glycerol and arabinose, nor synthetic mycolate esters of mannose and galactose are recognised. In addition, recognition is specific for the naturally occurring sugar linkage, since G-6-MM is recognised, whereas the synthetic isomer G-3-MM is not recognised. **c** Structure of mycobacterial glycosylphosphatidylinositols. Mycobacterial phosphatidyl inositol mannosides (PIMs), lipomannan (LM) and lipoarabinomannan (LAM) all share a phosphatidyl inositol core structure that anchors the lipid in the outer leaflet of the plasma membrane. The PIMs are a heterogenous group of antigens that vary in their degree of headgroup mannosylation. LM is formed by addition of mannan repeats (*bracketed*) to an existing PIM structure. LAM is formed by linkage of arabinan to an LM structure to form LAM, after which the headgroup can be capped with inositol phosphate, mannan, or may remain unmodified. **d** Structure of a mycobacterial sulfoglycolipid. The CD1b-restricted sulfoglycolipid A_2SGL (2-palmitoyl-3-hydroxy-phthioceranoyl-2′-sulfate-α-α′-D-trehalose) is derived from *M. tb*, and consists of a sulfated trehalose sugar esterified to two fatty acid chains

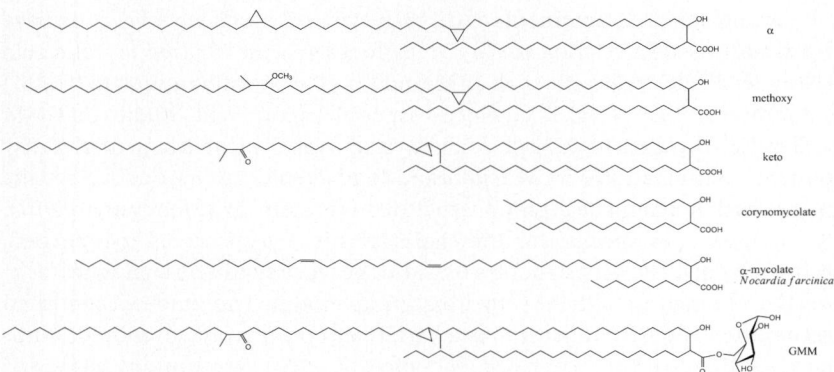

Fig. 3a (continued)

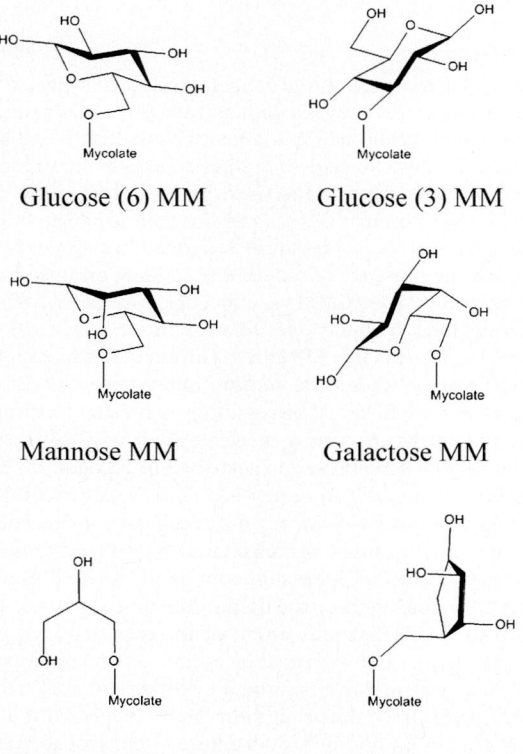

Glucose (6) MM   Glucose (3) MM

Mannose MM   Galactose MM

Monomycolylglycerol   Arabinose MM

Fig. 3b (continued)

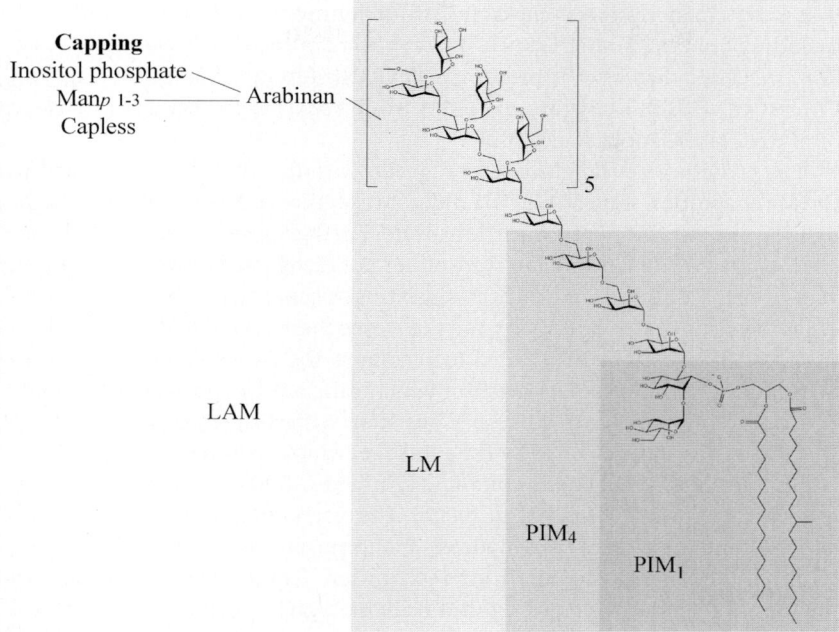

Capping
Inositol phosphate
   Man*p* 1-3 ———— Arabinan
   Capless

LAM

LM

PIM4

PIM1

Fig. 3c (continued)

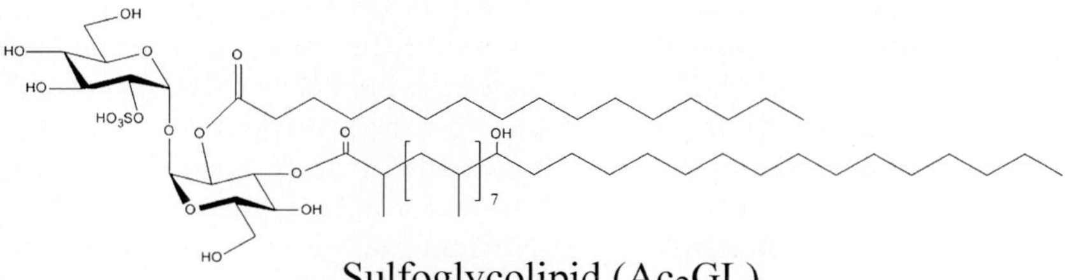

Sulfoglycolipid (Ac2GL)

Fig. 3d (continued)

M. bovis BCG, *M. fortuitum*, *M. smegmatis* and *M. phlei*. Even though mycolic acids from these species differ in chain length, presence or absence of R group substitutions, double bonds, and cyclopropane rings, recognition of GMM species was equivalent. This result indicates that naturally occurring variations in the lipid tail structure were not critical antigenic determinants for the LDN5 T cell clone, and highlights the possibility that GMM-specific T cells may play a role in responses to a relatively wide range of mycobacteria. Furthermore, recognition of a synthetic C_{32} GMM was also retained, suggesting that short-chain mycolates characteristic of nonmycobacterial actinomycetes, including human pathogens such as *Corynebacterium diphtheriae* and *Nocardia asteroides*, may also be presented by CD1b (Moody et al. 1997) (Fig. 3a). Consistent with this suggestion, GMM from *Nocardia farcinica* is known to bind to CD1b (Gadola et al. 2002).

The structure of the glucose headgroup was also found to be critical to GMM recognition (Fig. 3b). LDN5 did not recognise mycolic acid itself, highlighting the requirement for carbohydrate. Furthermore, other naturally occurring glycosylated mycolates were either not recognised or were recognised very poorly (Moody et al. 2000a), suggesting specificity for the glucose moiety. Indicative of fine specificity for the stereochemistry the glucose moiety, the LDN5 T cell clone also failed to recognise the stereoisomers mannose- or galactose-monomycolate, each of which differ in the position of a single hydroxyl group relative to glucose. Consistent with this, recognition was also specific for the natural carbohydrate linkage, which involves esterification of D-glucose via the 6-OH to mycolic acid (glucose-6-MM), since glucose-3-MM was not recognised (Moody et al. 2000a). The orientation of the lipid branches and the configuration of the β-hydroxy group specific to the natural mycobacterial GMM was also required for recognition. These data clearly support the idea that CD1-specific recognition can be highly specific for the exposed hydrophilic components of the lipid headgroup.

Studies on recognition of free mycolic acid by the DN1 T cell clone also confirmed the importance of the chemistry of the headgroup for recognition. Whereas mycolic acid was recognised, methyl esters of mycolic acid were not (Grant et al. 2002). This indicated the negatively charged carboxylate group was required for recognition, and strongly suggested methylation of this group abolished recognition by the DN1 TCR. Consistent with this, lipids with similar modifications, such as esterification to glucose as in GMM (Fig. 3a), were not recognised by the DN1 clone (Moody et al. 1997). However, recognition of mycolic acid by DN1 differed from that of GMM by LDN5 in that it was sensitive to structural differences in the meromycolate (longer) chain. In particular, *M. tuberculosis* mycolic acids can be classified as α, methoxy or keto based on the presence of distal cyclopropanol, methoxy or keto substitutions on the distal end of the meromycolate chain (Brennan and Nikaido 1995) (Fig. 3a). Recognition of methoxy and keto mycolic acid forms was observed, but α-mycolates failed to activate T cells, indicating that the presence of oxygen groups on the meromycolate chains is necessary for efficient recognition. The molecular mechanism underlying these differences remains unclear, but could conceivably involve indirect effects on TCR recognition mediated through lipid headgroup conformation, or inefficient loading or binding of α-mycolates onto CD1b (Grant et al. 2002).

Crystallographic studies of CD1b in complex with various lipids have shed light on the structural basis of mycobacterial mycolate presentation. Structures in complex with the self lipids phosphatidylinositol (PI) or ganglioside GM2 (GM2) (Gadola et al. 2002) revealed a complex network of hydrocarbon-filled hydrophobic channels radically different from the antigen-binding groove of MHC molecules, with a total volume of 2,200 $Å^3$. Two key features suggested structural adaptation of CD1b for binding lipids with long hydrocarbon tails. Firstly, unlike all other CD1 isoforms, three of the pockets within the larger CD1 groove, known as A′, T′ and F′ pockets, created an extended channel with the potential to accommodate lengthy meromycolate chains typical of mycobacterial mycolic acids. Secondly, the C′ channel, suggested to bind the α-branch chain of a mycolic acid, connected to an exit portal on the side of the CD1 molecule beneath the α2 helix. This feature, which also appears to be unique to CD1b, is likely to facilitate binding by lipids with α-branch chains longer than C_{16}, such as those of mycobacterial mycolates (Fig. 3a) (Cheng et al. 2006). The structure of CD1b in complex with GMM derived from the actinomycete *Nocardia farcinica* (Batuwangala et al. 2004) confirmed certain of these predictions. While the glucose moiety protruded from the antigen-binding surface between the α1 and α2 domains, the C_{49} meromycolate chain filled the A′T′F′ superchannel and protruded somewhat into the TCR recognition surface, and the relatively short (C8) α-branch was easily accommodated in the C′ channel, without egress from the C′ portal. Because the CD1b groove is unique among CD1 isoforms studied to date with regard to its size and presence of a second portal for lipid egress (Batuwangala et al. 2004; Gadola et al. 2002), these data provide some of the strongest evidence yet that different CD1 isoforms are evolutionarily adapted for binding to different subsets of lipid ligands. Consistent with CD1b being particularly well suited to presentation of long lipids, including those from pathogenic bacteria, experiments on CD1b lipid presentation by Moody et al. (2002) determined that the length of lipid alkyl chains has a dominant effect on presentation. In contrast to shorter lipids, long C80 mycolates were efficiently and preferentially loaded in endosomal compartments, resulting in T cell activation that was prolonged and more sensitive to lipid antigen. However, major questions remain. In particular, modelling studies based on the CD1b-GMM structure suggested that meromycolate chain substituents, including α, methoxy and keto variants, could be accommodated in the CD1b binding channel with only minor changes to side chain conformations and overall channel volume, leaving the question of how such substituents are distinguished in the context of mycolic acid unresolved (Grant et al. 2002).

Although TCR–lipid–CD1 complex structures are not currently available, studies on CD1b-restricted receptors have provided useful clues as to how lipid antigen recognition likely takes place. Early experiments established diverse TCR gene usage by group 1 CD1-restricted T cells, confirmed that the TCR itself was able to confer antigen specificity in a CD1-isoform restricted manner, and highlighted a propensity for positively charged residues in the CDR3 regions of receptors that recognised negatively charged organic acids or phosphate moieties (Grant et al. 1999). Also, extensive mutagenesis of CD1b supported recognition of the α1α2 peptide-binding platform and a diagonal orientation for mycolic acid and GMM-specific TCRs (Melian et al. 2000). Subsequent experiments on the DN1 TCR, which is specific for mycolic acid, established a key role for positively charged residues in CDR3β during antigen recognition, favouring the suggestion that the surface formed by the CDR loops of this TCR is directly involved in binding the lipid antigen and CD1-presenting molecule (Grant et al. 2002). Attempts to model TCR/CD1 complexes involving mycolic acid (Grant et al. 1999, 2002) or GMM (Batuwangala et al. 2004) based on TCR/MHC class I structures have suggested a broadly similar binding mode that would allow the CDR3 loops of the TCR to be positioned over the hydrophilic headgroup of the bound lipid, with CDR1 and CDR2 predicted to contact the CD1 α-helices and help orient the TCR. For the DN1 TCR, the CDR3β loop was hypothesised to protrude between the α1 and α2 helices, with its positively charged arginine residues predicted to directly contact the negatively charged headgroup of mycolic acid (Grant et al. 1999, 2002). Clearly further structural studies in this area will help to resolve these issues.

The production of the GMM antigen has also been a focus of study (Moody et al. 2000a). A range of mycobacteria, including *M. phlei*, *M. smegmatis* and *M. avium*, were unable to generate the GMM antigen de novo, unless an exogenous source of glucose was present. Production occurred at glucose concentrations that are appropriate for mammalian cells and therefore likely to be available to mycobacteria during tissue-based growth, and was efficient, since GMM comprised up to 2% of total cell wall extractable lipid. Furthermore, GMM was found to be produced in in vivo *M. leprae* infection at antigenically significant levels. This study suggests that mycobacteria produce GMM by acquiring exogenous glucose from either media or host tissues and esterifying it to mycobacterial mycolic acids. Since glucose is not likely to be present in mycobacterial growth environments other than infected tissues, an important implication is that GMM generation may be restricted to pathogenic mycobacteria capable of infecting host tissue, rather than environmental saprophytic bacteria. Such issues are relevant to immunity to mycobacteria, since humans are commonly exposed to environmental saprophytes but commonly do not mount strong cell-mediated immunity. Therefore, as a composite antigen generated from mycobacterial and host moieties, GMM may allow the immune system not only to discriminate self from non-self, but also pathogenic from innocuous non-self (Moody et al. 2000a).

3.2.2
Lipoarabinomannan, Lipomannan and Phosphatidylinositol Mannosides

Studies on T cell clones derived from either human leprosy skin lesions (LDN4) or from a healthy donor (BDN2) led to the identification of mycobacterial glycosylphosphatidylinositols as CD1b-restricted lipids (Sieling et al. 1995) (Fig. 3c). These antigens have at their core a phosphatidyl inositol structure homologous to that present in mammalian cells, and so are likely to bind to CD1b with their acyl chains occupying the A' and C' channels, as seen in the crystal structure of CD1b bound to phosphatidylinositol (Gadola et al. 2002). One subset, the phosphatidylinositol mannosides (PIMs), contain varying numbers of mannose residues, are restricted to actinomycetes (Brennan and Nikaido 1995) and are major components of the outer leaflet of the mycobacterial plasma membrane. Lipomannan (LM) and lipoarabino-mannan (LAM), which is essentially identical to the former but incorporates distal arabinose groups, are multiglycosylated extensions of the PIMs. LAM, a prominent component of the mycobacterial cell envelope, is heterogeneous in structure, with variation between different mycobacterial species in terms of whether and how the arabinose moieties possess a terminal mannose unit (Fig. 3c). LAM exerts a wide range of biological activities, including diverse effects on phagocyte chemotaxis and function, DC function and T cell migration and activation (Karakousis et al. 2004). In addition, both LAM and PIM have been shown to induce CD1 expression in human myeloid cells via TLR-2 (Roura-Mir et al. 2005), and a key unanswered question is whether LAM and PIM predominantly activate T cells via TLRs or by direct CD1-restricted presentation to the TCR (Moody 2006; Roura-Mir et al. 2005).

Analysis of the LDN4 and BDN2 clones led to the suggestion that specificity for hydrophilic determinants was a key feature of lipid antigen recognition by CD1-restricted T cells (Sieling et al. 1995). Experiments also highlighted specificity for mycobacterial carbohydrate structures since both clones were activated by mycobacterial lipoglycans, but lipoglycan moieties from other bacteria, such as either LPS from *Escherichia coli*, lipophosphoglycan (LPG) from *Leishmania major*, or LTAs from *Streptococcus pyogenes* did not induce responses (Sieling et al. 1995). However, further experiments indicated the clones had distinct specificities for the carbohydrate components of the lipoglycan. BDN2 was stimulated equivalently by LAM and LM, suggesting the arabinan component was not required for T cell activation. In contrast, LM was not as efficient as LAM in stimulating LDN4, suggesting the arabinan did affect recognition for this clone. Similarly, PIMs induced BDN2 to proliferate but stimulated LDN4 cells poorly. However, BDN2 showed poor recognition of PIM2, the minimal structural unit, and LDN4 recognition of LM was abrogated by prior α-mannosidase digestion of the antigen, suggesting that for both clones, the degree of mannosylation is important in recognition. In keeping with distinct specificities for the carbohydrate components, the two lines exhibited different species-specific recognition patterns. LDN4 recognised LAM from *M. leprae*, but did not respond to LAM from *M. tuberculosis*, whereas BDN2 cells recognised LAM from both species. One possible explanation for this was that LDN4 recognition required the entire mannan core, the structure of which differs in the number of mannose linkages and branching points between species, whereas BDN2 was able to recognise PIM6, an antigen conserved between different mycobacteria.

3.2.3
Sulfoglycolipids

Recently, mycobacterial sulfoglycolipids (SGL) have been identified as novel CD1b-restricted antigens recognised by *M. tuberculosis*-specific T cells (Gilleron et al. 2004). Mycobacterial SGL are cell envelope molecules that consist of a trehalose 2′ sulphate core, acylated by two to four fatty acids, which can be palmitic, stearic, hydroxyphthioceranoic, or phthioceranoic. They are thought to exert a range of biological activities, including antitumour activity (Yarkoni et al. 1979), and the extent of their expression in *M. tuberculosis* strains has been correlated with strain virulence in guinea pig models (Goren 1982). By combining fractionation of *M. tuberculosis* lipids with mass spectroscopy and T cell activation assays using CD8[+] *M. tuberculosis*-specific T cell clones derived from a healthy PPD[+] individual, a group of structurally related diacylated sulfoglycolipids (Ac$_2$SGL) containing hydroxyphthioceranoic and either palmitic (C_{16}) or stearic (C_{18}) acid chains, both attached to the glucose moiety lacking the sulphate group, were identified as the active antigenic species (Fig. 3d). This structure differs fundamentally from other CD1b-restricted mycolate antigens and lipoglycan antigens (based on a PI core structure), and it is unclear exactly how such SGL antigens are bound by CD1b. However, based on existing CD1b-lipid crystal structures (Batuwangala et al. 2004; Gadola et al. 2002) and the acyl chain lengths of the Ac$_2$SGLs (Gilleron et al. 2004), it seems most likely that the shorter palmitic (C_{16}) or stearic (C_{18}) chains are accommodated in the C′ pocket, with the longer hydroxyphthioceranoic (C_{32}) acid more suited to binding the A′T′F′ channel and the hydrophilic headgroup exposed for recognition by the TCR. Interestingly, removal of the sulphate group from the

Ac_2SGL antigen completely abrogated recognition by Ac_2SGL-specific T cell clones, a finding consistent with such a conserved mode of lipid binding and indicative of fine specificity of the TCR for the negatively charged SGL headgroup (Gilleron et al. 2004). Consistent with studies on other CD1-restricted antigens, presentation of Ac_2SGL was dependent on efficient endosomal loading. Studies on *M. tuberculosis*-infected cells also indicated that presentation of the Ac_2SGL antigen was relatively efficient during infection, and was sufficient to stimulate Ac_2SGL-specific T cell effector functions, which included production of IFN-γ and killing of intracellular bacteria in vitro. These data suggest that CD1b-restricted T cell responses to SGL selectively occur in *M. tuberculosis*-infected humans and could potentially contribute to immunity.

3.3
CD1c Presentation of Mycoketides

The first evidence that in addition to CD1b, CD1c could also restrict the T cell response to foreign antigens resulted from experiments on mycobacteria-specific T cell lines generated from healthy donor blood. The antigens recognised by these clones were shown to be both CD1-restricted and protease resistant, and therefore mycobacterial lipids were implicated (Beckman et al. 1996). Subsequent studies indicated that such CD1c-restricted clones could be CD8[+], proving that CD1-restricted populations specific for foreign lipids were not limited to CD4[-]CD8[-] T cell populations (Rosat et al. 1999).

The first CD1c-restricted antigens to be defined structurally were isolated from lipids in the cell wall of both *M. avium* and *M. tuberculosis* (Moody et al. 2000b) and shown to be closely related to mannosyl β-1-phosphomycoketides (MPMs). These antigens contain a single fully saturated alkyl chain that was similar to isoprenoid lipids, with methyl branches at every fourth carbon (Fig. 4), so that they are also referred to as mannosyl phosphoisoprenoids (MPIs). Their structures are therefore homologous to mannosyl phospho-dolichols (MPDs) that function as carbohydrate donors in glycan synthesis pathways, for example N-linked glycosylation in eukaryotes and cell wall assembly in prokaryotes. Subsequent studies have defined more comprehensively the species of bacteria that produce MPMs and clarified the biosynthetic pathways involved (Matsunaga et al. 2004). Firstly, the stimulatory MPM antigens were only present in cell wall extracts from mycobacteria and were restricted to species that could infect human cells including *M. avium*, *M. tuberculosis* (including clinical isolates from patients) and *M. bovis* BCG. In contrast, rapidly growing saprophytes incapable of infecting human cells, such as *M. phlei*, *M. fallax*, *M. smegmatis*, did not produce the antigen. Secondly,

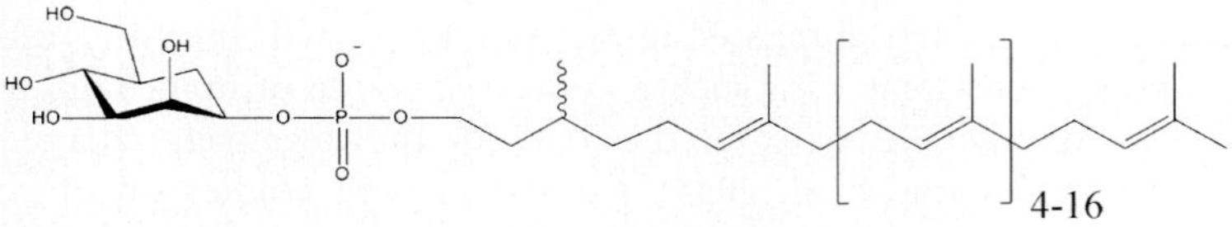

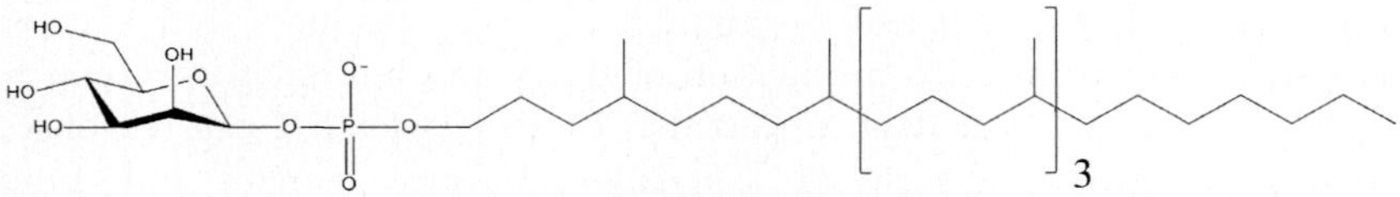

Fig. 4 CD1c-restricted Mycoketide antigens. The *upper panel* shows the structure of mannosyl-β-1-phosphodolichols (MPDs), true isoprenoid lipids that are present in a wide variety of species. The length of the dolichol portion varies between species due to different numbers of additional isoprenoid units (*bracketed*). Mammalian isoprenoids are long (e.g. *Homo sapiens*, $n=16$, C_{95} lipid chain) whereas protozoan isoprenoids are intermediate in length (e.g. *Plasmodium falciparum*, $n=9$, C_{60}). *Lower panel*: the mycobacterial lipid antigens that stimulated the CD1c-restricted clone CD8-1 (originally termed mannosyl-β-1-phosphoisoprenoids, MPIs) have an identical mannosyl-β-1 headgroup to mammalian MPDs but distinct saturated tail structures that are equivalent in length to MPDs with approximately four additional isoprenoid units (C_{35}), considerably shorter than those of mammals. Although these antigens are structural mimics of isoprenoids, their saturated tails are synthesised by a distinct polyketide mechanism, and they are now referred to as mannosyl-b-1-phosphomycoketides (MPMs). The *lower panel* shows the structure of an MPM with a C_{32} tail from *M. tb*

while these antigens are clearly isoprenoid-like in structure, characterisation of other closely related lipids has revealed structural diversity in the alkyl chains that cannot be accounted for by a true isoprenoid synthetic pathway based on condensation of C_5 IPP. Instead, biosynthesis of these MPM antigens was via a novel polyketide pathway involving the enzyme Pks12 and sequential condensation of C2 (malonate) and C3 (methylmalonate) units. MPMs therefore represent a novel set of single-chain alkane phospholipids that structurally mimic polyisoprenols but are synthesised using a polyketide mechanism, and are produced by mycobacterial pathogens that infect human tissue. The role of such mycoketides is unclear at present, but the fact they are only produced by infectious mycobacteria rather than saprophytes suggests they may play a role in intracellular growth. Also, the structural homology of MPMs with MPDs suggests that MPMs may also function as lipid intermediates in mannose transmembrane transport or transfer.

Experiments aiming to define the precise antigenic determinants of MPMs have allowed insight into factors affecting recognition of these antigens (Moody et al. 2000b). Experiments with synthetic lipids established that whereas the CD8-1 T cell line was able to recognise MPM analogues with mannose headgroups, those with a glucose moiety or lacking a sugar were not recognised. This indicated fine specificity for the carbohydrate headgroup of the MPM antigen, in common with other antigens restricted by other CD1 iso-forms. However, strikingly, the mannosyl-β-1-phosphate headgroup structure of MPMs is identical in mannosyl-β-1-phosphodolichols (MPDs) from mammalian cells (Matsunaga et al. 2004; Moody et al. 2000b) (Fig. 4). Not surprisingly therefore, the structure of the mycobacterial MPM alkyl chain was found to be important for recognition. Firstly, the presence of a saturated α-prenyl-like unit was required for recognition, and this effect was hypothesised to contribute to weaker recognition of structurally related but unsaturated mycobacterial phosphoisoprenoids, such as mannosyl-β1-phosphoheptaprenol (Moody et al. 2000b). Secondly, recognition of MPD dolichol analogues, identical to the natural mycobacterial antigens in their headgroup structure, was inversely proportional to length of the prenyl chain. Mannosyl phospho-dolichols (MPDs) with chain lengths similar to the mycobacterial antigens (C_{35}) were strongly recognised, whereas long chains typical of protozoa (C_{55}) or human MPDs (C_{95}) were not recognised (Matsunaga et al. 2004; Moody et al. 2000b) (Fig. 4). This indicates that, despite the identical headgroups present in MPMs and MPDs, mycobacterial MPMs are distinguished from mammalian MPDs and those from other species by the complete saturation and shorter length of their alkyl chains.

Studies on the CD1c-restricted mycobacterial MPM antigens have highlighted a number of important concepts relating to lipid antigen presentation and recognition in general. They suggest that CD1 molecules could present lipid antigens with single hydrocarbon tails, in contrast to previously defined antigens presented by CD1b and CD1d, which have two alkyl chains. Also, uniquely for CD1 antigens defined to date, the headgroups of MPMs are identical to mammalian MPD self antigens (Fig. 4). In contrast, the hydrophilic headgroups of other CD1-restricted lipids appear to be distinct from mammalian self lipid homologues. MPMs therefore provide the clearest example whereby distinctive chemical features of the hydrocarbon tails of the mycobacterial species, in particular the shorter length and fully saturated structure of MPM lipid moiety relative to mammalian equivalents, may play a role enabling CD1-restricted T cells to discriminate self from non-self. A likely explanation for this is that the structural features of CD1c enable preferential binding to mycobacterial MPMs compared to mammalian self-MPDs.

How these effects are manifest at a molecular level is currently unclear. Since CD1c is known to present self lipids with hydrophilic headgroups entirely different from MPMs (Shamshiev et al. 2000), it may be that MPM recognition often involves discrimination of headgroup features, as for the CD8-1 T cell clone. It seems quite likely that CD1c may bind MPMs in a broadly analogous fashion to CD1a binding to DDM, since the mycobactin lipid tail is accommodated in the A′ channel of the CD1a molecule, a region hypothesised to be structurally relatively conserved between CD1a and CD1c (Batuwangala et al. 2004). Furthermore, analysis of CD1c sequences (Batuwangala et al. 2004) in the context of CD1b (Batuwangala et al. 2004) and CD1a structures (Zajonc et al. 2003), suggests that CD1c shares similar amino acid substitutions to CD1a in the A′ channel, which would be broadly consistent with presentation of hydrocarbon tails of similar length to mycobacterial MPMs (C_{30-34}), but likely to exclude binding of considerably longer mammalian MPDs (C_{95}). Potentially the length of the A′ channel could affect whether MPDs derived from protozoa, which tend to be somewhat shorter ($\sim C_{55}$) than mammalian MPDs, are able to bind CD1c. In addition, decreases in the length and increases in the abundance of mammalian MPDs produced during cell senescence and transformation raise the possibility that such lipids might play a role as stress antigens for CD1c-restricted T cells in these scenarios (Crick et al. 1994; Edlund et al. 1992; Henry et al. 1991). In addition to discrimination via lipid length, it is also possible that CD1c may be specialised to bind the saturated tails of mycobacterial MPMs, since the curved nature of the lipid binding grooves would favour saturated structures vs the extensively unsaturated structures of dolichols, which would be more rigid.

4
Group 2 CD1-Restricted Lipid Antigens

4.1
CD1d Presentation of Bacterial and Protozoan Glycolipids

The group 2 CD1d molecule is recognised by T cells that are phenoytpically distinct from those restricted to group 1 CD1 molecules. CD1d-restricted T cells commonly express markers characteristic of natural killer (NK) cells, and are therefore referred to as natural killer T cells (NKT). They exhibit a restricted T cell receptor chain usage, with canonical iNKTs expressing a semi-invariant αβ TCR. In humans, NKTs predominantly use the Vα24 gene segment rearranged with Jα18 (formerly JαQ), and preferentially paired with Vβ11 chains. In mice, Vα14 (homologous to human Vα24) chains preferentially pair with Vβ8 (homologous to human Vβ11), Vβ7 or Vβ2 chains.

CD1d-restricted NKTs are overtly autoreactive in the sense that they can be stimulated by CD1d$^+$ APCs in the absence of foreign antigen (Bendelac et al. 1995; Exley et al. 1997; Porcelli et al. 1989). Both human and murine NKTs can be identified by recognition of α-galactosylceramide (Fig. 5a), a foreign glycosphingolipid that binds CD1d and was first identified in marine sponges (Natori et al. 1994). Although α-galactosylceramide has no known physiological function in mammalian immunity, it resembles mammalian ceramides in having a sphingosine base, an amide-like acyl chain, and an O-linked galactose sugar. However, the anomeric carbon of the sugar has an α (equatorial) linkage to oxygen, whereas in mammals, the corresponding linkage is β-anomeric (axial). NKT cells are not known to be activated by β-anomerically linked monoglycosyl ceramides, so that the α-linkage is crucial for recognition. Until recently, it was unclear how α-galactosylceramide related to either endogenous or foreign pathogen-derived antigens restricted to CD1d. However, NKT cells have been implicated as functionally important regulators of immune responses in a range of scenarios, including anti-tumour immunity, autoimmunity and allergic responses (Brigl and Brenner 2004). Similarly, there are also indications that NKT cells may be important in microbial immunity. In particular, mice treated with α-galactosylceramide have been shown to have increased resistance to infection by viruses, mycobacteria and trypanosomes. In addition, CD1d-deficient mice have increased susceptibility to bacterial, fungal and parasitic infection, suggesting CD1d-restricted cells are an important component of the pathogen-specific response. A key question is whether such effects are mediated by direct recognition of foreign microbial antigens, or altered regulation of endogenous lipid presentation in infection. Here we discuss recent studies that suggest both processes may be involved in CD1d-restricted responses.

4.1.1
Glycosyl Phosphatidylinositol-Like Lipids

Evidence from murine systems established that ubiquitous mammalian phospholipids including phosphatidyl inositol (PI) are endogenous ligands for CD1d and can be recognised by NKT hybridomas (De Silva et al. 2002; Gumperz et al. 2000; Joyce et al. 1998). Similarly, glycosylphosphatidyl inositol (GPI) has been eluted from CD1d and is thought to be a common natural CD1d-bound lipid (De Silva et al. 2002; Joyce et al. 1998). These studies provided a basis for identification of related foreign antigenic lipids. The first lipids reported to function as exogenous antigens for CD1d-restricted NKT cells were GPI structures linked to proteins derived from protozoan pathogens (Schofield et al. 1999). NKT recognition of GPIs was dependent

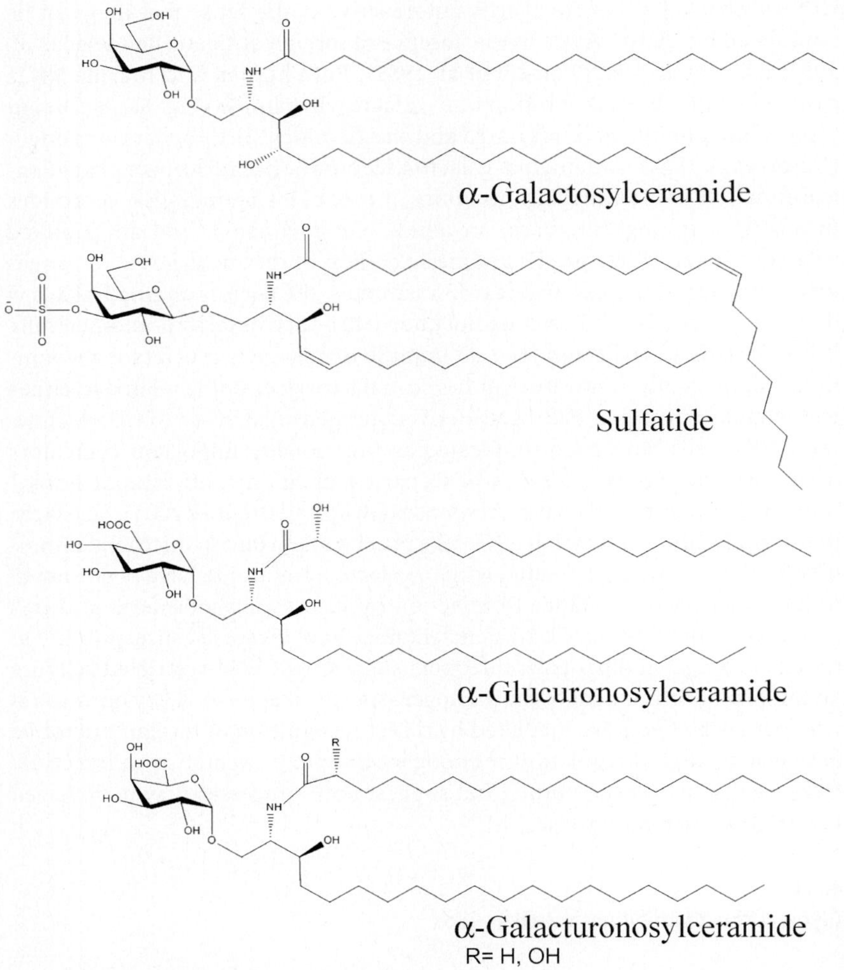

α-Galactosylceramide

Sulfatide

α-Glucuronosylceramide

α-Galacturonosylceramide
R= H, OH

Fig. 5a,b Foreign lipid antigens presented by CD1d. **a** Sphingolipid ligands presented by CD1d. *Upper two panels*: α-GalCer resembles mammalian ceramides such as sulfatide in having a sphingosine base, an amide-like acyl chain, and an O-linked galactose. However, the anomeric carbon of the sugar has an α (equatorial) linkage to oxygen, whereas in mammalian lipids such as sulfatide, the linkage is β-anomeric (axial). *Lower two panels*: structures of the *Sphingomonas* cell wall lipids α-glucuronosyl ceramide (*GSL-1*) and α-galacturonosylceramide (*GSL-1'*) are clearly closely related to α-GalCer and share similar α-anomeric linkages to the sugar headgroup. **b** Structure of lipophosphoglycan (*LPG*). The structure of LPG from *Leishmania*, with the phosphate–galactose–mannose repeating unit bracketed

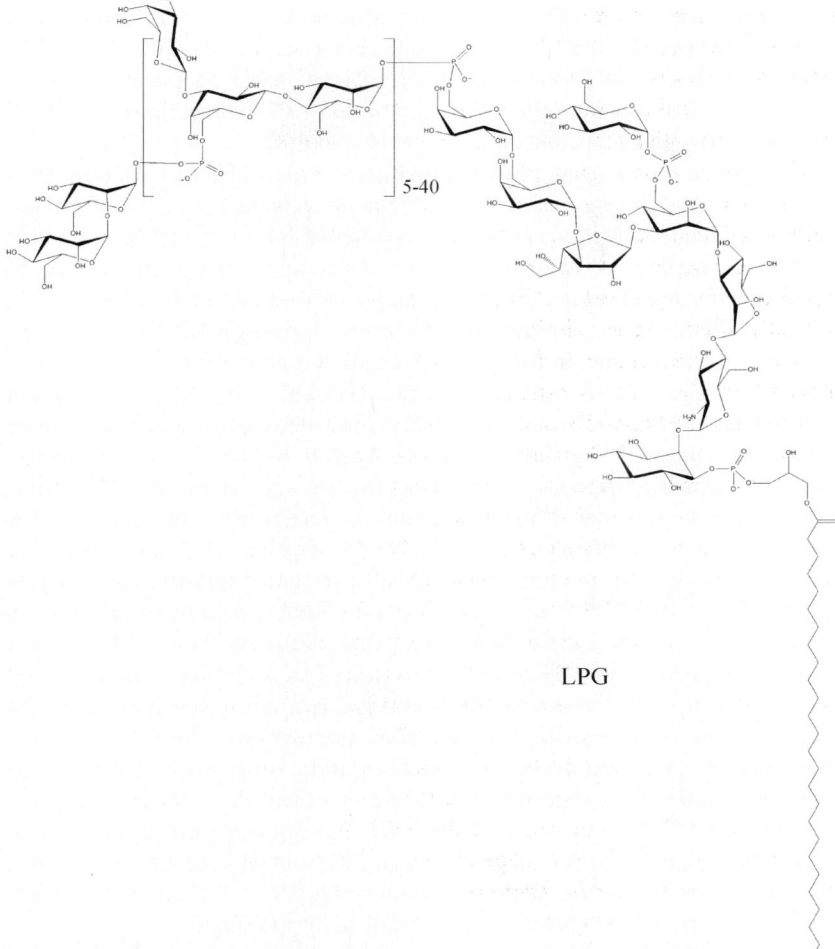

5-40

LPG

Fig. 5b (continued)

on the glycan headgroup, as PI itself was not stimulatory, and a range of mammalian self-GPIs were also reported to be stimulatory. Furthermore, recognition by murine NKTs of GPIs derived from *Plasmodium falciparum* and *Trypanosoma brucei* presented on the surface of B cells was proposed to provide CD1d-dependent B cell help, enabling IgG production to GPI-linked protozoan antigens (Schofield et al. 1999). However, subsequent studies have challenged these findings, indicating antibody responses were MHC class II-dependent rather than CD1d-restricted (Molano et al. 2000; Procopio et al. 2002; Romero et al. 2001). It is also unclear if endogenous GPIs act as self-antigens for NKTs (Schofield et al. 1999), as CD1d$^+$ APCs unable to synthesise GPIs were found to retain the ability to stimulate CD1d-restricted T cell hybridomas (De Silva et al. 2002; Molano et al. 2000).

Recently, mycobacterial phosphatidylinositol mannosides have been proposed as potential exogenous CD1d-restricted antigens (Fischer et al. 2004). Among *M. bovis* BCG lipids tested, only phosphatilylinositol tetramannoside (PIM$_4$) was capable of strong binding to CD1d. Interestingly, in addition to mycolic acids, mycobacterial lipids incapable of binding CD1d included LAM and LM, which share a similar core structure to phosphatidyl inositolmannosides. In vitro assays indicated PIM mediated activation of murine and human NKTs in a CD1d-restricted manner (Fischer et al. 2004). Comparison of the effect of PIM and PI on murine NKTs indicated similar amounts of IFNγ production, but no IL-4 production, in contrast to α-galactosylceramide. Experiments also highlighted a requirement for two acyl chains for CD1d binding, and the importance of the headgroup for recognition. In addition, PIM was also able to selectively expand Vα24Vβ11 human NKTs and sensitised target cells to lysis in in vitro assays. Finally, tetramer staining experiments indicated that PIM-CD1d tetramers stained a subset of human and mouse α-galactosylceramide-specific NKTs. In principle, these data might suggest that the mycobacterial PIM may be recognised in a similar manner to the endogenous lipid PI by murine NKTs and indicate a fine specificity for PIM within α-galactosylceramide-reactive NKT populations. However, the idea that α-galactosylceramide-reactive NKTs contain subpopulations with discrete specificities to a range of related foreign antigens does not easily explain the conserved TCR chain usage of the NKT TCR. In addition, an alternative hypothesis, that PIM is not a ligand for the TCR but instead activates TLR-2 on APCs leading to cellular responses that involve CD1d-TCR interactions but not CD1-restricted recognition of PIM, is difficult to exclude.

PI-related lipids derived from protozoan parasites of the genus *Leishmania* have also been suggested as foreign antigens restricted by CD1d (Amprey et al. 2004) (Fig. 5b). *Leishmania* protozoa infect millions of humans worldwide, causing a wide range of symptoms termed leishmaniasis. *Leishmania* are transmitted by infected sandflies, which transfer infectious protozoa to the host that differentiate inside the phagolysosomes of macrophages into replicative forms. The dense surface glycocalyx of *Leishmania*, formed by glycoinositol phospholipids (GIPLs) and related lipophosphoglycan (LPG) (Fig. 5b), is critical to resistance to such hydrolytic environments. CD1d$^{-/-}$ mice were found to have increased susceptibility to *Leishmania* infection, exhibiting a delay in the generation of protective immunity. This finding suggested that CD1d responses contribute to the development of a protective response. Consistent with this, CD1d$^{-/-}$ mice showed defective granuloma formation around infected macrophages, a TH1 process mediated by IFNγ. Experiments suggested that in CD1d$^+$ mice, *Leishmania* infection led to rapid production of IFN-γ by a small proportion of hepatic NKTs (3%–6%) and increases in their numbers, effects that were IL-12-independent. This led the authors to suggest that *Leishmania* glycolipids were directly recognised by NKTs through CD1d and that this contributed to subsequent responses involving classical T cells and NK cells. Consistent with this idea, in vitro assays showed that both GIPL and LPG, which share structural similarities to both PI and glycosphingolipids such as α-galactosylceramide, were able to bind CD1d. In support of direct recognition of *Leishmania* lipids, DCs pulsed with LPG-induced IFNγ production by hepatic lymphocytes from naïve mice, at levels broadly comparable with α-galactosylceramide, in a CD1d-restricted fashion. Interestingly, the LPG lipid tail was necessary but insufficient to induce such responses, suggesting that both lipid and glycan portions of the molecule were important. However, removal of the repeating units of phosphate-galactose and mannose had little effect. Consistent with activation of liver cells, direct injection of LPG led to IFNγ production by a minor subset (~1.5%) of α-galactosylceramide-reactive liver NKTs. These data link CD1d-dependent antimicrobial immunity in liver infection to the presentation of microbial lipoglycans by CD1d. They suggest an early role of *Leishmania*-responsive NKTs in establishing a protective TH1 response. However, they leave unresolved whether LPG is recognised in a CD1d-restricted manner by NKT cells, or whether alternatively its effects are mediated via effects on APCs. Interestingly, CD1d tetramers presenting LPG failed to identify responding populations, but this could either reflect indirect recognition mediated via alterations in self lipid presentation by CD1d, or alternatively, LPG could be directly recognised in a modified form. LPG is shed from the parasite surface into the lumen of the host cell phagosome during infection, where it could be processed by hydrolases and glycosidases prior to recognition by NKTs.

4.1.2
Bacterial Glycosphingolipids

In addition to phospholipids and GPIs, CD1d is also able to present bacterial sphingolipids that have α-anomeric linkages and are closely related to α-galactosylceramide for direct recognition by NKT cells (Fig. 5a). In a coculture system containing NKTs and DCs, IFNγ production in response to the LPS-positive bacteria *Salmonella* was TLR-dependent and weakly dependent on CD1d, whereas responses to the LPS-negative bacteria *Ehrlichia* and *Sphin*-

gomonas were drastically reduced in the absence of CD1d and did not involve TLRs (Mattner et al. 2005). This suggested that in response to *Salmonella*, IFNγ production was initiated after TLR signalling on the APCs. Furthermore, the use of mice deficient in synthesis of endogenous sphingolipids and blocking experiments using lectins specific for endogenous disaccharide linkages suggested NKT responses to *Salmonella* involved endogenous ligands. In contrast, the results suggested a direct role for CD1d-presented lipids in NKT activation in response to *Ehrlichia* and *Sphingomonas*. In support of this, glycosyl ceramides derived from the cell wall of *Sphingomonas* were identified that were found to strongly activate mouse and human NKT proliferation and IFNγ secretion. These compounds, α-glucuronosyl-ceramide (GSL-1) and α-galacturonosyl-ceramide (GSL-1′) (Fig. 5a), were naturally occurring bacterial sphingolipids closely related to α-galactosylceramide in that they contained α-anomeric linkages to the carbohydrate moiety and were previously found to substitute for LPS in the bacterial outer membrane (Kawahara et al. 2000). CD1d tetramers presenting GSL-1 stained all human NKTs, and a panel of 16 mouse NKT hybridomas responded directly to both compounds, suggesting that recognition of α-anomeric bacterial glycolipids may be a common property of conserved NKT TCRs. In support of a role for such recognition in vivo, NKT-deficient mice infected with *Sphingomonas* showed delayed bacterial clearance and higher bacterial load compared to controls, and were also unable to clear *Ehrlichia* infection. A parallel study also provided strong evidence for the importance of NKT cells after *Sphingomonas* infection, highlighting NKT activation after infection and defective bacterial clearance in NKT-deficient mice (Kinjo et al. 2005) and characterizing the same *Sphingomonas* lipids, GSL-1 and GSL-1′, as direct ligands for murine and human NKTs. Two further studies (Sriram et al. 2005; Wu et al. 2005) have also documented NKT recognition of glycosphingolipids from *Sphingomonas wittichii* and *Sphingomonas paucimobilis*, respectively.

These data underline the importance of NKTs as a key component of the innate immune response to microbial pathogens, and highlight their ability either to sense changes in presentation of endogenous CD1d-restricted lipids during infection, or alternatively to target pathogens lacking ligands for TLRs by directly responding to microbial lipids presented by CD1d. With respect to the latter mechanism, the finding that individual microbial lipids can potentially activate most or all invariant NKTs is consistent with use of a highly conserved TCR by such populations. Furthermore, the distinctive α-anomeric linkage of the *Sphingomonas* antigens could be considered a PAMP in an analogous fashion to TLR ligands, and the conserved NKT TCR a surrogate pattern recognition receptor (Kinjo et al. 2005). Although *Sphingomonas* is thought to be a relatively infrequent human pathogen, it is possible that direct activation of NKT cells by microbial lipids is a mechanism that also applies to related bacteria such as *Ehrlichia*, a natural human pathogen (Olano and Walker 2002), and *Rickettsiales*, which also lack LPS and are controlled by TLR-independent mechanisms (von Loewenich et al. 2004).

5
The Role of Group 1 CD1-Restricted T Cell Responses in Antimicrobial Immunity

The CD1a-, b- and c-restricted foreign antigens defined to date all derive from mycobacteria, suggesting a role for group 1 CD1-restricted responses in immunity to these pathogens. The T cell lines used to identify these antigens were generated from either the blood of healthy donors or from infected mycobacterial lesions, suggesting such T cells circulate in the peripheral repertoire and can also be recruited to infected tissues. Consistent with this suggestion, group 1 CD1 molecule expression is observed at the site of mycobacterial infection and has been correlated with effective host immune responses in leprosy patients (Narayanan et al. 1990; Sieling et al. 1999; Uehira et al. 2002). Furthermore, group 1 CD1 molecule expression is upregulated after exposure of myeloid cells to live *M. tuberculosis*, a process dependent on TLR-2 interactions with particular cell wall lipids (Roura-Mir et al. 2005). This is likely to represent an innate pattern recognition mechanism facilitating presentation of mycobacterial cell wall lipids by CD1a, CD1b and CD1c molecules and subsequent antigen-specific immunity.

The effector functions of antigen-specific T cells restricted to group 1 CD1 molecules also support a role in antimicrobial responses. Such cells generally secrete TH1 cytokines such as IFNγ and TNFα (Rosat et al. 1999; Sieling et al. 2000), contain perforin and are strongly cytotoxic (Ochoa et al. 2001; Rosat et al. 1999; Stenger et al. 1997, 1998a). In addition, human group 1 CD1-restricted T cells were able to kill *M. tuberculosis*-infected macrophages, and the cytotoxic granules of CD8$^+$ and CD4$^+$ single positive subsets contain granulysin, allowing direct killing of intracellular pathogens including *M. tuberculosis* (Gilleron et al. 2004; Stenger et al. 1997, 1998b). Consistent with such direct effector mechanisms, group 1 CD1 molecules have been shown to localise in the phagosomes of DCs infected with mycobacteria (Schaible et al. 2000). The significance of these effector functions could be considerable, since in *M. tuberculosis* infection, the ability to mount TH1 responses is thought to contribute to protective immunity in those resistant to disease and is likely to limit pathology in susceptible individuals (Casanova and Abel 2002; North and Jung 2004). In support of this, individuals with defects in IFNγ and IL-12 responses are susceptible to severe tuberculosis, and TH1 immunity is also thought to be important in granuloma formation in *M. tuberculosis* (Casanova and Abel 2002; Uehira et al. 2002). If recognition of foreign lipids in the context of group 1 CD1 molecules has the potential to limit mycobacterial growth, one expectation is that pathogens might evolve strategies to interfere with this pathway, as viruses interfere with MHC class I presentation. Consistent with such an immune evasion strategy, CD1a, b and c expression by DCs was downregulated after infection with live (but not heat-killed) *M. tuberculosis* (Mariotti et al. 2002; Stenger et al. 1998b). How the host immune system overcomes such a strategy is unclear, but it could involve uptake of mycobacterial antigens from apoptotic bodies that are released from macrophages by uninfected DCs that are capable of efficient antigen presentation (Schaible et al. 2003).

A number of studies have provided direct evidence that group 1 CD1-restricted responses to mycobacterial lipid antigens occur in vivo during human infection. Initially, CD1c-restricted responses to MPM were detected in patients infected with *M. tuberculosis* but not in healthy PPD-negative controls (Moody et al. 2000b). Subsequently, CD1b-restricted responses to GMM and to a sulfoglycolipid have also been demonstrated in *M. tuberculosis* patients (Gilleron et al. 2004; Ulrichs et al. 2003). Clearly, further studies are required in this area to address issues such as the kinetics and immunodominance of such lipid-specific responses, and to explore possible correlation with disease susceptibility. However, immunisation with mycobacterial lipids was found to reduce pulmonary pathology and bacterial burden in the guinea pig model of *M. tuberculosis* (Dascher et al. 2003). In addition, the major CD8[+] response that occurred after *M. bovis* BCG immunisation was found to be CD1-restricted (Kawashima et al. 2003). Consequently, lipid-specific T cell responses restricted by group 1 CD1 molecules are likely to contribute to protective immunity to mycobacteria, including *M. tuberculosis*, and these forms of immune recognition could form the basis of improved vaccine strategies.

6
The Role of Group 2 CD1-Restricted T Cell Responses in Antimicrobial Immunity

CD1d-restricted T cells have been implicated as contributing to antimicrobial responses to bacterial, parasite, viral and fungal infection from experiments in murine systems involving animals deficient in CD1d-restricted T cells, anti-CD1d mAbs, and α-galactosylceramide administration (Brigl and Brenner 2004). Recent data highlight two distinct mechanisms for such effects. The first

(Brigl et al. 2003; Mattner et al. 2005), proposed from studies on infection with the bacterium *Salmonella*, involves responses to CD1-restricted self antigens that are amplified by IL-12 produced by DCs in response to microbial products such as LPS. The second mechanism involves direct recognition of microbial products presented by CD1d and may be important for immunity to Gram-negative bacteria such as *Sphingomonas* that lack stimulatory ligands for TLRs on DCs (Kinjo et al. 2005; Mattner et al. 2005). Available data suggest both mechanisms are likely to lead to activation of CD1-restricted T cells early in infection, resulting in TH1-type effector responses including potent IFNγ secretion (Amprey et al. 2004; Brigl et al. 2003; Kinjo et al. 2005; Mattner et al. 2005). This favours a role for CD1d-restricted T cells in early innate immune recognition processes, consistent with the finding that NKT cells constitutively express IFNγ mRNA, suggesting they are poised for rapid effector responses (Stetson et al. 2003). Their role in direct presentation of mycobacterial cell wall lipids is less clear. Whereas expression of group 1 CD1 molecules on DCs is induced by exposure to *M. tuberculosis* cell wall components, CD1d expression is downregulated (Roura-Mir et al. 2005), suggesting distinct roles during mycobacterial infection. Furthermore, mice deficient in CD1d-restricted cells do not show impaired immunity to mycobacterial infection in certain mouse models (Brigl and Brenner 2004).

7
Concluding Remarks

T cell responses specific for foreign lipid antigens presented by CD1 molecules are potentially important components of the host response to microbial infection, especially for pathogens that have adapted to an intracellular existence in the endosomal compartment and are therefore poor targets for humoral immunity. Current evidence suggests CD1-restricted T cells participate in the immune response to medically important pathogens such as *M. tuberculosis*, and could potentially form the basis of improved vaccine strategies. Establishing the structures of such CD1-restricted lipid antigens and the molecular and immunological basis of their generation and recognition is a key step in the development of therapeutic approaches. The great structural diversity of microbial lipids and the limited number of defined antigens suggests we are at the start of this process. As more CD1-restricted microbial lipid antigens are discovered, an improved understanding of their relative immunodominance during infection, as well as the kinetics of lipid-specific T cell responses and their correlation with susceptibility to disease during human infection will become critical.

References

Amprey JL, Im JS, Turco SJ, Murray HW, Illarionov PA, Besra GS, Porcelli SA, Spath GF (2004) A subset of liver NKT cells is activated during *Leishmania donovani* infection by CD1d-bound lipophosphoglycan. J Exp Med 200:895–904

Batuwangala T, Shepherd D, Gadola SD, Gibson KJ, Zaccai NR, Fersht AR, Besra GS, Cerundolo V, Jones EY (2004) The crystal structure of human CD1b with a bound bacterial glycolipid. J Immunol 172:2382–2388

Beckman EM, Porcelli SA, Morita CT, Behar SM, Furlong ST, Brenner MB (1994) Recognition of a lipid antigen by CD1-restricted alpha beta+ T cells. Nature 372:691–694

Beckman EM, Melian A, Behar SM, Sieling PA, Chatterjee D, Furlong ST, Matsumoto R, Rosat JP, Modlin RL, Porcelli SA (1996) CD1c restricts responses of mycobacteria-specific T cells. Evidence for antigen presentation by a second member of the human CD1 family. J Immunol 157:2795–2803

Bendelac A, Lantz O, Quimby ME, Yewdell JW, Bennink JR, Brutkiewicz RR (1995) CD1 recognition by mouse NK1+ T lymphocytes. Science 268:863–865

Brennan PJ, Nikaido H (1995) The envelope of mycobacteria. Annu Rev Biochem 64:29–63

Brigl M, Brenner MB (2004) CD1: antigen presentation and T cell function. Annu Rev Immunol 22:817–890

Brigl M, Bry L, Kent SC, Gumperz JE, Brenner MB (2003) Mechanism of CD1d-restricted natural killer T cell activation during microbial infection. Nat Immunol 4:1230–1237

Briken V, Jackman RM, Watts GF, Rogers RA, Porcelli SA (2000) Human CD1b and CD1c isoforms survey different intracellular compartments for the presentation of microbial lipid antigens. J Exp Med 192:281–288

Brossay L, Tangri S, Bix M, Cardell S, Locksley R, Kronenberg M (1998) Mouse CD1-autoreactive T cells have diverse patterns of reactivity to CD1+ targets. J Immunol 160:3681–3688

Calabi F, Jarvis JM, Martin L, Milstein C (1989) Two classes of CD1 genes. Eur J Immunol 19:285–292

Card GL, Peterson NA, Smith CA, Rupp B, Schick BM, Baker EN (2005) The crystal structure of Rv1347c, a putative antibiotic resistance protein from *Mycobacterium tuberculosis*, reveals a GCN5-related fold and suggests an alternative function in siderophore biosynthesis. J Biol Chem 280:13978–13986

Casanova JL, Abel L (2002) Genetic dissection of immunity to mycobacteria: the human model. Annu Rev Immunol 20:581–620

Casey PJ (1995) Protein lipidation in cell signaling. Science 268:221–225

Crick DC, Scocca JR, Rush JS, Frank DW, Krag SS, Waechter CJ (1994) Induction of dolichyl-saccharide intermediate biosynthesis corresponds to increased long chain cis-isoprenyltransferase activity during the mitogenic response in mouse B cells. J Biol Chem 269:10559–10565

Dascher CC, Hiromatsu K, Xiong X, Morehouse C, Watts G, Liu G, McMurray DN, LeClair KP, Porcelli SA, Brenner MB (2003) Immunization with a mycobacterial lipid vaccine improves pulmonary pathology in the guinea pig model of tuberculosis. Int Immunol 15:915–925

De la Salle H, Mariotti S, Angenieux C, Gilleron M, Garcia-Alles LF, Malm D, Berg T, Paoletti S, Maitre B, Mourey L et al (2005) Assistance of microbial glycolipid antigen processing by CD1e. Science 310:1321–1324

De Silva AD, Park JJ, Matsuki N, Stanic AK, Brutkiewicz RR, Medof ME, Joyce S (2002) Lipid protein interactions: the assembly of CD1d1 with cellular phospholipids occurs in the endoplasmic reticulum. J Immunol 168:723–733

De Voss JJ, Rutter K, Schroeder BG, Su H, Zhu Y, Barry CE 3rd (2000) The salicylate-derived mycobactin siderophores of *Mycobacterium tuberculosis* are essential for growth in macrophages. Proc Natl Acad Sci U S A 97:1252–1257

Dussurget O, Timm J, Gomez M, Gold B, Yu S, Sabol SZ, Holmes RK, Jacobs WR Jr, Smith I (1999) Transcriptional control of the iron-responsive fxbA gene by the mycobacterial regulator IdeR. J Bacteriol 181:3402–3408

Dutronc Y, Porcelli SA (2002) The CD1 family and T cell recognition of lipid antigens. Tissue Antigens 60:337–353

Edlund C, Soderberg M, Kristensson K, Dallner G (1992) Ubiquinone, dolichol, and cholesterol metabolism in aging and Alzheimer's disease. Biochem Cell Biol 70:422–428

Ernst WA, Maher J, Cho S, Niazi KR, Chatterjee D, Moody DB, Besra GS, Watanabe Y, Jensen PE, Porcelli SA et al (1998) Molecular interaction of CD1b with lipoglycan antigens. Immunity 8:331–340

Exley M, Garcia J, Balk SP, Porcelli S (1997) Requirements for CD1d recognition by human invariant Valpha24+ CD4-CD8- T cells. J Exp Med 186:109–120

Fischer K, Scotet E, Niemeyer M, Koebernick H, Zerrahn J, Maillet S, Hurwitz R, Kursar M, Bonneville M, Kaufmann SH, Schaible UE (2004) Mycobacterial phosphatidylinositol mannoside is a natural antigen for CD1d-restricted T cells. Proc Natl Acad Sci U S A 101:10685–10690

Gadola SD, Zaccai NR, Harlos K, Shepherd D, Castro-Palomino JC, Ritter G, Schmidt RR, Jones EY, Cerundolo V (2002) Structure of human CD1b with bound ligands at 2.3. A, a maze for alkyl chains. Nat Immunol 3:721–726

Gilleron M, Stenger S, Mazorra Z, Wittke F, Mariotti S, Bohmer G, Prandi J, Mori L, Puzo G, De Libero G (2004) Diacylated sulfoglycolipids are novel mycobacterial antigens stimulating CD1-restricted T cells during infection with Mycobacterium tuberculosis. J Exp Med 199:649–659

Goren MB (1982) Immunoreactive substances of mycobacteria. Am Rev Respir Dis 125:50–69

Grant EP, Degano M, Rosat JP, Stenger S, Modlin RL, Wilson IA, Porcelli SA, Brenner MB (1999) Molecular recognition of lipid antigens by T cell receptors. J Exp Med 189:195–205

Grant EP, Beckman EM, Behar SM, Degano M, Frederique D, Besra GS, Wilson IA, Porcelli SA, Furlong ST, Brenner MB (2002) Fine specificity of TCR complementarity-determining region residues and lipid antigen hydrophilic moieties in the recognition of a CD1-lipid complex. J Immunol 168:3933–3940

Gumperz JE, Roy C, Makowska A, Lum D, Sugita M, Podrebarac T, Koezuka Y, Porcelli SA, Cardell S, Brenner MB, Behar SM (2000) Murine CD1d-restricted T cell recognition of cellular lipids. Immunity 12:211–221

Han M, Hannick LI, DiBrino M, Robinson MA (1999) Polymorphism of human CD1 genes. Tissue Antigens 54:122–127

Henry A, Stacpoole PW, Allen CM (1991) Dolichol biosynthesis in human malignant cells. Biochem J 278:741–747

Jahng A, Maricic I, Aguilera C, Cardell S, Halder RC, Kumar V (2004) Prevention of autoimmunity by targeting a distinct, noninvariant CD1d-reactive T cell population reactive to sulfatide. J Exp Med 199:947–957

Joyce S, Woods AS, Yewdell JW, Bennink JR, De Silva AD, Boesteanu A, Balk SP, Cotter RJ, Brutkiewicz RR (1998) Natural ligand of mouse CD1d1: cellular glycosylphosphatidylinositol. Science 279:1541–1544

Karakousis PC, Bishai WR, Dorman SE (2004) *Mycobacterium tuberculosis* cell envelope lipids and the host immune response. Cell Microbiol 6:105–116

Kaufmann SH (1995) Immunity to intracellular microbial pathogens. Immunol Today 16:338–342

Kawahara K, Moll H, Knirel YA, Seydel U, Zahringer U (2000) Structural analysis of two glycosphingolipids from the lipopolysaccharide-lacking bacterium *Sphingomonas capsulata*. Eur J Biochem 267:1837–1846

Kawashima T, Norose Y, Watanabe Y, Enomoto Y, Narazaki H, Watari E, Tanaka S, Takahashi H, Yano I, Brenner MB, Sugita M (2003) Cutting edge: major CD8. T cell response to live bacillus Calmette-Guerin is mediated by CD1 molecules. J Immunol 170:5345–5348

Kinjo Y, Wu D, Kim G, Xing GW, Poles MA, Ho DD, Tsuji M, Kawahara K, Wong CH, Kronenberg M (2005) Recognition of bacterial glycosphingolipids by natural killer T cells. Nature 434:520–525

LaMarca BB, Zhu W, Arceneaux JE, Byers BR, Lundrigan MD (2004) Participation of fad and mbt genes in synthesis of mycobactin in *Mycobacterium smegmatis*. J Bacteriol 186:374–382

Mariotti S, Teloni R, Iona E, Fattorini L, Giannoni F, Romagnoli G, Orefici G, Nisini R (2002) Mycobacterium tuberculosis subverts the differentiation of human monocytes into dendritic cells. Eur J Immunol 32:3050–3058

Matsunaga I, Bhatt A, Young DC, Cheng TY, Eyles SJ, Besra GS, Briken V, Porcelli SA, Costello CE, Jacobs WR Jr, Moody DB (2004) *Mycobacterium tuberculosis* pks12 produces a novel polyketide presented by CD1c to T cells. J Exp Med 200:1559–1569

Mattner J, Debord KL, Ismail N, Goff RD, Cantu C 3rd, Zhou D, Saint-Mezard P, Wang V, Gao Y, Yin N et al (2005) Exogenous and endogenous glycolipid antigens activate NKT cells during microbial infections. Nature 434:525–529

McMichael AJ, Pilch JR, Galfre G, Mason DY, Fabre JW, Milstein C (1979) A human thymocyte antigen defined by a hybrid myeloma monoclonal antibody. Eur J Immunol 9:205–210

Melian A, Watts GF, Shamshiev A, De Libero G, Clatworthy A, Vincent M, Brenner MB, Behar S, Niazi K, Modlin RL et al (2000) Molecular recognition of human CD1b antigen complexes: evidence for a common pattern of interaction with alpha beta TCRs. J Immunol 165:4494–4504

Molano A, Park SH, Chiu YH, Nosseir S, Bendelac A, Tsuji M (2000) Cutting edge: the IgG response to the circumsporozoite protein is MHC class II-dependent and CD1d-independent: exploring the role of GPIs in NKT cell activation and antimalarial responses. J Immunol 164:5005–5009

Moody DB, Reinhold BB, Guy MR, Beckman EM, Frederique DE, Furlong ST, Ye S, Reinhold VN, Sieling PA, Modlin RL et al (1997) Structural requirements for glycolipid antigen recognition by CD1b-restricted T cells. Science 278:283–286

Moody DB, Guy MR, Grant E, Cheng TY, Brenner MB, Besra GS, Porcelli SA (2000a) CD1b-mediated T cell recognition of a glycolipid antigen generated from mycobacterial lipid and host carbohydrate during infection. J Exp Med 192:965–976

Moody DB, Ulrichs T, Muhlecker W, Young DC, Gurcha SS, Grant E, Rosat JP, Brenner MB, Costello CE, Besra GS, Porcelli SA (2000b) CD1c-mediated T-cell recognition of isoprenoid glycolipids in *Mycobacterium tuberculosis* infection. Nature 404:884–888

Moody DB, Briken V, Cheng TY, Roura-Mir C, Guy MR, Geho DH, Tykocinski ML, Besra GS, Porcelli SA (2002) Lipid length controls antigen entry into endosomal and nonendosomal pathways for CD1b presentation. Nat Immunol 3:435–442

Moody DB, Young DC, Cheng TY, Rosat JP, Roura-Mir C, O'Connor PB, Zajonc DM, Walz A, Miller MJ, Levery SB et al (2004) T cell activation by lipopeptide antigens. Science 303:527–531

Narayanan RB, Girdhar A, Girdhar BK (1990) CD1-positive epidermal Langerhans cells in regressed tuberculoid and lepromatous leprosy lesions. Int Arch Allergy Appl Immunol 92:94–96

Natori T, Morita M, Akimoto K, Koezuka Y (1994) Agelasphins novel antitumor and immunostimulatory cerebrosides from the marine sponge Agelas-Mauritianus. Tetrahedron 50:2711–2784

North RJ, Jung YJ (2004) Immunity to tuberculosis. Annu Rev Immunol 22:599–623

Ochoa MT, Stenger S, Sieling PA, Thoma-Uszynski S, Sabet S, Cho S, Krensky AM, Rollinghoff M, Nunes Sarno E, Burdick AE et al (2001) T-cell release of granulysin contributes to host defense in leprosy. Nat Med 7:174–179

Olano JP, Walker DH (2002) Human ehrlichioses. Med Clin North Am 86:375–392

Porcelli S, Brenner MB, Greenstein JL, Balk SP, Terhorst C, Bleicher PA (1989) Recognition of cluster of differentiation 1 antigens by human CD4-CD8-cytolytic T lymphocytes. Nature 341:447–450

Porcelli S, Morita CT, Brenner MB (1992) CD1b restricts the response of human CD4-8- T lymphocytes to a microbial antigen. Nature 360:593–597

Procopio DO, Almeida IC, Torrecilhas AC, Cardoso JE, Teyton L, Travassos LR, Bendelac A, Gazzinelli RT (2002) Glycosylphosphatidylinositol-anchored mucin-like glycoproteins from *Trypanosoma cruzi* bind to CD1d but do not elicit dominant innate or adaptive immune responses via the CD1d/NKT cell pathway. J Immunol 169:3926–3933

Pukel CS, Lloyd KO, Travassos LR, Dippold WG, Oettgen HF, Old LJ (1982) GD3, a prominent ganglioside of human melanoma. Detection and characterisation by mouse monoclonal antibody. J Exp Med 155:1133–1147

Quadri LE, Sello J, Keating TA, Weinreb PH, Walsh CT (1998) Identification of a *Mycobacterium tuberculosis* gene cluster encoding the biosynthetic enzymes for assembly of the virulence-conferring siderophore mycobactin. Chem Biol 5:631–645

Ratledge C, Dover LG (2000) Iron metabolism in pathogenic bacteria. Annu Rev Microbiol 54:881–941

Ratledge C, Snow GA (1974) Isolation and structure of nocobactin NA, a lipid-soluble iron-binding compound from *Nocardia asteroides*. Biochem J 139:407–413

Romero JF, Eberl G, MacDonald HR, Corradin G (2001) CD1d-restricted NKT cells are dispensable for specific antibody responses and protective immunity against liver stage malaria infection in mice. Parasite Immunol 23:267–269

Rosat JP, Grant EP, Beckman EM, Dascher CC, Sieling PA, Frederique D, Modlin RL, Porcelli SA, Furlong ST, Brenner MB (1999) CD1-restricted microbial lipid antigen-specific recognition found in the CD8+ alpha beta T cell pool. J Immunol 162:366–371

Roura-Mir C, Wang L, Cheng TY, Matsunaga I, Dascher CC, Peng SL, Fenton MJ, Kirschning C, Moody DB (2005) *Mycobacterium tuberculosis* regulates CD1 antigen presentation pathways through TLR-2. J Immunol 175:1758–1766

Schaible UE, Hagens K, Fischer K, Collins HL, Kaufmann SH (2000) Intersection of group ICD1 molecules and mycobacteria in different intracellular compartments of dendritic cells. J Immunol 164:4843–4852

Schaible UE, Winau F, Sieling PA, Fischer K, Collins HL, Hagens K, Modlin RL, Brinkmann V, Kaufmann SH (2003) Apoptosis facilitates antigen presentation to T lymphocytes through MHC-I and CD1 in tuberculosis. Nat Med 9:1039–1046

Schofield L, McConville MJ, Hansen D, Campbell AS, Fraser-Reid B, Grusby MJ, Tachado SD (1999) CD1d-restricted immunoglobulin G formation to GPI-anchored antigens mediated by NKT cells. Science 283:225–229

Shamshiev A, Donda A, Prigozy TI, Mori L, Chigorno V, Benedict CA, Kappos L, Sonnino S, Kronenberg M, De Libero G (2000) The alphabeta T cell response to self-glycolipids shows a novel mechanism of CD1b loading and a requirement for complex oligosaccharides. Immunity 13:255–264

Sieling PA, Chatterjee D, Porcelli SA, Prigozy TI, Mazzaccaro RJ, Soriano T, Bloom BR, Brenner MB, Kronenberg M, Brennan PJ et al (1995) CD1-restricted T cell recognition of microbial lipoglycan antigens. Science 269:227–230

Sieling PA, Jullien D, Dahlem M, Tedder TF, Rea TH, Modlin RL, Porcelli SA (1999) CD1 expression by dendritic cells in human leprosy lesions: correlation with effective host immunity. J Immunol 162:1851–1858

Sieling PA, Ochoa MT, Jullien D, Leslie DS, Sabet S, Rosat JP, Burdick AE, Rea TH, Brenner MB, Porcelli SA, Modlin RL (2000) Evidence for human CD4+ T cells in the CD1-restricted repertoire: derivation of mycobacteria-reactive T cells from leprosy lesions. J Immunol 164:4790–4796

Snow GA (1970) Mycobactins: iron-chelating growth factors from mycobacteria. Bacterio Rev 34:99–125

Sriram V, Du W, Gervay-Hague J, Brutkiewicz RR (2005) Cell wall glycosphingolipids of *Sphingomonas paucimobilis* are CD1d-specific ligands for NKT cells. Eur J Immunol 35:1692–1701

Stenger S, Mazzaccaro RJ, Uyemura K, Cho S, Barnes PF, Rosat JP, Sette A, Brenner MB, Porcelli SA, Bloom BR, Modlin RL (1997) Differential effects of cytolytic T cell subsets on intracellular infection. Science 276:1684–1687

Stenger S, Hanson DA, Teitelbaum R, Dewan P, Niazi KR, Froelich CJ, Ganz T, Thoma-Uszynski S, Melian A, Bogdan C et al (1998a) An antimicrobial activity of cytolytic T cells mediated by granulysin. Science 282:121–125

Stenger S, Niazi KR, Modlin RL (1998b) Down-regulation of CD1 on antigen-presenting cells by infection with *Mycobacterium tuberculosis*. J Immunol 161:3582–3588

Stetson DB, Mohrs M, Reinhardt RL, Baron JL, Wang ZE, Gapin L, Kronenberg M, Locksley RM (2003) Constitutive cytokine mRNAs mark natural killer (NK) and NKT cells poised for rapid effector function. J Exp Med 198:1069–1076

Sugita M, Jackman RM, van Donselaar E, Behar SM, Rogers RA, Peters PJ, Brenner MB, Porcelli SA (1996) Cytoplasmic tail-dependent localization of CD1b antigen-presenting molecules to MIICs. Science 273:349–352

Sugita M, Grant EP, van Donselaar E, Hsu VW, Rogers RA, Peters PJ, Brenner MB (1999) Separate pathways for antigen presentation by CD1 molecules. Immunity 11:743–752

Uehira K, Amakawa R, Ito T, Tajima K, Naitoh S, Ozaki Y, Shimizu T, Yamaguchi K, Uemura Y, Kitajima H et al (2002) Dendritic cells are decreased in blood and accumulated in granuloma in tuberculosis. Clin Immunol 105:296–303

Ulrichs T, Moody DB, Grant E, Kaufmann SH, Porcelli SA (2003) T-cell responses to CD1-presented lipid antigens in humans with *Mycobacterium tuberculosis* infection. Infect Immun 71:3076–3087

Von Loewenich FD, Scorpio DG, Reischl U, Dumler JS, Bogdan C (2004) Frontline: control of *Anaplasma phagocytophilum*, an obligate intracellular pathogen, in the absence of inducible nitric oxide synthase, phagocyte NADPH oxidase, tumor necrosis factor Toll-like receptor (TLR)2 and TLR4, or the TLR adaptor molecule MyD88. Eur J Immunol 34:1789–1797

Wooldridge KG, Williams PH (1993) Iron uptake mechanisms of pathogenic bacteria. FEMS Microbiol Rev 12:325–348

Wu DY, Segal NH, Sidobre S, Kronenberg M, Chapman PB (2003) Cross-presentation of disialoganglioside GD3 to natural killer T cells. J Exp Med 198:173–181

Wu D, Xing GW, Poles MA, Horowitz A, Kinjo Y, Sullivan B, Bodmer-Narkevitch V, Plettenburg O, Kronenberg M, Tsuji M et al (2005) Bacterial glycolipids and analogs as antigens for CD1d-restricted NKT cells. Proc Natl Acad Sci U S A 102:1351–1356

Wu D, Zajonc DM, Fujio M, Sullivan BA, Kinjo Y, Kronenberg M, Wilson IA, Wong CH (2006) Design of natural killer T cell activators: structure and function of a microbial glycosphingolipid bound to mouse CD1d. Proc Natl Acad Sci U S A 103:3972–3977

Yarkoni E, Goren MB, Rapp HJ (1979) Regression of a transplanted guinea pig hepatoma after intralesional injection of an emulsified mixture of endotoxin and mycobacterial sulfolipid. Infect Immun 24:357–362

Zajonc DM, Elsliger MA, Teyton L, Wilson IA (2003) Crystal structure of CD1a in complex with a sulfatide self antigen at a resolution of 2.15 A. Nat Immunol 4:808–815

Zajonc DM, Crispin MD, Bowden TA, Young DC, Cheng TY, Hu J, Costello CE, Rudd PM, Dwek RA, Miller MJ et al (2005a) Molecular mechanism of lipopeptide presentation by CD1a. Immunity 22:209–219

Zajonc DM, Maricic I, Wu D, Halder R, Roy K, Wong CH, Kumar V, Wilson IA (2005b) Structural basis for CD1d presentation of a sulfatide derived from myelin and its implications for autoimmunity. J Exp Med 202:1517–1526

Zeng Z, Castano AR, Segelke BW, Stura EA, Peterson PA, Wilson IA (1997) Crystal structure of mouse CD1: an MHC-like fold with a large hydrophobic binding groove. Science 277:339–345

Zhou D, Mattner J, Cantu C 3rd, Schrantz N, Yin N, Gao Y, Sagiv Y, Hudspeth K, Wu YP, Yamashita T et al (2004) Lysosomal glycosphingolipid recognition by NKT cells. Science 306:1786–1789

Section II
Cellular Biology

CTMI (2007) 314:113–141
© Springer-Verlag Berlin Heidelberg 2007

CD1 Expression on Antigen-Presenting Cells

S. K. Dougan · A. Kaser · R. S. Blumberg (✉)

Gastroenterology Division, Department of Medicine, Brigham and Women's
Hospital, 75 Francis St, Thorn 1415, Boston, MA 02115, USA
rblumberg@partners.org

Abstract CD1 proteins present self and microbial glycolipids to CD1-restricted T cells,
or in the case of CD1d, to NKT cells. The CD1 family in humans consists of group
I proteins CD1a, CD1b, CD1c, and CD1e and the group II protein CD1d. Rodents
express only CD1d, but as CD1d is broadly expressed and traffics to all endosomal
compartments, this single CD1 family member is thereby able to acquire antigens in

many subcellular compartments. A complete understanding of the CD1 family requires an appreciation of which cells express CD1 and how CD1 contributes to the unique function of each cell type. While group I CD1 expression is limited to thymocytes and professional APCs, CD1d has a wider tissue distribution and can be found on many nonhematopoietic cells. The expression and regulation of CD1 are presented here with particular emphasis on the function of CD1 in thymocytes, B cells, monocytes and macrophages, dendritic cells (DCs), and intestinal epithelial cells (IECs). Altered expression of CD1 in cancer, autoimmunity, and infectious disease is well documented, and the implication of CD1 expression in these diseases is discussed.

1
Tissue Distribution of CD1a, CD1b, CD1c, and CD1e

CD1 proteins were first identified by a monoclonal antibody (NA1/34; CD1a) generated by immunization of mice with human thymocytes (McMichael et al. 1979). CD1a, CD1b, and CD1c molecules are asparagine-glycosylated and have a molecular weight of 49, 45, and 43 kDa, respectively; the polypeptide backbones of all three molecules have a molecular weight of 33 kDa (Knowles and Bodmer 1982; van de Rijn et al. 1983; Olive et al. 1984; Lerch et al. 1986). CD1a, CD1b, and CD1c are heterodimers of the CD1 heavy chain and β_2-microglobulin (β_2-m). The ratio of β_2-m to CD1 molecules is not as constant as β_2-m to MHC class I, suggesting that CD1 heterodimers can dissociate (Knowles and Bodmer 1982; Olive et al. 1984).

Group 1 CD1 molecules are almost exclusively found on professional antigen-presenting cells (APCs) and thymocytes. They are expressed on double-positive (CD4$^+$CD8$^+$) cortical thymocytes and with less intensity on CD4$^+$ and CD8$^+$ single-positive thymocytes (Fainboim and Salamone Mdel 2002). Langerhans cells express CD1c and more prominently CD1a (Pena-Cruz et al. 2003). In addition to CD207$^+$CD14$^-$CD1a^{high} dermal Langerhans cells, a CD207$^-$CD14$^-$CD1a^{mid} antigen-presenting cell population has recently been described that expresses the chemokine receptor CCR7 and migrates in response to the chemokines CCL19 and CCL21 (Angel et al. 2006). Dermal DCs and lymph node interdigitating DCs express CD1b and CD1c (McMichael 1987). While CD1a and CD1b peripheral expression is restricted to DCs, CD1c is expressed on DCs and a subset of B cells (Small et al. 1987; Plebani et al. 1993). CD1c is found in lymph node mantle zones and germinal centers (McMichael 1987; Smith et al. 1988; Roura-Mir et al. 2005a), on marginal zone B cells in the spleen (Smith et al. 1988), as well as on a subpopulation of circulating peripheral B cells (Small et al. 1987; Plebani et al. 1993). CD1c can be induced by B cell activation, and CD1c has been proposed as a marker for distinguishing B cell populations, in particular mantle zone B cells (Delia et al. 1988). Unlike other CD1 molecules, CD1e localizes to the Golgi and is not expressed on the cell surface of DCs, thus excluding a direct interaction with T cells (Angenieux et al. 2005). Upon DC maturation, CD1e traffics to lysosomes, where it is cleaved into a soluble form capable of binding glycolipids (Angenieux et al. 2005). Mycobacterial hexamannosylated phosphatidyl-*myo*-inositols (PIM_6) stimulate CD1b-restricted T cells after partial digestion of the oligomannose moiety by a lysosomal α-mannosidase, and soluble CD1e is required for this degradation (de la Salle et al. 2005). This suggests that CD1e is involved in glycolipid editing, thereby expanding the repertoire of glycolipid T cell antigens (de la Salle et al. 2005).

DCs differentiated from $CD14^+$ monocytes with interleukin-4 (IL-4) and granulocyte-monocyte colony stimulating factor (GM-CSF) express CD1a, CD1b, and CD1c when cultured in fetal calf serum, but human serum inhibits CD1a expression (Duperrier et al. 2000; Pietschmann et al. 2000; Xia and Kao 2002). Interestingly, *Bordetella pertussis* toxin treatment of monocyte-derived DCs selectively inhibits expression of CD1a, while CD1b and CD1c expression is retained (Martino et al. 2006). When DCs are differentiated from $CD34^+$ hematopoietic progenitor cells by culture with GM-CSF and tumor necrosis factor (TNF), two separate DC lineages form: one subset is $CD1a^+$ and lacks expression of CD14 (Caux et al. 1992, 1996); the $CD14^+CD1a^-$ subset further differentiates to a subset expressing CD1a, CD1b, and CD1c (Caux et al. 1996; Banchereau et al. 2000). The former shows characteristics of epidermal Langerhans cells, while the latter resembles interdigitating DCs and DCs in nonlymphoid tissues.

CD1 expression during DC maturation differs from MHC class II regulation. In immature DCs, CD1b and MHC class II are present in multilamellar lysosomes, but while CD1b is found on the limiting membrane, MHC class II is located in the internal membranes (Sugita et al. 1996; van der Wel et al. 2003). CD1b and CD1c expression on the surface of DCs do not change during maturation; CD1a expression decreases slightly (Cao et al. 2002; van der Wel et al. 2003). In sharp contrast, MHC class II is redistributed to the plasma membrane upon maturation (van der Wel et al. 2003). As a consequence, although DC maturation greatly enhances presentation of peptide antigens, CD1-restricted antigens are presented on immature and mature DCs with equal efficiency (Cao et al. 2002).

Serum lipids bind to and promote stable surface expression of CD1a, as suggested by a report showing decreased CD1a detection by conformation dependent antibodies on MOLT-4 cells cultured under low serum conditions (Manolova et al. 2006). This apparent reduction in expression likely involved unfolding of surface CD1a molecules because detection could be restored by addition of CD1a lipid ligands, which presumably stabilized the CD1a structure. A similar increase in CD1a detection by conformation-dependent antibodies was observed on freshly isolated Langerhans cells exposed to sulfatide (Manolova et al. 2006), suggesting the lipid ligands of CD1a regulate its conformation.

Cellular infection with *Mycobacterium tuberculosis* upregulates CD1a, CD1b, and CD1c expression in CD1⁻ myeloid precursors, while CD1d expression is downregulated (Roura-Mir et al. 2005b). This CD1-inducing property involved polar lipids derived from *M. tuberculosis* and required TLR2, which suggests that mycobacterial cell wall lipids provide two distinct signals for the activation of lipid-reactive T cells: lipid adjuvants that activate APCs through TLR2 and the actual lipid antigen recognized by the T cell receptor (Roura-Mir et al. 2005b).

2
Isoforms of Group I CD1 Molecules

Messenger RNA splicing complexity has been described for group 1 CD1 molecules (Woolfson and Milstein 1994). CD1a transfected cell lines secreted a CD1a isoform derived from an unspliced transcript (Woolfson and Milstein 1994). However, this isoform was not found in the thymus. In the case of CD1c, complex intrathymic splicing generates a secreted CD1c isoform, which can be detected from cell culture supernatants (Woolfson and Milstein 1994). Complex splicing of CD1e was reported in thymocytes and DCs (Woolfson and Milstein 1994; Angenieux et al. 2000). Both of these differentially spliced CD1e isoforms slowly leave the endoplasmic reticulum (ER) due to the presence of atypical dilysine motifs in the cytoplasmic tail (Angenieux et al. 2000). These molecules are associated with β2-m and accumulate in late Golgi and late endosomal compartments (Angenieux et al. 2000).

3
Group 1 CD1 Expression in Disease

In leprosy, patients with the tuberculoid form of the disease, a clinical pattern associated with active cellular immunity toward *Mycobacterium leprae*, show induction of CD1a, CD1b, and CD1c on DCs in dermal granulomas, whereas patients with lepromatous form do not show induction of CD1 molecules (Sieling et al. 1999). Downregulation of CD1 molecules might constitute an immune evasion strategy of microorganisms.

With regard to noninfectious diseases, CD1a and CD1c have been reported on DCs in the inflamed synovium of rheumatoid arthritis (Page et al. 2002). Expression of CD1a, CD1b, CD1c, and CD1d has been demonstrated in CD68$^+$ lipid-laden foam cells in atherosclerotic lesions, and these cells can present exogenous antigens to T cells, while normal arterial specimens do not express CD1 molecules (Melian et al. 1999). CD1b expression was also prominently found on perivascular inflammatory cells of chronic-active multiple sclerosis (MS) lesions, whereas macrophages within the lesion showed little staining (Battistini et al. 1996). At the lesion edge, CD1b was found on hypertrophic astrocytes. In chronic-silent MS lesions, CD1b expression was found on only a few perivascular astrocytic foot processes and the occasional perivascular macrophage, which suggests that CD1b-restricted antigen presentation could have a role specifically in active disease. In autoimmune thyroiditis, CD1 bearing DCs and CD1c-positive B cells were detected in inflamed thyroid tissue, and CD1a-restricted and CD1c-restricted T cell lines could be derived from patient thyroid glands (Roura-Mir et al. 2005a).

Altered expression of group I CD1 proteins has been reported for several types of cancer. In human breast cancer, tumor-infiltrating CD1-positive DCs have been reported, and their presence correlated with prognosis (Bell et al. 1999; Iwamoto et al. 2003). In mycosis fungoides, a cutaneous T cell lymphoma, CD1b and CD1c expression was increased (Fivenson and Nickoloff 1995). In contrast, in B chronic lymphocytic leukemia, CD1c is strongly downregulated, possibly as an immune evasion strategy (Zheng et al. 2002).

4
Tissue Distribution of Human CD1d

CD1d was originally cloned from human neonatal thymus (Calabi et al. 1986) and CD1d mRNA is detectable by Northern blot of thymic RNA (Balk et al. 1989). Thymic expression of CD1d protein was first identified by monoclonal antibodies raised against murine CD1d, named 3C11 and 1H1, which showed positive staining of human thymus (Canchis et al. 1993).

In peripheral blood, CD1d is expressed on B cells, monocytes and activated T cells (Exley et al. 2000). CD1d was first found on B cells by flow cytometry, and CD1d could be immunoprecipitated from an Epstein-Barr virus (EBV)-transformed B cell line using the 1H1 antibody (Blumberg et al. 1991). Although cortical thymocytes express CD1d, expression is downregulated in medullary thymocytes and absent on naïve peripheral T cells (Exley et al. 2000). CD1d is re-expressed upon activation, and this accounts for the 3–15% of peripheral blood T cells that are positive for CD1d (Ulanova et al.

2000a; Salamone et al. 2001). CD1d is also present at low levels on monocyte-derived macrophages, monocyte-derived DCs, and dermal DCs (Spada et al. 2000; Gerlini et al. 2001). In the lymph node, CD1d is prominently expressed on DCs in the paracortical T cell zones and on mantle zone B cells, but not on any cells of the germinal center (Exley et al. 2000; Yang et al. 2000).

CD1d is expressed broadly outside of the hematopoietic compartment. Using the 3C11 and 1H1 antibodies, strong CD1d staining was detected in epithelial cells of the small bowel and colon, and 1H1 could immunoprecipitate a 48 kDa, β2-m associated glycoprotein from colonic epithelium (Blumberg et al. 1991). A more extensive screen of human tissue sections revealed CD1d staining on hepatocytes, bile duct epithelium, pancreas, kidney, endometrium, testis, epididymis, conjunctiva, breast, skin, and weakly in tonsils (Canchis et al. 1993). Vascular smooth muscle cells in all of these tissues were stained brightly by 3C11 (Canchis et al. 1993). In the skin, CD1d can be found on keratinocytes, endothelium, eccrine ducts, acrosyringium, and the pilosebaceous unit except for dermal papillae and hair matrix cells (Bonish et al. 2000). Anagen phase growing hair, but not resting or involution stage hair, strongly expresses CD1d (Adly et al. 2005). CD1d positive spindle-shaped cells are found underlying the oral epithelium in noninflamed sections of periodontal biopsies (Yamazaki et al. 2001). CD1d is expressed on the trophoblast where it may play a role in maintaining tolerance at the maternal–fetal interface (Jenkinson et al. 1999). Hepatocytes weakly express CD1d but can upregulate their expression level during viral infection (Tsuneyama et al. 1998; Durante-Mangoni et al. 2004). Human intestinal epithelial cells (IEC) express multiple isoforms of CD1d and can present glycolipid antigens to NKT cells (Balk et al. 1994; Somnay-Wadgaonkar et al. 1999; van de Wal et al. 2003). Within the intestine, CD1d is on epithelial cells from the jejunum and colon (Blumberg et al. 1991; Somnay-Wadgaonkar et al. 1999), but has not been found on epithelial cells from duodenal biopsies (Somnay-Wadgaonkar et al. 1999; Ulanova et al. 2000b; Lin et al. 2005). The wide tissue distribution of CD1d and its location on many parenchymal and endothelial cells is markedly different from the group I CD1 proteins.

5
Tissue Distribution of Rodent CD1d

The tissue distribution of mouse CD1d was first analyzed by RNase protection assays, which showed CD1d mRNA in thymus, liver, spleen, myeloid cells, B and T cell lines and weakly in kidney and brain (Bradbury et al. 1988). The first monoclonal antibodies against mouse CD1d, 1H1, and 3C11 found

CD1d by immunohistochemistry in thymus, lymph node, and liver but not in brain, skin, heart, skeletal muscle, kidney, lung, or esophagus. Very bright staining was observed on the epithelium of the stomach, small intestine, and colon (Bleicher et al. 1990). A second group generated polyclonal antisera to CD1d and showed by immunoblotting that mouse CD1d was present in all fetal organs but only in thymus, spleen, liver, and lung of adult mice (Mosser et al. 1991). Flow cytometry and immunohistochemistry with monoclonal antibodies named 1B1 and 9C7 showed staining for CD1d on T cells, B cells, macrophages, and hepatocytes, but not on epithelial cells of the small intestine (Brossay et al. 1997). Another study using two independently generated monoclonal antibodies, 3H3 and 5C6, found CD1d staining by flow cytometry on mouse thymocytes, splenocytes, lymph node cells, bone marrow, intraepithelial lymphocytes, macrophages, DCs, and a thymic epithelial cell line. Staining was not observed on IECs, but was observed in the liver beginning at embryonic day 14 and remained fairly constant throughout development (Mandal et al. 1998).

The initial characterizations of mouse CD1d revealed consistent results, with one notable exception. IECs were the brightest staining cells detected by antibodies 1H1 and 3C11, but IECs appeared negative using all other anti-CD1d antibodies. Furthermore, in situ hybridization of mouse intestine showed abundant CD1d mRNA in Paneth cells, but not in epithelial cells (Lacasse and Martin 1992). The lack of detectable mRNA in IECs is likely due to a relatively low transcription rate and long protein half-life of CD1d. Indeed, pulse chase metabolic labeling studies have detected CD1d as long as 4 days after initial labeling (Kim et al. 2000). The discrepancy in antibody staining could be due to intestine-specific isoforms of CD1d, which are not recognized by most anti-CD1d antibodies. In fact, evidence suggests that 3C11 recognizes a particular isoform of CD1d since this antibody selectively immunoprecipitates the human 37-kDa nonglycosylated, but not the 48-kDa fully glycosylated form of CD1d (Somnay-Wadgaonkar et al. 1999). Also, 3C11 brightly stains smooth muscle vasculature in wild type and β2-m$^{-/-}$ mice, suggesting that 3C11 can recognize a noncanonical CD1d that does not require β2-m association (Amano et al. 1998).

Despite questions about recognition by most CD1d-specific antibodies, CD1d on mouse IECs is functional and can present a glycolipid antigen, α-galactosyl ceramide (α-galcer) to NKT cells. For example, a mouse intestinal epithelial line, MODE-K, shows negligible surface expression of CD1d by flow cytometry, but MODE-K cells present α-galcer to NKT cells in dose-dependent fashion, and this presentation is blocked by addition of anti-CD1d antibodies (van de Wal et al. 2003). In a clever effort to visualize CD1d, fluorescently labeled α-galcer was injected intravenously into wild type or CD1d$^{-/-}$

mice. The intestines of wild type, but not the CD1d$^{-/-}$ mice, clearly showed fluorescent α-galcer lining the lumenal surface of IECs (Saubermann et al. 2000). A recent study of colitis used both quantitative PCR and immunohistochemistry with the 1B1 antibody showed faint CD1d expression on colonic epithelial cells in Balb/c mice, which greatly increased during disease progression (Hornung et al. 2006).

Further analysis of the mouse hematopoietic compartment identified CD1d expression in multiple lineages, including B cells, T cells, macrophages, CD11c$^+$ DCs, thymocytes, thymic stromal cells, and thymic DCs (Roark et al. 1998; Chun et al. 2003). Splenic marginal zone B cells have the highest constitutive surface expression of CD1d of any cell type, and CD1d is commonly used as a marker to identify this subset of B cells (Amano et al. 1998; Roark et al. 1998; Makowska et al. 1999). Unlike human T cells, which generally downregulate expression of CD1d in the periphery, mouse peripheral T cells continue to express CD1d, albeit at lower levels than that found on thymocytes (Roark et al. 1998).

Like human CD1d, mouse CD1d is expressed outside the hematopoietic system, particularly on hepatocytes and intestinal epithelial cells (Bleicher et al. 1990; Trobonjaca et al. 2001a, 2001b). Mouse CD1d is also present on endometrial endothelial cells of the cervix and fallopian tubes (Sallinen et al. 2000). CD1d can be found on collecting ducts and blood vessels of the pancreas (Ylinen et al. 2000).

Rat CD1d has similar tissue distribution to that seen in mouse. Rat CD1d transcripts have been detected in liver, kidney, heart, lung, intestine, thymus, lymph nodes, and spleen (Ichimiya et al. 1994), and CD1d protein was found by immunohistochemistry on rat hepatocytes and intestinal epithelial cells (Burke et al. 1994). Further analysis of rat intestine revealed that crypt enterocytes expressed CD1d mRNA but not protein, while enterocytes in the villi expressed CD1d protein, but not transcripts (Kasai et al. 1997). Thus, CD1d expression in rat enterocytes is upregulated during migration-associated differentiation.

6
Isoforms and Splice Variants of CD1d

Several splice variants of human CD1d have been described. In one study, human trophoblasts were found to express two CD1d transcripts, one encoding the full length protein, and one with a deletion of exon 4 (Jenkinson et al. 1999). Exon 4 encodes the α3 domain that is responsible for β2-m association, and the splice variant could yield a functional truncated protein consisting of just the lipid-binding groove. Such a protein product has not been reported, but the exon 4 deleted transcript and six other splice variants were described in a second study (Kojo et al. 2000). It is possible that CD1d is prone to aberrant splicing; mouse thymic CD1d mRNA is often incompletely spliced (Bradbury et al. 1990). Without clear evidence of a protein product, it is difficult to discern the role of alternate splicing in CD1d regulation. Activated protein C receptor is structurally similar to CD1d, but does not associate with β2-m, suggesting that a β2m nonassociating splice variant of CD1d could be functional (Simmonds and Lane 1999).

The mouse genome contains two CD1d genes, CD1d1.1 and CD1d1.2, which are 95% identical. CD1d1.2, however, lacks a conserved cysteine in the α2 domain, which, based on the crystal structure of CD1d1.1, is critical for forming a disulfide bond (Bradbury et al. 1988; Zeng et al. 1997). Nevertheless, CD1d can be found on CD1d1.1-deficient thymocytes by flow cytometry, indicating that CD1d1.2 encodes a protein that can be expressed on the cell surface and recognized by anti-CD1d antibodies (Chen et al. 1999). Furthermore, cells transfected with CD1d1.2 can activate certain NKT cell hybridomas (Chen et al. 1999). CD1d1.1 and CD1d1.2 mRNA are expressed in equal abundance in the thymus, but Northern blot analysis of other tissues shows that CD1d1.1 is the predominant transcript (Bradbury et al. 1988). B6 mice harbor a frameshift mutation in CD1d1.2, rendering it nonfunctional in this mouse strain (Park et al. 1998). Given that B6 mice exhibit no obvious defects in CD1d antigen presentation or NKT cell function, CD1d.1 must be sufficient for in vivo function. To definitively address whether or not CD1d1.2 was sufficient to present antigen and select NKT cells in vivo, mice that expressed only CD1d1.2 on a mixed 129/B6 background were compared to mice deficient in both CD1d genes. NKT cells were not present in either mouse, and NKT cell hybridomas did not respond to thymocytes or splenocytes from the CD1d1.2 mouse (Chen et al. 1999). Therefore, although CD1d1.2 on transfected cells may stimulate NKT cells in vitro, CD1d1.2 likely plays little role in vivo.

CD1d contains four sites for N-linked glycosylation. While the amino acid sequence predicts a 37-kDa protein, CD1d is often reported as a smear or multiple bands on SDS-PAGE, ranging in molecular weight from 37 to 55 kDa. The higher-molecular-weight species can be reduced to 37 kDa by treatment with N-glycanase, indicating that these bands are glycosylated CD1d (Mosser et al. 1991). Tissue-specific isoforms of CD1d have been postulated because APCs isolated from different organs display distinctly different abilities to activate mouse NKT cell hybridomas. NKT hybridoma recognition depends somewhat on the tissue origin of the NKT cell; hybridomas derived from thymocytes were more likely to be activated by thymocytes than splenocytes, whereas hybridomas derived from splenocytes displayed the reverse pattern (Park et al. 1998). When the same CD1d construct was transfected into a thymoma, a B cell lymphoma and a macrophage tumor line, the three transfectants displayed equally high CD1d surface expression, but markedly different abilities to activate a panel of NKT cell hybridomas (Brossay et al. 1998). While differences in co-stimulation could account for the variation in NKT cell activation, hybridomas have been shown to be insensitive to co-stimulation; thus, it is more likely that the CD1d transfectants expressed CD1d with different bound lipids or different glycosylation patterns. Different glycosylation patterns of CD1d can be detected by immunoblot. Mouse thymocytes, for example, express a heavily glycosylated, high-molecular-weight form of CD1d not present in other tissues (Mosser et al. 1991).

Human thymocytes express a unique isoform of CD1d. When solubilized in non-ionic detergents, thymocyte CD1d loses epitopes recognized by antibodies 51.1 and 42.1 as shown by a loss of immunoprecipitable protein. CD1d transfected C1R cells, by comparison, do not show this loss of epitopes. An NKT cell hybridoma, which recognized CD1d transfected C1R and CHO cells, failed to recognize CD1d on human thymocytes. Finally, human thymocytes are not stained by antibodies 3C11 and 1H1, indicating that the epitopes recognized by these antibodies are not expressed on thymocytes (Exley et al. 2000).

Human CD1d on IECs exists as two distinct isoforms. The major isoform is a glycosylated 48-kDa form that associates with β2m and is expressed basally and apically (Somnay-Wadgaonkar et al. 1999). The second isoform is 37 kDa, lacks carbohydrates, does not associate with β2-m, tends to form trimers, and is primarily distributed on the apical surface of polarized epithelial cells (Balk et al. 1994; Somnay-Wadgaonkar et al. 1999). CD1d associates with prolyl-4 hydroxylase (P4H) during its biogenesis in the ER, and protein sequencing of the 48- and 37-kDa isoforms revealed that only the 37-kDa form of CD1d contains hydroxyproline residues (Kim et al. 2000). Therefore, at least in human IECs, a portion of the nascent CD1d is hydroxyprolinated by P4H, does not bind β2-m, escapes glycosylation, and traffics to the apical surface. The purpose of this pathway, which accounts for less than 10% of CD1d molecules in IECs, is still unclear, but it is possible that this unique isoform affects NKT cell regulation in the gut mucosa. Human IECs activate CD8[+] intraepithelial lymphocytes through CD1d and the carcinoembryonic antigen-related cell adhesion molecule (CEACAM) homolog glycoprotein 180 (gp180) (Campbell et al. 1999). This function can be performed by the β2-m nonassociated isoform; when transfected into β2-m-negative FO-1 cells, human CD1d could interact with gp180 at the cell surface and activate CD8[+] T cells (Campbell et al. 1999; Kim et al. 2000). The 37-kDa CD1d isoform might play a role in identifying abnormal epithelium since its expression would not be affected by loss of β2-m, as frequently occurs in human colon cancers

(Goepel et al. 1991). Although a β2-m nonassociated form of CD1d has not been found on normal human B cells, metabolic labeling of CD1d transfected B cell lymphoma lines has shown that mature CD1d can exit the ER without β2-m association (Kang and Cresswell 2002).

A mouse β2-m nonassociated form of CD1d has been postulated to exist. Mouse CD1d transfected into β2-m$^{-/-}$ cell lines results in cell surface expression of CD1d, although this finding has been contested (Balk et al. 1994; Brutkiewicz et al. 1995; Teitell et al. 1997). Examination of β2-m$^{-/-}$ mice has revealed that these mice do not support NKT cell selection (Bendelac et al. 1994). Furthermore, CD1d cannot be detected on any β2-m$^{-/-}$ cell type by flow cytometry or by immunofluorescent staining with multiple anti-CD1d antibodies, with the exception of some vascular endothelial cells stained by the 3C11 antibody (Bendelac et al. 1994; Teitell et al. 1997; Amano et al. 1998). On the other hand, splenic LPS blasts from β2-m$^{-/-}$ mice could activate a CD1d-restricted T cell clone, and this activation was abrogated by blocking antibodies to CD1d (Amano et al. 1998). Another group derived NKT cell hybridomas from MHC II-deficient mice and showed that two hybridomas could recognize β2-m$^{-/-}$ splenocytes in CD1d-restricted fashion (Cardell et al. 1995). These hybridomas were verified to recognize β2-m$^{-/-}$ B cells but not β2-m$^{-/-}$ T cells (Brossay et al. 1997). Given the available evidence, it is probable that mouse CD1d can be expressed at the cell surface in the absence of β2-m, but that this occurs at such low frequency that it cannot be detected by flow cytometry or immunofluorescence.

7
Regulation of CD1d Expression During Cellular Differentiation and Infection

Human CD1d is controlled by two TATA boxless promoters, one proximal (−106 to +24) and one distal (−665 to −202) to the transcription start site (Chen and Jackson 2004). Specificity protein 1 (SP-1) binds to the proximal promoter in two places; the SP-1 site closest to the transcription start is required for CD1d expression, possibly as a mechanism of recruiting RNA polymerase II in the absence of a TATA box. The second SP-1 site greatly enhances gene expression, although it is not absolutely required. The distal promoter contains an LEF-1 site that binds a negative regulator. Several γ-IRE-CS, NF-IL-6, and TCF-1 sites were also predicted from sequence analysis, suggesting a role for IFNγ and IL-6 in CD1d regulation. Human CD1d is regulated by cell type-specific factors since promoter constructs showed varied activity when transfected into different cell lines (Chen and Jackson 2004).

Analysis of the human CD1d promoter also revealed a putative retinoic acid response element. Retinoic acid (RA) treatment induced CD1d transcription in the human monocyte cell line THP-1, and ligation of the RA-inducible cell-surface receptor CD38 resulted in an increase in intracellular and surface CD1d protein (Q. Chen and A.C. Ross, personal communication).

Mouse CD1d also lacks a TATA box; however, no SP-1 sites were identified in a 200-base pair promoter region (Geng et al. 2005). Instead, an ETS binding site was shown to be critical for activity, and the ETS family transcription factors Elf1 and PU.1 were shown to bind to this site. Elf1 positively regulates CD1d expression in B cells but not other cell types as Elf1-deficient mice have decreased expression of CD1d only on B lineage cells. On the other hand, PU.1 negatively regulates CD1d expression since activation of PU.1 in a myeloid cell line resulted in a decrease in CD1d surface levels. Mouse CD1d mRNA levels correlate well with surface protein expression, indicating that transcriptional regulation modulates surface concentrations of CD1d (Geng et al. 2005).

In contrast to the regulation of Group 1 CD1 proteins, surface levels of mouse and human CD1d remain constant over a wide range of experimental conditions (Mandal et al. 1998; Exley et al. 2000). Surface CD1d on human monocytes is constitutively low and remains fairly constant during differentiation into DCs. Although immunoblotting for CD1d revealed that DCs contain more CD1d protein on a per cell basis than monocytes, immunofluorescent staining showed this was due to a larger intracellular pool (Spada et al. 2000). Unlike the group I CD1 proteins, CD1d on DCs is not upregulated by GM-CSF, IL-4, immunization with tetanus toxin, or infection by mycobacteria (Ulanova et al. 2000a). Expression is moderately downregulated by TGF-β and seen by a decrease in CD1d transcription and surface expression on human monocyte-derived DCs (Ronger-Savle et al. 2005). CD1d disappears from monocyte-derived DCs during culture in media containing fetal calf serum, but when cultured in media supplemented with human serum, CD1d expression is unchanged (Gerlini et al. 2001).

Some evidence for regulation of CD1d levels exists. Human immature DCs infected with *Leishmania infantum* or cultured with purified *Leishmania* lipophosphoglycan upregulate surface CD1d expression, which renders infected DCs more sensitive to NKT cell-mediated lysis (Campos-Martin et al. 2006). Infection with mycobacteria does not affect surface CD1d expression by mouse DCs (Feng et al. 2001), but mouse macrophages upregulate CD1d during infection (Skold et al. 2005). Human IEC lines express low levels of CD1d, which can be moderately increased by culture with IFNγ or LPS, but not by culture with IL-2, IL-4, or TNFα (Colgan et al. 1996; Fuss et al. 2004). IEC cell lines generally express much lower levels of CD1d than IECs freshly isolated from human colon (Colgan et al. 2003). This phenomenon was explained by the discovery that heat shock protein (HSP) 110, a soluble protein found in mouse and human intestinal luminal fluid, upregulates CD1d expression on IEC cell lines. HSP110 had no effect on CD1d on fresh IECs, indicating that this pathway is already saturated and contributes to the constitutive expression of CD1d in the intestine (Colgan et al. 2003). As keratinocytes migrate from the basal layer through the stratum corneum, they increase expression of CD1d, and CD1d protein redistributes from a primarily intracellular location in undifferentiated cells to the plasma membrane in differentiated cells (Fishelevich et al. 2006). CD1d can be induced on keratinocytes by culture with IFNγ or by skin exposure to poison ivy (Bonish et al. 2000).

Viral infection has long been known to regulate MHC class I and II expression; antigen-presenting molecules are prime targets for viral immunoevasion strategies. Likewise, CD1d had been shown to be downregulated by certain viruses. The human immunodeficiency virus (HIV) nuclear envelope factor (Nef) causes a reduction in surface CD1d due to increased CD1d internalization and an increased retention of CD1d in the trans-Golgi network (Chen et al. 2006). Karposi's sarcoma-associated herpes virus (KSHV) protein modulator of immune recognition 1 and 2 (MIR1 and MIR2) are known to downregulate MHC I and B7-1 by increased proteasomal degradation. Even though MIR1 and MIR2 ubiquitinate the CD1d cytoplasmic tail, CD1d is not targeted for degradation. Instead, CD1d is internalized, resulting in greatly diminished surface levels and decreased NKT cell recognition of the infected cells (Sanchez et al. 2005). Herpes simplex virus type 1 (HSV-1) interferes with the normal recycling pattern of surface CD1d in infected cells by redistributing CD1d to the limiting membrane of lysosomes and preventing its reappearance on the cell surface after endocytosis. This effectively reduces surface CD1d levels and decreases the ability of HSV-1 infected cells to be recognized by NKT cells (Yuan et al. 2006). By contrast, cells may upregulate CD1d as an antiviral defense mechanism since liver biopsies of hepatitis C-infected patients show increased expression of CD1d on hepatocytes (Durante-Mangoni et al. 2004).

A study of vaccina and vesicular stomatitis viral infections of CD1d-transfected fibroblasts showed that viral infection could impair NKT cell recognition without affecting surface levels of CD1d by preventing CD1d lysosomal trafficking (Renukaradhya et al. 2005). Lysosomal trafficking is necessary for interaction with antigenic lipids and lipid-editing enzymes, such as saposins (Zhou et al. 2004). Altering CD1d trafficking away from lysosomes even without affecting surface expression could be a viral strategy for evading recognition by NKT cells. All in all, viral infections that affect CD1d function imply a role for NKT cells in the immune response to these pathogens.

Microsomal triglyceride transfer protein (MTP), an ER-resident chaperone and lipid transfer protein, loads endogenous lipids onto nascent CD1d (Brozovic et al. 2004; Dougan SK 2005). Purified MTP can transfer phospholipid to recombinant CD1d in vitro, and MTP silencing or chemical inhibition in APCs causes a decrease in their ability to activate NKT cells. MTP regulates CD1d expression; inhibiting MTP lipid transfer activity in primary cells causes an average 20%–30% reduction in CD1d surface levels, possibly by retaining CD1d in the ER (Dougan SK 2005).

8
CD1d Expression and Function on Thymocytes

CD1d is expressed on both mouse and human thymocytes. In the mouse, CD1d is most highly expressed on CD4CD8-expressing and CD4-expressing thymocytes with a twofold decrease in CD1d expression on CD8 cells. Upon exit to the periphery, mouse T cells further decrease CD1d expression, although the relative difference between CD4$^+$ and CD8$^+$ T cells is maintained (Roark et al. 1998). In humans, CD1d is present on cortical thymocytes but is rarely found on medullary thymocytes (Exley et al. 2000). This downregulation of CD1d during thymic development leads to low expression on small numbers of human peripheral T cells. CD1d is upregulated on activated T cells; human peripheral blood occasionally contains a small population of CD1d$^+$ CD69$^+$ T cells, which are not present in samples taken from the same donor at later time points (Exley et al. 2000). Phytohemagglutinin (PHA) stimulation of peripheral blood mononuclear cells increases CD1d transcription, resulting in CD1d surface expression on activated T cells (Salamone et al. 2001). Apart from the critical role of thymocytes in NKT cell selection, it is not yet clear whether T lineage cells can function as CD1d-restricted APCs. Mouse thymocytes, unlike most other freshly isolated CD1d$^+$ cells in the absence of exogenous antigen, are susceptible to lysis by mouse liver iNKT cells (Osman et al. 2000). In addition, a CD1d^{high}, NK1.1$^-$ population of mouse splenic NKT cells has been shown to present α-galcer to other cells in the same population, indicating that NKT cells themselves can present antigen on CD1d (Hameg et al. 2000).

9
CD1d Expression and Function on B Cells

Mouse B cells express CD1d; in fact, the highest level of peripheral CD1d expression in a mouse is found on marginal zone (MZ) B cells (Roark et al.

1998). This population of CD21^{high}, CD23^{low}, IgM^{high}, IgD^{low}, CD1d^{high} cells appears after approximately 3 weeks of age (Makowska et al. 1999). CD1d-expressing MZ B cells develop in germ-free mice, MHC II$^{-/-}$ mice and TCRβ$^{-/-}$ mice, suggesting that neither antigen nor T cell help is required for their development. Nonetheless, a significant portion of CD1d high MZ B cells contain somatic hypermutations indicating that a subset of these cells are antigen-experienced. CD1d high MZ B cells fail to develop in CD19$^{-/-}$ mice probably due to weaker signaling through the B cell receptor in these mice. CD19$^{-/-}$ mice have a normal compartment of follicular B cells, suggesting that CD1d-expressing MZ B cells are more reliant on BCR signaling than follicular B cells for their development (Makowska et al. 1999; Pillai et al. 2005).

NKT cells can provide help to both mouse and human B cells. Mice transgenic for the invariant NKT cell receptor had elevated basal levels of IgG1 and IgE (Bendelac et al. 1996). In a mouse malaria model, it was shown that production of antibodies against glycosyl phosphatidylinositol (GPI)-anchored proteins is dependent on NKT cells and that NKT cells can recognize GPI-pulsed APCs in a CD1d-restricted manner (Schofield et al. 1999). This finding was contested in a later paper showing that NKT cells were dispensable for overall malaria protection, but production of a particular malaria-specific antibody was NKT cell-dependent (Romero et al. 2001; Hansen et al. 2003). Furthermore, Ig production was documented in a memory recall model in MHC class II-deficient mice, suggesting that antibody production is due to NKT cell help because no other CD4$^+$ cells are present in these mice (Hansen et al. 2003).

Human NKT cells upregulate lymphoid tissue homing receptors CCR7 and CD62 ligand upon activation, allowing them to traffic to the lymph nodes and spleen where they can encounter B cells (Galli et al. 2003). Activated NKT cells cause B cell proliferation and IgM production, which is dependent on IL-4 and IL-13 but not CD40. Although NKT cells are more strongly activated by B cells presenting α-galcer, B cells in the absence of exogenous antigen activate NKT cells. This low level activation is abolished in the presence of CD1d blocking antibodies, strongly indicating that NKT cells can recognize an endogenous ligand on B cells (Galli et al. 2003).

Transgenic mice expressing CD11c promoter-driven diphtheria toxin receptor and B cell-deficient (μT$^{-/-}$) mice were used to parse out the roles of each APC type in NKT cell activation (Bezbradica et al. 2005). B cells could present α-galcer in vivo, but were less stimulatory than DCs. However, mice containing DCs but no B cells showed increased levels of NKT cell activation, and adoptive transfer of wild type but not CD1d$^{-/-}$ B cells dampened DC presentation of α-galcer down to normal levels. Thus B cells, in a CD1d-depedent manner, can suppress the ability of DCs to activate NKT cells.

10
CD1d Expression and Function on Monocytes and Macrophages

Both mouse and human monocytes and macrophages express CD1d, but activate NKT cells only weakly. However, mouse macrophages infected with mycobacteria upregulate CD1d and become highly potent at stimulating NKT cells (Skold et al. 2005). Unlike DCs, which are highly stimulatory even when expressing barely detectable surface levels of CD1d, a macrophage's ability to present antigen is directly dependent on the number of molecules of CD1d on the cell surface (Skold et al. 2005).

Mouse liver resident macrophages, or Kupffer cells, can also upregulate CD1d in response to mycobacterial lipids (Ryll et al. 2001). Furthermore, depletion of mouse liver dendritic cells prior to injection of α-galcer had no effect on the number of IL-4 and IFN-γ-producing liver NKT cells, but depletion of Kupffer cells severely diminished these populations (Schmieg et al. 2005).

In humans, macrophage-like foam cells in atherosclerotic plaques express CD1d, and foam cells differentiated from macrophages in tissue culture present lipid antigens to NKT cells (Melian et al. 1999). Ligation of CD1d on fresh peripheral blood monocytes with cross-linking antibodies stimulates IL-12 production (Yue et al. 2005).

11
CD1d Expression and Function on Dendritic Cells

Of all APC types, DCs are the most effective in activating NKT cells. Despite low surface levels of CD1d, DCs can stimulate NKT cell proliferation and production of both IFN-γ and IL-4 (Spada et al. 2000). Human Vα24+ NKT cells are cytolytic against myeloid and monocyte derived DCs, but not against B cells, T cells, monocytes, or leukemic cells, and destruction of APCs may be important in counter-regulating NKT cell responses (Nicol et al. 2000; Yang et al. 2000). Cytolysis of human DCs is partially due to CD40–CD40 ligand interactions since ligation of CD40 on DCs induces apoptosis (Nieda et al. 2001). CD11c+ human myeloid DCs express CD1d while CD11c− plasmacytoid DCs do not. Nonetheless, plasmacytoid DCs (PDC) can synergistically activate NKT cells through OX40–OX40 ligand interactions and production of IFNα (Marschner et al. 2005). CD40 interactions with CD40 ligand are necessary for mouse DC presentation of α-galcer; administration of CD40L-blocking antibodies diminishes DC production of IL-12 and NKT cell production of IFN-γ in response to α-galcer injection (Kitamura et al. 1999; Nishimura et al. 2000).

12
CD1d Expression and Function on Epithelial Cells

Intestinal epithelial cells express glycosylated CD1d and a unique 37-kDa unglycosylated isoform that does not associate with β2m (Bleicher et al. 1990; Balk et al. 1994; Somnay-Wadgaonkar et al. 1999; Kim et al. 2000). Ligation of CD1d on human IECs causes IL-10 secretion via signaling through the cytoplasmic tail, and IEC production of IL-10 can counteract IFN-γ-induced loss of barrier function (Colgan et al. 1999). Intestinal CD1d may regulate luminal bacteria as colonization of germ-free CD1d$^{-/-}$ mice occurs more rapidly than in germ-free wild type mice. CD1d$^{-/-}$ mice also show an increase in colonization of the lung by *Pseudomonas aeruginosa* (Nieuwenhuis et al. 2002). Thus, CD1d plays a role in natural host defense against bacterial colonization and invasion at the mucosal barrier.

13
CD1d in Disease

MHC class I and II molecules are extensively regulated during inflammation and their surface expression exhibits a broad range of concentrations during various disease states. Although CD1d expression does not vary as widely, its important role in presenting antigen to NKT cells makes CD1d an ideal target for regulation during diseases involving this particular T cell subset. Early studies of immunoperoxidase stainings of human colonic sections suggested that CD1d was more abundantly expressed on the colonic epithelium of patients with inflammatory bowel disease (Canchis et al. 1993). This observation was later substantiated by immunoprecipitation studies showing that increased CD1d protein was present in the affected tissues of patients with Crohn's disease and ulcerative colitis (Page et al. 2000). Mouse models of colitis have shown both protective and pathological roles for NKT cells, but which APC is responsible for activating the NKT cells for these distinct responses remains an unanswered question (Saubermann et al. 2000; Heller et al. 2002). Given that CD1d cross-linking causes intestinal epithelial cells and DCs to secrete IL-10 and IL-12, respectively, it is possible that epithelial cells and dendritic cell interactions with NKT cells provide protection against and activation of colitis (Colgan et al. 1999; Yue et al. 2005). Expression of CD1d on colonic epithelium increases during colitis induced by adoptive transfer of CD62L$^+$ CD4$^+$ cells into SCID Balb/c mice (Hornung et al. 2006).

The liver is an abundant source of NKT cells in rodents and humans, and several liver diseases involve alterations in CD1d expression (Bleicher et al. 1990; Canchis et al. 1993; Burke et al. 1994). In humans, CD1d is expressed in epithelioid granuloma cells in both primary biliary cirrhosis and sarcoidosis. Early-stage PBC patients express CD1d on epithelial cells of the small bile duct, whereas this staining is observed neither in late-stage PBC patients nor in healthy controls (Tsuneyama et al. 1998). Hepatocytes constitutively express low levels of surface CD1d but are highly effective antigen-presenting cells (Bleicher et al. 1990; Trobonjaca et al. 2001b; Durante-Mangoni et al. 2004). Furthermore, human CD1d is strongly upregulated on hepatocytes infected with hepatitis C virus. This upregulation can lead to alterations in the cytokine profile of liver-resident NKT cells since intrahepatic lymphocytes (IHLs) isolated from healthy livers tend to produce IFN-γ upon stimulation, while IHLs from severely diseased livers secrete IL-4 and IL-13 (Durante-Mangoni et al. 2004).

Psoriasis is another disease influenced by aberrantly activated NKT cells, as suggested by studies showing that an NKT cell line derived from psoriatic patients produces IFN-γ and IL-13 in response to CD1d bearing keratinocytes and that this same NKT cell line is capable of creating a psoriatic plaque when injected into human skin grafted onto an immunocompromised mouse (Nickoloff et al. 1999, 2000). CD1d is expressed by human keratinocytes and is upregulated in psoriatic lesions (Canchis et al. 1993; Bonish et al. 2000).

In experimental autoimmune encephalomyelitis (EAE), CD1d is upregulated on microglia, macrophages and infiltrating T cells in inflamed CNS tissue (Busshoff et al. 2001). Guinea pigs also show upregulation of CD1 molecules during EAE, particularly on astrocytes and infiltrating B cells and macrophages (Cipriani et al. 2003).

Infiltrating CD1d$^+$ cells have been correlated with several disease states, although it is unclear whether these CD1d$^+$ cells migrated in response to inflammation or whether B cells or DCs already present in the affected tissues increased their expression of CD1d. Nevertheless, increased numbers of CD1d$^+$ B cells have been found by immunohistochemistry in periodontal lesions, and an increased infiltration of CD1d$^+$ cells, likely B cells and DCs, has been observed in the lamina propria of the small intestine in patients with cow's milk hypersensitivity (Ulanova et al. 2000b; Amanuma et al. 2006).

One infiltrating CD1d$^+$ cell type is the regulatory B cell. This population, described in the TCR$\alpha^{-/-}$ mouse model of colitis, is likely derived from a marginal zone B cell precursor, which upregulates CD1d expression, migrates to the mesenteric lymph nodes, and secretes immunosuppressive IL-10 (Mizoguchi and Bhan 2006). These so-called Bregs function independently of NKT cells since they suppress colitis in a mouse lacking T and NKT cells. However, CD1d is critical to Breg's suppressive function since adoptive transfer of wild type B cells, but not CD1d$^{-/-}$ B cells, into TCR$\alpha^{-/-}$ μT$^{-/-}$ double-deficient mice ameliorates colitis (Mizoguchi et al. 2002). It is likely that ligation of

CD1d on Bregs, similar to ligation of CD1d on IECs, signals production of IL-10 (Colgan et al. 1999). Subsequent studies confirmed the presence of intestinal regulatory B cells and showed that B cells from mesenteric lymph nodes, but not from spleen, conferred protection from colitis (Wei et al. 2005).

The role of CD1d in cancer has been the subject of intense research ever since the CD1d ligand α-galactosylceramide was isolated while screening for anti-tumor compounds (Morita et al. 1995). Many tumors express CD1d so that NKT cells not only secrete IFN-γ and other anti-tumor cytokines but also directly cause tumor lysis (Metelitsa et al. 2003; Takahashi et al. 2003; Dhodapkar et al. 2004; Fais et al. 2004). CD1d is expressed on acute myeloid leukemias (AML), juvenile myelomonocytic leukemias (JMML), acute lymphoblastic leukemias (ALL), B cell chronic lymphocytic leukemias (B-CLL), and gliomas and brain tumor vasculature (Metelitsa et al. 2003; Takahashi et al. 2003; Dhodapkar et al. 2004; Fais et al. 2004). A study of human myeloma patients found that although myelomas express CD1d and can be lysed by α-galcer expanded iNKT lines, fresh iNKT from myeloma patients are hyporesponsive. The defects in proliferation, production of IFN-γ and tumor lysis could be reversed by short-term in vitro culture of the patients' iNKT cells, suggesting that CD1d$^+$ myelomas temporarily suppress NKT cell function (Dhodapkar et al. 2003).

Tumors may express CD1d above normal levels. Microarray analysis of cutaneous T cell lymphomas (CTCL) found that CD1d was consistently up-regulated (Nebozhyn et al. 2006). However, surface expression of CD1d on a panel of mouse tumor cell lines did not vary in response to cytokines or other stimuli, indicating that although tumors may express CD1d, the expression pattern of CD1d does not tend to change (Fiedler et al. 2002).

From the tumor immunologist's point of view, the most intriguing question regarding CD1d is whether tumor antigens, in particular the ever-elusive tumor rejection antigens without which the tumor cannot survive, can be presented on CD1d. At least one tumor antigen, ganglioside GD3 from human melanoma, can be presented on CD1d. Injection of a human melanoma cell line into mice resulted in GD3-loaded CD1d tetramer-positive NKT cells, which produced IL-4 and IFN-γ in response to GD3 pulsed APCs (Wu et al. 2003). CD1d$^+$ DCs are critical for generation of tumor immunity in a mouse melanoma model. Wild type mice injected with B16 melanoma cells engineered to secrete GM-CSF do not develop tumors upon subsequent challenge with B16; however, CD1d$^{-/-}$ mice do succumb to tumors in this model. Further investigation showed that vaccination generates a large population of CD8α$^-$ CD1d^{high} splenic dendritic cells, which produce MIP-2 and are associated with increased splenic NKT cells (Gillessen et al. 2003). A corresponding population of B7-1$^+$ CD1a$^+$ DCs can be found at the vaccination sites of human patients injected with autologous, irradiated GM-CSF-secreting tumor vaccines, and many of these patients develop anti-tumor responses (Mach et al. 2000).

14
Concluding Remarks

CD1 has long been considered the third way of antigen presentation. However, unlike MHC class I and II, the range of CD1-presented antigens was initially limited. Recent work has greatly expanded the range of self and foreign antigens presented by all CD1 family members, particularly CD1d. It is now clear that CD1d, at least on DCs, plays a role in infectious disease both directly by presentation of microbial lipids and indirectly by NKT cell recognition of self lipid in the context of inflammation. Understanding the expression and function of CD1 on particular cell types is critical to understanding the presentation of lipid antigens and the role of self versus foreign lipids in immune regulation.

References

Adly MA, Assaf HA, Hussein M (2005) Expression of CD1d in human scalp skin and hair follicles: hair cycle related alterations. J Clin Pathol 58:1278–1282

Amano M et al (1998) CD1 expression defines subsets of follicular and marginal zone B cells in the spleen: beta 2-microglobulin-dependent and independent forms. J Immunol 161:1710–1717

Amanuma R, Nakajima T, Yoshie H, Yamazaki K (2006) Increased infiltration of CD1d and natural killer T cells in periodontal disease tissues. J Periodontal Res 41:73–79

Angel CE, George E, Brooks AE, Ostrovsky LL, Brown TL, Dunbar PR (2006) Cutting edge: CD1a+ antigen-presenting cells in human dermis respond rapidly to CCR7 ligands. J Immunol 176:5730–5734

Angenieux C, Salamero J, Fricker D, Cazenave JP, Goud B, Hanau D, de La Salle H (2000) Characterization of CD1e, a third type of CD1 molecule expressed in dendritic cells. J Biol Chem 275:37757–37764

Angenieux C, Fraisier V, Maitre B, Racine V, van der Wel N, Fricker D, Proamer F, Sachse M, Cazenave JP, Peters P, Goud B, Hanau D, Sibarita JB, Salamero J, de la Salle H (2005) The cellular pathway of CD1e in immature and maturing dendritic cells. Traffic 6:286–302

Balk SP, Bleicher PA, Terhorst C (1989) Isolation and characterization of a cDNA and gene coding for a fourth CD1 molecule. Proc Natl Acad Sci U S A 86:252–256

Balk SP et al (1994) Beta 2-microglobulin-independent MHC class Ib molecule expressed by human intestinal epithelium. Science 265:259–262

Banchereau J et al (2000) Immunobiology of dendritic cells. Annu Rev Immunol 18:767–811

Battistini L, Fischer FR, Raine CS, Brosnan CF (1996) CD1b is expressed in multiple sclerosis lesions. J Neuroimmunol 67:145–151

Bell D et al (1999) In breast carcinoma tissue, immature dendritic cells reside within the tumor, whereas mature dendritic cells are located in peritumoral areas. J Exp Med 190:1417–1426

Bendelac A, Killeen N, Littman DR, Schwartz RH (1994) A subset of CD4+ thymocytes selected by MHC class I molecules. Science 263:1774–1778

Bendelac A, Hunziker RD, Lantz O (1996) Increased interleukin 4 and immunoglobulin E production in transgenic mice overexpressing NK1 T cells. J Exp Med 184:1285–1293

Bezbradica JS, Stanic AK, Matsuki N et al (2005) Distinct roles of dendritic cells and B cells in Va14Ja18 natural T cell activation in vivo. J Immunol 174:4696–4705

Bleicher PA, Balk SP, Hagen SJ, Blumberg RS, Flotte TJ, Terhorst C (1990) Expression of murine CD1 on gastrointestinal epithelium. Science 250:679–682

Blumberg RS, Turnhorst C, Bleicher P et al (1991) Expression of a nonpolymorphic MHC class I-like molecule CD1D, by human intestinal epithelial cells. J Immunol 147:2518–2524

Bonish B, Jullien D, Dutronc Y et al (2000) Overexpression of CD1d by keratinocytes in psoriasis and CD1d-dependent IFN-gamma production by NK-T cells. J Immunol 165:4076–4085

Bradbury A, Belt KT, Neri TM, Milstein C, Calabi F (1988) Mouse CD1 is distinct from and co-exists with TL in the same thymus. EMBO J 7:3081–3086

Bradbury A, Calabi F, Milstein C (1990) Expression of CD1 in the mouse thymus. Eur J Immunol 20:1831–1836

Brossay L, Jullien D, Cardell S et al (1997) Mouse CD1 is mainly expressed on hemopoietic-derived cells. J Immunol 159:1216–1224

Brossay L, Tangri S, Bix M, Cardell S, Locksley R, Kronenberg M (1998) Mouse CD1-autoreactive T cells have diverse patterns of reactivity to CD1+ targets. J Immunol 160:3681–3688

Brozovic S, Nagaishi T, Yoshida M, Betz S, Salas A, Chen D, Kaser A, Glickman J, Kuo T, Little A, Morrison J, Corazza N, Kim JY, Colgan SP, Young SG, Exley M, Blumberg RS (2004) CD1d function is regulated by microsomal triglyceride transfer protein. Nat Med 10:535–539

Brutkiewicz RR, Bennink JR, Yewdell JW, Bendelac A (1995) TAP-independent, beta 2-microglobulin-dependent surface expression of functional mouse CD1.1. J Exp Med 182:1913–1919

Burke S, Landau S, Green R et al (1994) Rat cluster of differentiation 1 molecule: expression on the surface of intestinal epithelial cells and hepatocytes. Gastroenterology 106:1143–1149

Busshoff U, Hein A, Iglesias A, Dorries R, Regnier-Vigouroux A (2001) CD1 expression is differentially regulated by microglia, macrophages and T cells in the central nervous system upon inflammation and demyelination. J Neuroimmunol 113:220–230

Campbell NA, Kim HS, Blumberg RS, Mayer L (1999) The nonclassical class I molecule CD1d associates with the novel CD8 ligand gp180 on intestinal epithelial cells. J Biol Chem 274:26259–26265

Campos-Martin Y, Colmenares M, Gozalbo-Lopez B, Lopez-Nunez M, Savage PB, Martinez-Naves E (2006) Immature human dendritic cells infected with *Leishmania infantum* are resistant to NK-mediated cytolysis but are efficiently recognized by NKT cells. J Immunol 176:6172–6179

Canchis PW, Bhan AK, Landau SB, Yang L, Balk SP, Blumberg RS (1993) Tissue distribution of the non-polymorphic major histocompatibility complex class I-like molecule CD1d. Immunology 80:561–565

Cao X, Sugita M, Van der Wel N et al (2002) CD1 molecules efficiently present antigen in immature dendritic cells and traffic independently of MHC class II during dendritic cell maturation. J Immunol 169:4770–4777

Cardell S, Tangri S, Chan S, Kronenberg M, Benoist C, Mathis D (1995) CD1-restricted CD4+ T cells in major histocompatibility complex class II-deficient mice. J Exp Med 182:993–1004

Caux C, Dezutter-Dambuyant C, Schmitt D, Banchereau J (1992) GM-CSF and TNF-alpha cooperate in the generation of dendritic Langerhans cells. Nature 360:258–261

Caux C, Vanbervliet B, Massacrier C et al (1996) CD34+ hematopoietic progenitors from human cord blood differentiate along two independent dendritic cell pathways in response to GM-CSF+TNF alpha. J Exp Med 184:695–706

Chen N et al (2006) HIV-1 down-regulates the expression of CD1d via Nef. Eur J Immunol 36:278–286

Chen QY, Jackson N (2004) Human CD1D gene has TATA boxless dual promoters: an SP1-binding element determines the function of the proximal promoter. J Immunol 172:5512–5521

Chen YH, Wang B, Chun T et al (1999) Expression of CD1d2 on thymocytes is not sufficient for the development of NKT cells in CD1d1-deficient mice. J Immunol 162:4560–4566

Chun T, Page MJ, Gapin L et al (2003) CD1d-expressing dendritic cells but not thymic epithelial cells can mediate negative selection of NKT cells. J Exp Med 197:907–918

Cipriani B, Chen L, Hiromatsu K et al (2003) Upregulation of group 1. CD1 antigen presenting molecules in guinea pigs with experimental autoimmune encephalomyelitis: an immunohistochemical study. Brain Pathol 13:1–9

Colgan SP, Morales VM, Madara JL, Polischuk JE, Balk SP, Blumberg RS (1996) IFN-gamma modulates CD1d surface expression on intestinal epithelia. Am J Physiol 271:C276–C283

Colgan SP, Hershberg RM, Furuta GT, Blumberg RS (1999) Ligation of intestinal epithelial CD1d induces bioactive IL-10: critical role of the cytoplasmic tail in autocrine signaling. Proc Natl Acad Sci U S A 96:13938–13943

Colgan SP et al (2003) Intestinal heat shock protein 110 regulates expression of CD1d on intestinal epithelial cells. J Clin Invest 112:745–754

De la Salle HMariotti S, Angenieux C, Gilleron M, Garcia-Alles LF, Malm D et al (2005) Assistance of microbial glycolipid antigen processing by CD1e. Science 310:1321–1324

Delia D, Cattoretti G, Polli N et al (1988) CD1c but neither CD1a nor CD1b molecules are expressed on normal, activated, and malignant human B cells: identification of a new B-cell subset. Blood 72:241–247

Dhodapkar KM, Cirignano B, Chamian F et al (2004) Invariant natural killer T cells are preserved in patients with glioma and exhibit antitumor lytic activity following dendritic cell-mediated expansion. Int J Cancer 109:893–899

Dhodapkar MV, Geller MD, Chang DH et al (2003) A reversible defect in natural killer T cell function characterizes the progression of premalignant to malignant multiple myeloma. J Exp Med 197:1667–1676

Dougan SKSA, Rava P, Agyemang A, Kaser A, Morrison J, Khurana A, Kronenberg M, Johnson C, Exley M, Hussain MM, Blumberg RS (2005) Microsomal triglyceride transfer protein lipidation and control of CD1d on antigen-presenting cells. J Exp Med 202:529–539

Duperrier K, Eljaafari H, Dezutter-Dambuyant C et al (2000) Distinct subsets of dendritic cells resembling dermal DCs can be generated in vitro from monocytes, in the presence of different serum supplements. J Immunol Methods 238:119–131

Durante-Mangoni E et al (2004) Hepatic CD1d expression in hepatitis C virus infection and recognition by resident proinflammatory CD1d-reactive T cells. J Immunol 173:2159–2166

Exley M, Garcia J, Wilson SB et al (2000) CD1d structure and regulation on human thymocytes, peripheral blood T cells B cells and monocytes. Immunology 100:37–47

Fainboim L, Salamone Mdel C (2002) CD1: a family of glycolypid-presenting molecules or also immunoregulatory proteins? J Biol Regul Homeost Agents 16:125–135

Fais F, Morabito F, Stelitano C et al (2004) CD1d is expressed on B-chronic lymphocytic leukemia cells and mediates alpha-galactosylceramide presentation to natural killer T lymphocytes. Int J Cancer 109:402–411

Feng CG, Demangel C, Kamath AT, Macdonald M, Britton WJ (2001) Dendritic cells infected with *Mycobacterium bovis* bacillus Calmette Guerin activate CD8(+) T cells with specificity for a novel mycobacterial epitope. Int Immunol 13:451–458

Fiedler T, Walter W, Reichert TE, Maeurer MJ (2002) Regulation of CD1d expression by murine tumor cells: escape from immunosurveillance or alternate target molecules? Int J Cancer 98:389–397

Fishelevich R, Malalina A, Luzina I et al (2006) Ceramide-dependent regulation of human epidermal keratinocyte CD1d expression during terminal differentiation. J Immunol 176:2590–2599

Fivenson DP, Nickoloff BJ (1995) Distinctive dendritic cell subsets expressing factor XIIIa CD1a CD1b and CD1c in mycosis fungoides and psoriasis. J Cutan Pathol 22:223–228

Fuss IJ, Heller F, Boirivant M et al (2004) Nonclassical CD1d-restricted NKT cells that produce IL-13 characterize an atypical Th2 response in ulcerative colitis. J Clin Invest 113:1490–1497

Galli G, Nuti S, Tavarini S et al (2003) CD1d-restricted help to B cells by human invariant natural killer T lymphocytes. J Exp Med 197:1051–1057

Geng Y, Laslo P, Barton K, Wang CR (2005) Transcriptional regulation of CD1D1 by Ets family transcription factors. J Immunol 175:1022–1029

Gerlini G, Hefti HP, Kleinhans M, Nickoloff BJ, Burg G, Nestle FO (2001) Cd1d is expressed on dermal dendritic cells and monocyte-derived dendritic cells. J Invest Dermatol 117:576–582

Gillessen S, Naumov YN, Niuwenhuis EE et al (2003) CD1d-restricted T cells regulate dendritic cell function and antitumor immunity in a granulocyte-macrophage colony-stimulating factor-dependent fashion. Proc Natl Acad Sci U S A 100:8874–8879

Goepel JR, Rees RC, Rogers K, Stoddard CJ, Thomas WE, Shepherd L (1991) Loss of monomorphic and polymorphic HLA antigens in metastatic breast and colon carcinoma. Br J Cancer 64:880–883

Hameg A, Apostolu I, Leite-De-Moraes M et al (2000) A subset of NKT cells that lacks the NK1.1 marker, expresses CD1d molecules, and autopresents the alpha-galactosylceramide antigen. J Immunol 165:4917–4926

Hansen DS, Siomos MA, De Koning-Ward T, Buckingham L, Crabb BS, Schofield L (2003) CD1d-restricted NKT cells contribute to malarial splenomegaly and enhance parasite-specific antibody responses. Eur J Immunol 33:2588–2598

Heller F, Fuss IJ, Nieuwenhuis EE, Blumberg RS, Strober W (2002) Oxazolone colitis, a Th2 colitis model resembling ulcerative colitis, is mediated by IL-13-producing NK-T cells. Immunity 17:629–638

Hornung M, Farkas SA, Sattler C, Schlitt HJ, Geissler EK (2006) DX5(+)NKT cells induce the death of colitis-associated cells: involvement of programmed death ligand-1. Eur J Immunol 36:1210–1221

Ichimiya S, Kikuchi K, Matsuura A (1994) Structural analysis of the rat homologue of CD1. Evidence for evolutionary conservation of the CD1D class and widespread transcription by rat cells. J Immunol 153:1112–1123

Iwamoto M et al (2003) Prognostic value of tumor-infiltrating dendritic cells expressing CD83 in human breast carcinomas. Int J Cancer 104:92–97

Jenkinson HJ, Wainwright SD, Simpson KL, Perry AC, Fotiadou P, Holmes CH (1999) Expression of CD1D mRNA transcripts in human choriocarcinoma cell lines and placentally derived trophoblast cells. Immunology 96:649–655

Kang SJ, Cresswell P (2002) Calnexin, calreticulin, and ERp57 cooperate in disulfide bond formation in human CD1d heavy chain. J Biol Chem 277:44838–44844

Kasai K, Matsuura A, Kikuchi K, Hashimoto Y, Ichimiya S (1997) Localization of rat CD1 transcripts and protein in rat tissues–an analysis of rat CD1 expression by in situ hybridization and immunohistochemistry. Clin Exp Immunol 109:317–322

Kim HS, Colgan SP, Pitman R, Hershberg RM, Blumberg RS (2000) Human CD1d associates with prolyl-4-hydroxylase during its biosynthesis. Mol Immunol 37:861–868

Kitamura H, Iwakabe A, Yahata T et al (1999) The natural killer T (NKT) cell ligand alpha-galactosylceramide demonstrates its immunopotentiating effect by inducing interleukin (IL)-12 production by dendritic cells and IL-12 receptor expression on NKT cells. J Exp Med 189:1121–1128

Knowles RW, Bodmer WF (1982) A monoclonal antibody recognizing a human thymus leukemia-like antigen associated with beta 2-microglobulin. Eur J Immunol 12:676–681

Kojo S, Adachi Y, Tsutsumi A, Sumida T (2000) Alternative splicing forms of the human CD1D gene in mononuclear cells. Biochem Biophys Res Commun 276:107–111

Lacasse J, Martin LH (1992) Detection of CD1 mRNA in Paneth cells of the mouse intestine by in situ hybridization. J Histochem Cytochem 40:1527–1534

Lerch PG, van de Rijn M, Smart JE, Knowles RW, Terhorst C (1986) Isolation and purification of the human thymocyte antigens T6 and M241. Mol Immunol 23:131–139

Lin Y, Roberts TJ, Spence PM, Brutkiewicz RR (2005) Reduction in CD1d expression on dendritic cells and macrophages by an acute virus infection. J Leukoc Biol 77:151–158

Mach N, Gillessen S, Wilson SB, Sheehan C, Mihm M, Dranoff G (2000) Differences in dendritic cells stimulated in vivo by tumors engineered to secrete granulocyte-macrophage colony-stimulating factor or Flt3-ligand. Cancer Res 60:3239–3246

Makowska A, Faizunnessa NN, Anderson P, Midtvedt T, Cardell S (1999) CD1high B cells: a population of mixed origin. Eur J Immunol 29:3285–3294

Mandal M, Chen XR, Alegre ML et al (1998) Tissue distribution, regulation and intracellular localization of murine CD1 molecules. Mol Immunol 35:525–536

Manolova V, Kistoska M, Paoletti S et al (2006) Functional CD1a is stabilized by exogenous lipids. Eur J Immunol 36:1083–1092

Marschner A, Rothenfusser S, Hornung V et al (2005) CpGODN enhance antigen-specific NKT cell activation via plasmacytoid dendritic cells. Eur J Immunol 35:2347–2357

Martino A, Volpe E, Auricchio G, Colizzi V, Baldini PM (2006) Influence of *Pertussis* toxin on CD1a isoform expression in human dendritic cells. J Clin Immunol 26:153–159

McMichael AJ (1987) Leucocyte typing III: white cell differentiation antigens. Oxford University Press Oxford, New York

McMichael AJ, Pilch JR, Galfre G, Mason DY, Fabre JW, Milstein C (1979) A human thymocyte antigen defined by a hybrid myeloma monoclonal antibody. Eur J Immunol 9:205–210

Melian A, Geng YJ, Sukhova GK, Libby P, Porcelli SA (1999) CD1 expression in human atherosclerosis. A potential mechanism for T cell activation by foam cells. Am J Pathol 155:775–786

Metelitsa LS, Weinberg KI, Emanuel PD, Seeger RC (2003) Expression of CD1d by myelomonocytic leukemias provides a target for cytotoxic NKT cells. Leukemia 17:1068–1077

Mizoguchi A, Mizoguchi E, Takedatsu H, Blumberg RS, Bhan AK (2002) Chronic intestinal inflammatory condition generates IL-10-producing regulatory B cell subset characterized by CD1d upregulation. Immunity 16:219–230

Mizoguchi A, Bhan AK (2006) A case for regulatory B cells. J Immunol 176:705–710

Morita M, Motoki K, Akimoto K et al (1995) Structure-activity relationship of alpha-galactosylceramides against B16-bearing mice. J Med Chem 38:2176–2187

Mosser DD, Duchaine J, Martin LH (1991) Biochemical and developmental characterization of the murine cluster of differentiation 1 antigen. Immunology 73:298–303

Nebozhyn M, Loboda A, Kari L et al (2006) Quantitative PCR on 5 genes reliably identifies CTCL patients with 5% to 99% circulating tumor cells with 90% accuracy. Blood 107:3189–3196

Nickoloff BJ, Wrone-Smith T, Bonish B, Porcelli SA (1999) Response of murine and normal human skin to injection of allogeneic blood-derived psoriatic immunocytes: detection of T cells expressing receptors typically present on natural killer cells, including CD94, CD158, and CD161. Arch Dermatol 135:546–552

Nickoloff BJ, Bonish B, Huang BB, Porcelli SA (2000) Characterization of a T cell line bearing natural killer receptors and capable of creating psoriasis in a SCID mouse model system. J Dermatol Sci 24:212–225

Nicol A et al (2000) Dendritic cells are targets for human invariant Valpha24+ natural killer T-cell cytotoxic activity: an important immune regulatory function. Exp Hematol 28:276–282

Nieda M, Nicol A, Koezuka Y et al (2001) TRAIL expression by activated human CD4(+)V alpha 24NKT cells induces in vitro and in vivo apoptosis of human acute myeloid leukemia cells. Blood 97:2067–2074

Nieuwenhuis EE, Matsumoto T, Exley M et al (2002) CD1d-dependent macrophage-mediated clearance of *Pseudomonas aeruginosa* from lung. Nat Med 8:588–593

Nishimura T, Kitamura H, Iwakabe A et al (2000) The interface between innate and acquired immunity: glycolipid antigen presentation by CD1d-expressing dendritic cells to NKT cells induces the differentiation of antigen-specific cytotoxic T lymphocytes. Int Immunol 12:987–994

Olive D, Dubreuil P, Mawas C (1984) Two distinct TL-like molecular subsets defined by monoclonal antibodies on the surface of human thymocytes with different expression on leukemia lines. Immunogenetics 20:253–264

Osman Y, Kawamura T, Naito T et al (2000) Activation of hepatic NKT cells and subsequent liver injury following administration of alpha-galactosylceramide. Eur J Immunol 30:1919–1928

Page G, Lebecque S, Miossec P (2002) Anatomic localization of immature and mature dendritic cells in an ectopic lymphoid organ: correlation with selective chemokine expression in rheumatoid synovium. J Immunol 168:5333–5341

Page MJ, Poritz LS, Tilberg AF, Zhang WJ, Chorney MJ, Koltun WA (2000) Cd1d-restricted cellular lysis by peripheral blood lymphocytes: relevance to the inflammatory bowel diseases. J Surg Res 92:214–221

Park SH, Roark JH, Bendelac A (1998) Tissue-specific recognition of mouse CD1 molecules. J Immunol 160:3128–3134

Pena-Cruz V, Ito S, Dascher CC, Brenner MB, Sugita M (2003) Epidermal Langerhans cells efficiently mediate CD1a-dependent presentation of microbial lipid antigens to T cells. J Invest Dermatol 121:517–521

Pietschmann P, Stockl J, Draxler S, Majdic O, Knapp W (2000) Functional and phenotypic characteristics of dendritic cells generated in human plasma supplemented medium. Scand J Immunol 51:377–383

Pillai S, Cariappa A, Moran ST (2005) Marginal zone B cells. Annu Rev Immunol 23:161–196

Plebani A, Proserpio AR, Guarneri D, Buscaglia M, Cattoretti G (1993) B and T lymphocyte subsets in fetal and cord blood: age-related modulation of CD1c expression. Biol Neonate 63:1–7

Renukaradhya GJ et al (2005) Virus-induced inhibition of CD1d1-mediated antigen presentation: reciprocal regulation by p38 and ERK. J Immunol 175:4301–4308

Roark JH, Park SH, Jayawardena J, Kavita U, Shannon M, Bendelac A (1998) CD1.1 expression by mouse antigen-presenting cells and marginal zone B cells. J Immunol 160:3121–3127

Romero JF, Eberl G, MacDonald HR, Corradin G (2001) CD1d-restricted NKT cells are dispensable for specific antibody responses and protective immunity against liver stage malaria infection in mice. Parasite Immunol 23:267–269

Ronger-Savle S et al (2005) TGFbeta inhibits CD1d expression on dendritic cells. J Invest Dermatol 124:116–118

Roura-Mir C, Catalfamo M, Cheng TY et al (2005a) CD1a and CD1c activate intrathyroidal T cells during Graves' disease and Hashimoto's thyroiditis. J Immunol 174:3773–3780

Roura-Mir C, Wang L, Cheng TY et al (2005b) *Mycobacterium tuberculosis* regulates CD1 antigen presentation pathways through TLR-2. J Immunol 175:1758–1766

Ryll R, Watanabe K, Fujiwara N et al (2001) Mycobacterial cord factor, but not sulfolipid, causes depletion of NKT cells and upregulation of CD1d1 on murine macrophages. Microbes Infect 3:611–619

Salamone MC, Rabinovich GA, Mendiguren AK, Salamone GV, Fainboim L (2001) Activation-induced expression of CD1d antigen on mature T cells. J Leukoc Biol 69:207–214

Sallinen K, Verajankorva E, Pollanen P (2000) Expression of antigens involved in the presentation of lipid antigens and induction of clonal anergy in the female reproductive tract. J Reprod Immunol 46:91–101

Sanchez DJ, Gumperz JE, Ganem D (2005) Regulation of CD1d expression and function by a herpesvirus infection. J Clin Invest 115:1369–1378

Saubermann LJ et al (2000) Activation of natural killer T cells by alpha-galactosylceramide in the presence of CD1d provides protection against colitis in mice. Gastroenterology 119:119–128

Schmieg J, Yang G, Franck RW, Van Rooijen N, Tsuji M (2005) Glycolipid presentation to natural killer T cells differs in an organ-dependent fashion. Proc Natl Acad Sci U S A 102:1127–1132

Schofield L et al (1999) CD1d-restricted immunoglobulin G formation to GPI-anchored antigens mediated by NKT cells. Science 283:225–229

Sieling PA et al (1999) CD1 expression by dendritic cells in human leprosy lesions: correlation with effective host immunity. J Immunol 162:1851–1858

Simmonds RE, Lane DA (1999) Structural and functional implications of the intron/exon organization of the human endothelial cell protein C/activated protein C receptor (EPCR) gene: comparison with the structure of CD1/major histocompatibility complex alpha1 and alpha2 domains. Blood 94:632–641

Skold M, Xiong X, Illarionov PA, Besra GS, Behar SM (2005) Interplay of cytokines and microbial signals in regulation of CD1d expression and NKT cell activation. J Immunol 175:3584–3593

Small TN et al (1987) M241 (CD1) expression on B lymphocytes. J Immunol 138:2864–2868

Smith ME, Thomas JA, Bodmer WF (1988) CD1c antigens are present in normal and neoplastic B-cells. J Pathol 156:169–177

Somnay-Wadgaonkar K et al (1999) Immunolocalization of CD1d in human intestinal epithelial cells and identification of a beta2-microglobulin-associated form. Int Immunol 11:383–392

Spada FM, Borriello F, Sugita M, Watts GF, Koezuka Y, Porcelli SA (2000) Low expression level but potent antigen presenting function of CD1d on monocyte lineage cells. Eur J Immunol 30:3468–3477

Sugita M et al (1996) Cytoplasmic tail-dependent localization of CD1b antigen-presenting molecules to MIICs. Science 273:349–352

Takahashi T, Haraguchi K, Chiba S, Yasukawa M, Shibata Y, Hirai H (2003) Valpha24+ natural killer T-cell responses against T-acute lymphoblastic leukaemia cells: implications for immunotherapy. Br J Haematol 122:231–239

Teitell M et al (1997) Nonclassical behavior of the mouse CD1 class I-like molecule. J Immunol 158:2143–2149

Trobonjaca Z, Leithauser F, Moller P, Bluethmann H et al (2001a) MHC-II-independent CD4+ T cells induce colitis in immunodeficient RAG$^{-/-}$ hosts. J Immunol 166:3804–3812

Trobonjaca Z, Leithauser F, Moller P, Schirmbeck R, Reimann J (2001b) Activating immunity in the liver. I. Liver dendritic cells (but not hepatocytes) are potent activators of IFN-gamma release by liver NKT cells. J Immunol 167:1413–1422

Tsuneyama K, Yasoshima M, Harada K, Hiramatsu K, Gershwin ME, Nakanuma Y (1998) Increased CD1d expression on small bile duct epithelium and epithelioid granuloma in livers in primary biliary cirrhosis. Hepatology 28:620–623

Ulanova M, Tarkowski A, Porcelli SA, Hanson LA (2000a) Antigen-specific regulation of CD1 expression in humans. J Clin Immunol 20:203–211

Ulanova M, Torebring M, Porcelli SA et al (2000b) Expression of CD1d in the duodenum of patients with cow's milk hypersensitivity. Scand J Immunol 52:609–617

Van de Rijn M, Lerch PG, Knowles RW, Terhorst C (1983) The thymic differentiation markers T6 and M241 are two unusual MHC class I antigens. J Immunol 131:851–855

Van de Wal Y et al (2003) Delineation of a CD1d-restricted antigen presentation pathway associated with human and mouse intestinal epithelial cells. Gastroenterology 124:1420–1431

Van der Wel NN et al (2003) CD1 and major histocompatibility complex II molecules follow a different course during dendritic cell maturation. Mol Biol Cell 14:3378–3388

Wei B et al (2005) Mesenteric B cells centrally inhibit CD4+ T cell colitis through interaction with regulatory T cell subsets. Proc Natl Acad Sci U S A 102:2010–2015

Woolfson A, Milstein C (1994) Alternative splicing generates secretory isoforms of human CD1. Proc Natl Acad Sci U S A 91:6683–6687

Wu DY, Segal NH, Sidobre S, Kronenberg M, Chapman PB (2003) Cross-presentation of disialoganglioside GD3 to natural killer T cells. J Exp Med 198:173–181

Xia CQ, Kao KJ (2002) Heparin induces differentiation of CD1a+ dendritic cells from monocytes: phenotypic and functional characterization. J Immunol 168:1131–1138

Yamazaki K, Ohsawa Y, Yoshie H (2001) Elevated proportion of natural killer T cells in periodontitis lesions: a common feature of chronic inflammatory diseases. Am J Pathol 158:1391–1398

Yang OO et al (2000) CD1d on myeloid dendritic cells stimulates cytokine secretion from and cytolytic activity of V alpha 24 J alpha QT cells: a feedback mechanism for immune regulation. J Immunol 165:3756–3762

Ylinen L et al (2000) The role of lipid antigen presentation, cytokine balance, and major histocompatibility complex in a novel murine model of adoptive transfer of insulitis. Pancreas 20:197–205

Yuan W, Dasgupta A, Cresswell P (2006) Herpes simplex virus evades natural killer T cell recognition by suppressing CD1d recycling. Nat Immunol 7:835–842

Yue SC, Shaulov A, Wang R, Balk SP, Exley MA (2005) CD1d ligation on human monocytes directly signals rapid NF-kappaB activation and production of bioactive IL-12. Proc Natl Acad Sci U S A 102:11811–11816

Zeng Z, Castano AR, Segelke BW, Stura EA, Peterson PA, Wilson IA (1997) Crystal structure of mouse CD1: an MHC-like fold with a large hydrophobic binding groove. Science 277:339–345

Zheng Z, Venkatapathy S, Rao G, Harrington CA (2002) Expression profiling of B cell chronic lymphocytic leukemia suggests deficient CD1-mediated immunity, polarized cytokine response, altered adhesion and increased intracellular protein transport and processing of leukemic cells. Leukemia 16:2429–2437

Zhou D, Cantu C 3rd, Sagiv Y, Schrantz N, Kulkarni AB, Qi X, Mahuran DJ, Morales CR, Grabowski GA, Benlagha K, Savage P, Bendelac A, Teyton L (2004) Editing of CD1d-bound lipid antigens by endosomal lipid transfer proteins. Science 303:523–527

CTMI (2007) 314:143–164

Pathways of CD1 and Lipid Antigen Delivery, Trafficking, Processing, Loading, and Presentation

M. Sugita[1] (✉) · D. C. Barral[2] · M. B. Brenner[2]

[1]Division of Cell Regulation, Institute for Virus Research, Kyoto University, Kyoto, Japan
msugita@virus.kyoto-u.ac.jp

[2]Division of Rheumatology, Immunology and Allergy, Brigham and Women's Hospital, Harvard Medical School, Boston, MA, USA

Abstract Specific T cell responses to a variety of self and microbial lipids depend on proper assembly and intracellular trafficking of CD1 molecules that intersect with and load processed lipid antigens. These pathways involve unique membrane trafficking and chaperones that are distinct from those utilized for major histocompatibility complex (MHC)-mediated presentation of peptide antigens, and thus define unique lipid antigen presentation pathways. Furthermore, recent studies have identified components of lipid metabolism that participate in lipid delivery, uptake, processing and loading onto CD1 molecules. Defects in these pathways result in impaired T cell development and function, underscoring their critical role in the lipid-specific T cell immune responses.

1
Introduction

Studies on antigen presentation by CD1 have led to new chapters in the textbooks of immunology and microbiology and hold great promise for biotechnology and medicine. As outlined in other articles of this volume of *Current Topics*, the fact that the antigens presented are self and foreign lipids anticipates that many specialized and unique features participate in antigen presentation by CD1. In this chapter, we describe the pathways of CD1-based lipid antigen presentation. We will outline the intracellular trafficking of the CD1a, CD1b, CD1c, and CD1d molecules from their assembly in the endoplasmic reticulum (ER), along a route that delivers them to the plasma membrane followed by their internalization and sorting into specific endosomes, where they load or exchange specific lipid antigens. These CD1 pathways intersect with lipid trafficking pathways involving the delivery of exogenous lipid antigens to antigen-presenting cells (APCs) and the localization of self and foreign lipid antigens in intracellular compartments of APCs. These processes involve cellular machinery shared with lipid metabolism including the apolipoproteins, lipoprotein receptors, saposins, and other lipid transfer proteins These lipid antigen co-factors share certain functions with hallmark examples from studies of protein antigen presentation by MHC class I and class II, but generally differ in their biophysical properties, which allow binding to hydrophobic lipids. Lipid antigens may be loaded in CD1 within endosomes after uptake from exogenous sources, from microbes in phagosomes, from self lipids in the ER and from both self and foreign lipids in the late endosomes and lysosomes where the necessary conditions for processing and loading onto CD1 can be accomplished.

2
CD1 Assembly in the Endoplasmic Reticulum

2.1
Association with β2-Microglobulin and Chaperones

Strictly regulated assembly processes in the ER are monitored by quality control mechanisms that are essential for ensuring the proper function of antigen-presenting molecules. In the case of MHC class I, newly synthesized heavy chains first bind calnexin in the ER via specific interactions between the monoglucosylated N-linked glycan of MHC class I heavy chains and the lectin domain of calnexin (Diedrich et al. 2001; Sugita and Brenner 1994). Subsequently, a homologous ER-retained soluble lectin domain-containing chaperone, calreticulin, replaces calnexin when assembly with β2-microglobulin (β2m) occurs (Sadasivan et al. 1996). These protein-folding chaperones also recruit the thiol oxidoreductase ERp57 to promote disulfide bond formation in the associated MHC class I heavy chains (Hughes and Cresswell 1998; Morrice and Powis 1998). The calreticulin-bound, β2m-associated class I heavy chains are then recruited to become part of a multisubunit peptide loading complex that also contains the transporter associated with antigen processing (TAP) and tapasin (Ortmann et al. 1994; Sadasivan et al. 1996). Following peptide binding, the fully assembled trimolecular complex composed of class I heavy chains, β2m, and peptide finally exits the ER and reaches the plasma membrane where T cell recognition occurs.

CD1 heavy chains share structural similarities with MHC class I in terms of their domain organization, as both are a heavy chain with α1, α2, and α3 extracellular domains and associate with β2m. CD1 molecules utilize some of the same chaperones as do MHC class I molecules, but CD1 folding and assembly reveal both subtle and dramatic differences compared to MHC class I. Both calnexin and calreticulin preferentially bind β2m-free, but not β2m-bound, CD1d heavy chains, and disulfide bond formation is mediated by the associated ERp57 (Kang and Cresswell 2002). The fully oxidized CD1d heavy chains dissociate from these chaperones, and the majority of CD1d heavy chains then bind β2m before exiting the ER. Notably, a small but significant fraction of CD1d heavy chains is also able to exit the ER without association with β2m and reach the plasma membrane (Balk et al. 1994; Kim et al. 1999). These β2m-free CD1d heavy chains could potentially mediate antigen presentation (Amano et al. 1998), and thus, association with β2m is not an absolute requirement for CD1d transport and function. In contrast, CD1b heavy chains are retained in the ER in β2m-deficient cells (Huttinger et al. 1999; Sugita et al. 1997), suggesting that CD1 isoforms may differ in their strict requirement for β2m association before exiting the ER.

2.2
Binding of Endogenous Phospholipids in the ER

Peptide loading onto MHC class I in the ER is an essential step for its transport and function, as evidenced by TAP-deficient cells in which the surface expression and function of MHC class I are severely impaired (York and Rock 1996). Several lines of evidence suggest that CD1 molecules acquire self-lipid ligands in the ER, which influences their surface expression and antigen presentation function. Phosphatidylinositol-containing compounds including glycosyl-phosphatidylinositol (GPI) were eluted from CD1d molecules expressed in TAP-deficient cells (Joyce et al. 1998). In the same study, a truncated soluble form of CD1d that follows a secretory route without intersecting the endocytic pathway has also been shown to associate with GPI, indicating that GPI binding can occur in the secretory pathway. A subsequent study detected association of phosphatidylinositol (PI) with a soluble form of CD1d containing the KDEL ER retention signal (De Silva et al. 2002). Because GPI and PI are abundantly expressed in the ER, these data suggest that assembly of CD1d with cellular phospholipids occurs in the ER (Park et al. 2004).

2.3
Role for Microsomal Triglyceride Transfer Protein

One mechanism of cellular lipid loading onto CD1d in the ER has recently been identified. Microsomal triglyceride transfer protein (MTP) is a lipid transfer protein that is essential for lipidation of apolipoprotein B (ApoB), and thus is required for assembly of ApoB-containing very-low-density lipoproteins (VLDL) and chylomicrons by the liver and by the intestine, respectively (Gordon and Jamil 2000). Transfer of several lipid species, including PI and triglyceride, is known to be mediated by MTP (Jamil et al. 1995), and both hepatocytes and intestinal epithelial cells express endogenous CD1d proteins, suggesting the possibility that MTP may also be involved in cellular lipid loading onto CD1d in the ER (Fig. 1). Indeed, physical association of CD1d with MTP has been detected in hepatocytes, and in the absence of MTP, CD1d cell-surface expression and antigen presentation function are significantly reduced, while CD1d expression in the ER is increased (Brozovic et al. 2004). Further, MTP expression is also detected in CD1d-expressing professional APCs, such as B cells, macrophages, and dendritic cells, and their ability to activate NKT cells is impaired by treatment with a specific MTP inhibitor (Dougan et al. 2005). These data suggest a critical role for MTP in proper assembly and antigen presentation function of CD1d. Despite clear evidence that CD1 molecules bind lipids in the ER, it is not yet clear if bound lipids function as chaperones that dictate folding of the CD1d heavy chain and its association with β2m.

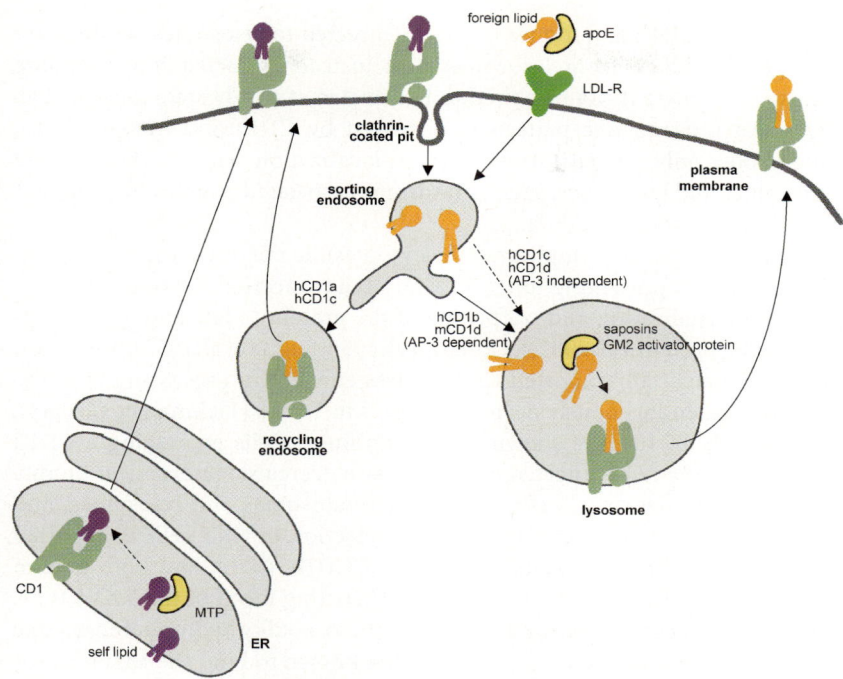

Fig. 1 Components of the lipid metabolism are utilized for CD1 lipid antigen-presentation pathways. CD1 molecules are assembled and loaded with self lipids in the ER. MTP plays a critical role in CD1d function and might be involved directly in the loading of self lipids onto CD1d. After trafficking to the plasma membrane via the secretory pathway, CD1 molecules are internalized in clathrin-coated pits and follow different routes from the early/sorting endosome. ApoE plays an important role in the uptake of exogenous lipids into the endocytic pathway, via the LDL-R. Saposins/GM2 activator protein can assist CD1 lipid loading in late endocytic compartments. After loading occurs in these compartments, CD1 molecules can traffic back to the plasma membrane and present antigens to T cells

3
CD1 Trafficking in the Endocytic Pathway

3.1
Internalization from the Plasma Membrane

Following assembly in the ER, the majority of CD1 molecules follow a secretory route and traffic directly to the plasma membrane (Fig. 1). The CD1 molecules are then internalized and enter the endocytic pathway, where each CD1 isoform penetrates the endosomal network to a varying extent.

For instance, CD1b and mouse CD1d are directed to lysosomes, while CD1a is largely excluded from lysosomes and instead is sorted into recycling endosomes, where it can be abundantly detected at steady state (Sugita et al. 1999). An intermediate pattern is displayed by CD1c and human CD1d, which show only partial intracellular co-localization with markers of late endosomes and lysosomes, such as lysosome associated membrane protein-1 (LAMP-1) (Sugita et al. 2002).

Several studies have implicated the cytoplasmic tail of CD1 in its trafficking and antigen-presenting function. CD1b tail truncation has been shown to abolish internalization and trafficking of the protein to late endocytic compartments (Briken et al. 2002; Jackman et al. 1998; Sugita et al. 1996). Moreover, the cytoplasmic tail-truncated CD1b is less efficient in presenting both exogenous and endogenously derived antigens to T cells (Jackman et al. 1998). Studies with CD1d have shown similar findings. Cells expressing a CD1d heavy chain as a tail-truncated mutant show a decreased internalization rate of the protein, deficient trafficking to late endosomes and lysosomes, and the presentation of antigens and positive selection of NKT cells is impaired (Chiu et al. 2002). The cytoplasmic tails of CD1b, CD1c, and both human and murine CD1d contain a tyrosine-based sorting motif of the YXXφ type, where Y is a tyrosine, X is any amino acid, and φ a bulky hydrophobic residue (Table 1). Tyrosine-based sorting motifs are known to bind the adaptor protein complex-2 (AP-2) at the plasma membrane, which allows sorting of CD1 and other transmembrane cargo proteins into clathrin-coated pits. By surface plasmon resonance, CD1b and CD1c tail peptides have been shown to bind AP-2 with similar affinities (Briken et al. 2002). Indeed, both CD1b and CD1c have been detected in clathrin-coated pits and clathrin-coated vesicles by immunogold-labeled electron microscopy (immuno-EM) (Sugita et al. 1996, 2000). Using a dominant-negative mutant of dynamin, a molecule involved in clathrin-mediated endocytosis, the internalization of CD1b has been shown to be dynamin-dependent (Briken et al. 2002).

In contrast to other CD1 isoforms, CD1a does not contain any apparent sorting motifs in its cytoplasmic tail (Table 1). Nevertheless, CD1a was found in clathrin-coated pits and clathrin-coated vesicles in in vitro-derived den-

Table 1 Cytoplasmic domains of different CD1 isoforms (tyrosine-based motifs are in bold)

CD1a	RKRCFC
CD1b	RRR**SYQ**NIP
CD1c	KKHC**SYQ**DIL
CD1d	KRQT**SYQ**GVL

dritic cells (DCs) and freshly isolated Langerhans cells, a type of dendritic cells resident in the epidermis (Salamero et al. 2001; Sugita et al. 1999). However, the mechanism of CD1a internalization is not known.

3.2
Trafficking to Early Recycling Endosomes

After internalization, both CD1a and CD1c co-localize with a dominant-negative form of the small GTPase ARF6 (ARF6 T27N) in the early recycling compartment (ERC) (Sugita et al. 1999, 2000) (Fig. 1). In contrast, CD1b is almost absent from this compartment (Sugita et al. 1999). Moreover, CD1a has been shown to co-localize prominently with Rab11, a marker for the ERC, and to recycle back to the plasma membrane from an internal pool, in freshly isolated Langerhans cells (Salamero et al. 2001).

3.3
Trafficking to Late Endosomes and Lysosomes

A critical role for the AP-3 adaptor protein complex in the lysosomal trafficking of human CD1b and murine CD1d has been established in vitro and in vivo. The AP-3 complex, composed of δ, $\beta 3$, $\mu 3$, and $\sigma 3$ subunits, specifically binds the cytosolic tyrosine-based motifs in integral membrane proteins, such as LAMP-1 and LAMP-3 (CD63), which localize primarily to late endosomes and lysosomes (Dell'Angelica et al. 1999). It was proposed previously that AP-3 is expressed both at the trans-Golgi network (TGN) and at the sorting endosomes of the early endocytic system, to mediate delivery of cargo proteins to late endosomes and lysosomes, but recent immuno-EM analysis using an antibody specific for the AP-3 δ subunit has identified AP-3-concentrated membrane buds originating from the tubular sorting endosomes as the primary site for its expression (Bonifacino 2004; Peden et al. 2004). These AP-3 budding profiles also contain LAMP-1 and LAMP-2, implicating AP-3 in the sorting of specific lysosomal proteins at these tubular sorting endosomes.

   A yeast two-hybrid analysis has shown that, among human CD1 isoforms, only the cytoplasmic tyrosine-based motif of CD1b is capable of binding AP-3 (Sugita et al. 2002). This finding leads to the speculation that, following internalization from the plasma membrane, CD1b deviates from the default recycling pathway by virtue of specific interaction with AP-3 and traffics deeply into late endosomes and lysosomes. Indeed, in AP-3-deficient cells derived from patients with Hermansky-Pudlak syndrome type 2 (HPS-2), CD1b is scarcely expressed in LAMP-1$^+$ late endosomes and lysosomes and, instead, accumulates in the transferrin receptor-containing early recycling pathway and on the plasma membrane. Failure of CD1b to traffic to acidic late endosomes and lysosomes in these cells results in profound defects in antigen presentation, underscoring a key role for AP-3 in supporting CD1b function (Sugita et al. 2002). Both CD1b and MHC class II sample antigens in late endosomes and lysosomes, but, unlike CD1b, MHC class II traffics normally and functions efficiently in AP-3-deficient cells, owing to MHC class II association with invariant chain, as discussed below (Caplan et al. 2000; Sevilla et al. 2001). Of note, patients with HPS-2 often suffer from recurrent bacterial infections. The impaired function of CD1b in these patients may contribute to their immunodeficiency.

Although human CD1c also contains a similar cytoplasmic tyrosine-based motif, it failed to bind AP-3 in yeast two-hybrid assays (Sugita et al. 2002). CD1c appears to survey antigens more broadly in the endocytic system, which includes both the early recycling compartment (ERC) and lysosomes, suggesting that an AP-3 independent pathway for CD1 trafficking to lysosomes also exists (Sugita et al. 2000). In dendritic cell lysosomes with a typical appearance of multilamellar structure, whereas CD1b is preferentially localized to the most external limiting membrane, CD1c is expressed more abundantly in the inner membranes (van der Wel et al. 2003). Thus, some lipids that are localized selectively to the inner membranes of lysosomes (Kobayashi et al. 1998b), may be sampled preferentially by CD1c, rather than CD1b.

Like human CD1b, murine CD1d molecules are prominently localized in lysosomes, and their lysosomal trafficking is mediated by at least two separate mechanisms, namely interaction of their cytoplasmic tyrosine-based motif with AP-3 and their assembly with the MHC class II-associated invariant chain (Ii). The importance of AP-3 in murine CD1d trafficking and function has been fully appreciated, using mice with AP-3 dysfunction (Cernadas et al. 2003; Chui et al. 2002; Elewaut et al. 2003). In these mice, redistribution of CD1d from lysosomes to the cell surface is observed, and development of the $V\alpha14^+$ invariant T cell receptor (TCR) NKT cells is impaired. These mice exhibit normal MHC class II expression and function; and thus, the differential binding affinity to AP-3 sharply dissects pathways for peptide and lipid antigen presentation.

In the ER, at least a fraction of murine CD1d heavy chains can associate with the MHC class II–Ii complex and traffic to lysosomes (Kang and Cresswell 2002). The impact of this interaction on CD1d trafficking is observed in cells expressing a CD1d mutant molecule that lacks the cytoplasmic tail and thus is unable to bind adaptor protein complexes (Jayawardena-Wolf et al. 2001). While this tail-deleted form of CD1d fails to gain access to lysosomes in cells that lack Ii, CD1ds lysosomal localization is readily detected when Ii is available. Further, deficiencies in the cathepsins responsible for Ii processing in late endosomes and lysosomes result in impaired development of the invariant $V\alpha14^+$ NKT cells, suggesting a role for Ii in CD1d function (Honey et al. 2002; Riese et al. 2001). On the other hand, mice bearing a germ line deletion of the cytoplasmic tail of CD1d, in which the expressed CD1d protein interacts with Ii, but not with AP-3, show a much more striking impairment of the invariant $V\alpha14^+$ NKT cell development, indicating that the Ii-dependent delivery of CD1d to lysosomes alone is not sufficient for its proper function (Chiu et al. 2002). It is still possible that the relative importance of AP-3 and Ii in CD1d function may differ in various cell types.

3.4
Impact of Dendritic Cell Maturation in CD1 Trafficking

In immature DCs, MHC class II can be found in late endosomal and lysosomal compartments, referred to as the MHC class II compartments (MIIC), where it co-localizes with specific markers, such as LAMP-3 and LAMP-1 (Nijman et al. 1995). DC maturation stimuli, such as tumor necrosis factor-α (TNF-α) and lipopolysaccharide (LPS) both downregulate macropinocytosis in DCs and trigger transport of MHC class II molecules from the MIICs to the plasma membrane, leading to an increase in their surface levels (Cella et al. 1997; Pierre et al. 1997; Sallusto et al. 1995). In contrast, DCs matured by treatment with TNF-α or LPS do not show significant changes in surface expression of CD1b, CD1c, and CD1d, and show a small decrease in surface CD1a (Cao et al. 2002; van der Wel et al. 2003). Moreover, the intracellular pool of CD1b and CD1c is maintained, while CD1a shows a decrease in the surface to intracellular ratio, consistent with its decrease in surface expression (Cao et al. 2002; van der Wel et al. 2003). When the internalization of CD1b was analyzed, no changes in uptake after DC maturation could be detected, similar to the transferrin receptor (van der Wel et al. 2003). This indicates that, contrary to MHC class II, CD1b as well as the transferrin receptor continue to be internalized and recycled in mature DCs, and therefore not all molecules decrease their internalization rate in mature DCs. Interestingly, whereas CD1b is mainly localized to the limiting membrane of MIICs, MHC class II was detected in the internal membranes (van der Wel et al. 2003). Upon LPS-induced maturation, CD1b segregates from MHC class II, and the MIICs undergo major structural changes, resulting in a new compartment called the mature DC lysosome or MDL, which contains CD1b but virtually no MHC class II (van der Wel et al. 2003). Consistent with these trafficking differences in MHC class II and CD1 between immature and mature DCs, the presentation of a CD1b-restricted antigen, glucose monomycolate (GMM), was equally effective in both immature and mature DCs, contrary to MHC class II-restricted protein antigen presentation, which is markedly enhanced by DC maturation (Cao et al. 2002).

4
Mechanisms for Lipid Uptake by Antigen-Presenting Cells

Macropinocytosis is used extensively in the uptake of fluid phase antigens by DCs, a process that works efficiently for soluble antigens. However, as many lipids specifically bind to cell-surface receptors, and new studies have shown that a variety of other mechanisms might play a role in their uptake by APCs. These mechanisms might include:

1. Cell-surface receptors that bind lipid particles such as the low-density lipoprotein receptor (LDL-R), the LDL-R-like protein (LRP), and scavenger receptors (SR, CD34, SR-A, SR-B)

2. Cell-surface receptors that bind glycans such as C-type lectins

3. Mechanisms that internalize plasma membrane itself such as rafts, caveolae, and other membranes carried in endocytic processes

4.1
Apolipoproteins and Lipoprotein Receptors

One example of high relevance to the delivery of exogenous lipid antigens to APCs is that of apolipoproteins. A majority of the lipids in the circulation are transported as soluble complexes bound to lipoproteins (Willnow et al. 1999). These proteins help to organize lipids for transport into lipoprotein particles that contain varying amounts of dietary lipids, resulting in different sedimentation densities and a nomenclature based on density: very-low-density lipoprotein (VLDL), low-density lipoprotein (LDL), and high-density lipoprotein (HDL). The core of these particles is largely composed of triglycerides and cholesteryl esters as well as some sphingolipids and fat-soluble vitamins, all of which are normally thought of as lipids for metabolic needs. It has recently been shown, however, that exogenous lipid antigens destined to be presented by CD1 molecules are also captured in these particles (van den Elzen et al. 2005). Apolipoprotein E (ApoE), derived either from human serum or recombinant sources, markedly enhanced lipid uptake by human monocyte-derived DCs. When a model antigen, galactose ($\alpha1\rightarrow2$)galactosylceramide, (αGalGalCer) was added to serum, it was distributed in the VLDL fraction and bound ApoE. When αGalGalCer or microbial antigens such as GMM or mannosyl phosphomycoketides (MPM) were used to pulse DCs, the efficiency of presentation in the presence of ApoE was many times greater than in its absence (van den Elzen et al. 2005). Moreover, lipid antigens of microbial or synthetic origin were taken up within 2 min, a short time frame consistent with receptor-mediated uptake, and these antigens were delivered specifically into the endosomal compartments in an ApoE-associated form (Fig. 1). ApoE can not only deliver lipids via the circulation from distant sources in the host, but importantly also can be secreted and recaptured locally by DCs or macrophages as a means of sampling their tissue milieu for lipid antigens, much as macropinocytosis is used to sample the local milieu for soluble protein antigens. It seems likely that other lipoproteins that participate in general lipid metabolism may also be co-opted for lipid antigen delivery.

4.2
Scavenger Receptors

Several cell-surface receptors play major roles in normal lipid metabolism and may potentially also play roles in CD1 lipid antigen uptake. In the ApoE-mediated lipid antigen delivery system noted above, uptake by the APC was predominantely mediated by the LDL-R (van den Elzen et al. 2005). LRP, which is structurally similar to the LDL-R, can also bind ApoE and saposins (see below) and is implicated in lipoprotein metabolism (Herz and Strickland 2001). LRP and other receptors, initially identified based upon their ability to bind lipoproteins, are now increasingly appreciated to play broader roles in biology. Scavenger receptors were named to distinguish their ability to take up modified forms of LDL (compared to the classical LDL-R) (Brown and Goldstein 1983). It is now recognized that a number of structurally distinct scavenger receptors interact with a range of physiologically relevant ligands (Greaves and Gordon 2005). Scavenger receptors expressed on macrophages and myeloid cells include the class B scavenger receptor CD36, which binds modified LDL, oxidized choline glycerophospholipids, and long chain fatty acids. This receptor is also well known for its role in uptake of apoptotic cells. The class B scavenger receptor (SR-B1) binds native HDL as well as oxidized LDL, acetyl-LDL, ionic phospholipids, and apoptotic cells. The class A scavenger receptors are also implicated in the uptake of oxidized LDL, acetyl-LDL, the lipid-A moiety of LPS, and other ligands (Greaves and Gordon 2005). These and other scavenger receptors such as CD68 and LOX-1 have not yet been implicated in CD1-based antigen uptake, but they are attractive candidates. Overall, it seems likely that many of the molecules involved in the uptake of lipids for metabolic and housekeeping needs may be utilized by specific antigens for uptake into CD1-bearing APCs.

4.3
Lectins

Several glycan-binding receptors may mediate the uptake of glycolipids. Lipoarabinomannan (LAM), a mannose-containing glycolipid, can be taken up into APCs by the macrophage mannose receptor (MMR), a C-type lectin expressed on macrophages and many DCs (Prigozy et al. 1997). Following binding to the MMR, the lipid antigens are delivered into the endocytic system of the APCs where CD1 molecules are distributed. Langerin, a type II membrane-associated C-type lectin expressed on CD1a$^+$ epidermal Langerhans cells, is another example that participates in CD1 antigen presentation. Blockade of the receptor-ligand interaction with specific antibodies resulted in failure in CD1a, but not CD1b, antigen presentation, emphasizing its role in uptake of CD1a-presented glycolipid antigens (Hunger et al. 2004). Following internalization, langerin is transported to specific early endocytic compartments, called Birbeck granules, where CD1a is also abundantly expressed, suggesting that CD1a antigen loading may occur in these intracellular compartments (Sugita et al. 1999). Other C-type lectins, such as DC-SIGN, DEC205, DCIR, BDCA-2, and others may serve similar functions on DCs if their specificity allows binding to amphipathic lipids (Figdor et al. 2002). Recently, a lectin specific for beta-galactosides, galectin-3, was implicated in the uptake of mycolic acids derived from mycobacteria (Barboni et al. 2005). Lipids that can bind the LPS binding protein (LBP) also might be taken up by the APC for presentation by CD1.

4.4
Receptor-Independent Pathways

Besides surface receptors, the uptake of lipids into the endocytic system of APCs may also occur based on their incorporation into the plasma membrane that is then taken up as part of general endocytic processes (Conner and Schmid 2003). Thus, phagocytosis, macropinocytosis, pinocytosis that is clathrin-mediated or -independent, all result in uptake of the plasma membrane that may have incorporated lipid antigens. The cholesterol- and sphingolipid-rich microdomains (rafts) of the plasma membrane are known to differentially incorporate proteins and may also differentially incorporate lipid antigens based on the resident lipid composition of the microdomain (Ikonen 2001). Both rafts and caveolae (caveolin-containing subdomains of glycolipid rafts) are internalized (Nabi and Le 2003), providing further means of delivering lipid antigens incorporated in these microdomains to CD1-loading endosomal compartments.

The internalization of lipids at the plasma membrane can also occur by a class of proteins that facilitate the transfer of lipids from one leaflet of the membrane bilayer to the other. The ABC transporters are proteins that are members of the family of pumps also involved in transporting drugs, bile salts, and other amphipathic molecules. They can be involved in flipping lipids across the bilayer (Raggers et al. 2000). Other proteins have been found that also mediate uptake of long chain fatty acids (FAT and FATP) (Ehehalt et al. 2006; Schaffer and Lodish 1994). It is not known yet if any of these classes of transport or translocation proteins play a role in CD1-mediated antigen presentation.

4.5
Apoptotic Vesicles

Another important mechanism for lipid-antigen uptake involves uptake of apoptotic vesicles from infected cells. Many cell types infected with microbes may not express CD1 proteins. If the infectious agent eventually induces apoptosis of the infected cells, the resultant apoptotic bodies may be taken up by uninfected APCs that express CD1 for presentation to T cells (Schaible et al. 2003).

5
Intracellular Trafficking of Lipid Antigens

5.1
Role of Membrane Microdomains

While much has been learned about the intracellular trafficking of proteins with specific sorting motifs, much less is known about cellular mechanisms that control intracellular lipid trafficking. The early concept that membranes are a homogeneous, passive substrate has changed, and it is now known that membranes show regulated changes in their density within a single membrane and differing membrane lipid compositions within individual organelles. As lipids do not display recognized targeting motifs, it seems likely that their chemical and physical properties play a key role in controlling their distribution (Kobayashi et al. 1998a; Mukherjee and Maxfield 2000). Major lipids of cellular membranes include glycerophospholipids, which are composed of a glycerol backbone with two hydrocarbon tails and a polar headgroup, and sphingolipids, which contain a sphingosine base and one N-linked acyl chain. Interestingly, many of the bacterial and self-lipid antigens presented by CD1 fall into one of these two lipid groups. In addition, lipid-modified proteins (GPI-anchored), acylated proteins, and isoprene-linked proteins also insert into membranes and bear structural features similar to several defined CD1-presented lipid antigens. Thus, membrane microdomains defined by the differential lipid composition may potentially contribute to sorting lipid antigens (Nabi and Le 2003).

5.2
Differential Endocytic Trafficking Based on Tail Structure

Once internalized, lipids may sort based on their physical properties. In some cases, localization in cholesterol or sphingolipid-rich microdomains as occurs in the plasma membrane may be retained as membranes rich in these components in the ERC. Further, some lipids appear to sort based on their physical characteristics even if defined microdomains are not apparent. For example, lipid analogs that differ only in the length and saturation of their tails were shown to sort distinctly (Mukherjee et al. 1999). The authors found that one analog with long, fully saturated lipid tails moved from sorting endosomes into late endosomes and lysosomes, while the counterpart molecule having the same polar headgroup but with shorter and partially unsaturated tails, instead moved rapidly from sorting endosomes to the ERC. Indeed, efficient sorting of lipids with long, but not short, alkyl chains to lysosomes has been observed for glucose monomycolate, a CD1b-presented microbial antigen (Moody et al 2002). Also, in contrast to the cholesterol and sphingolipid-rich membranes of the ERC, late endosomal and lysosomal compartments are enriched in neutral lipids such as triglycerides and cholesterol esters and certain phospholipids (Kobayashi et al. 1998a). Interestingly, this separation in lipid trafficking between the ERC and late endosomes and lysosomes is paralleled by the differential trafficking of human CD1a (ERC) and human CD1b or mouse CD1d (late endosomes and lysosomes) (Sugita et al. 1999). While these CD1 isoforms distribute in highly localized fashion, CD1c is distributed more promiscuously throughout the endocytic system. Thus, the differential trafficking would enable CD1 molecules to survey a range of endosomal compartments to which relevant CD1-presented lipid antigens traffic. To the extent that each of these subcellular compartments differ in their lipid composition, this could be a means to more broadly acquire and present diverse lipids or a means to direct CD1 to the compartment in which key self or foreign antigens localize.

6
Antigen Processing and Loading onto CD1

6.1
Lysosomal Glycosidases and CD1e

Pathways involved in intracellular cleavage of precursors to generate antigens that bind to CD1 proteins have not been comprehensively established, but a model system in which a CD1d-presented glycosphingolipid is processed and recognized by the invariant $V\alpha14^+$ NKT cells has been studied as a molecular model. Interaction of exogenous αGalCer with CD1d can take place either in lysosomes, after endocytosis, or on the plasma membrane, resulting in activation of the invariant $V\alpha14^+$ NKT cells (Prigozy et al. 2001). By contrast, the related disaccharide glycosphingolipid αGalGalCer requires endocytosis and subsequent endosomal processing into αGalCer for successful stimulation of NKT cells (Prigozy et al. 2001). This glycolipid antigen processing step is mediated specifically by a lysosomal enzyme, α-galactosidase A, that functions only at low pH. Thus, unlike αGalCer, presentation of αGalGalCer to NKT cells depends on vesicular acidification as well as the cytoplasmic tail-mediated delivery of CD1d to lysosomes (Prigozy et al. 2001).

An apparently parallel model of lipid antigen processing has also been proposed for human CD1b-dependent presentation of a mycobacterial hexamannosylated phosphatidyl-*myo*-inositols (PIM_6) (de la Salle et al. 2005). For presentation to specific CD1b-restricted T cells, PIM_6 containing six α-D-Man$p$ units must be processed in the endocytic pathway into PIM_2 containing only two α-D-Man$p$ units, which is catalyzed by the lysosomal enzyme α-mannosidase. Notably, processing of PIM_6 into PIM_2 in lysosomes requires the function of a special member of the CD1 family, CD1e (de la Salle et al. 2005). Unlike other human CD1 molecules, CD1e is not expressed at detectable levels on the plasma membrane. Instead, the majority of the integral membrane CD1e proteins accumulate in the TGN of immature dendritic cells, with a minor fraction expressed in late endosomes and lysosomes (Angenieux et al. 2005). After dendritic cell maturation, CD1e redistributes primarily to late endosomes and lysosomes, where it is cleaved to generate a soluble form (Angenieux et al. 2000). It has been proposed that the soluble CD1e captures PIM_6, a process facilitated at low pH, and assists the α-mannosidase-mediated digestion of PIM_6 to PIM_2 (de la Salle et al. 2005). In contrast, the endosomal processing of αGalGalCer described above apparently does not depend on the function of CD1e because it occurs in mice, which along with certain other mammals, lack a human CD1e ortholog. Further studies are needed to establish whether CD1e function is required for the presentation of a variety of glycolipid antigens and whether CD1e may be critical for the subsequent lipid loading step onto CD1.

6.2
Saposins and the GM2 Activator Protein

Both endogenous lipids and endocytosed exogenous lipids with alkyl chains can be inserted into the lipid bilayers of endocytic vesicles, raising the question of how they might be transferred to the solvent exposed antigen-binding groove of CD1 molecules. Recently, sphingolipid activator proteins (SAPs), such as saposins and the GM2 activator protein, have been shown to play such a role (Kang and Cresswell 2004; Winau et al. 2004; Zhou et al. 2004). Saposins A, B, C, and D are enzymatically inactive glycoproteins generated by endosomal proteolytic cleavage of the precursor prosaposin, while the GM2 activator protein is encoded on a separate gene. These products localize to late endosomes and lysosomes to assist glycosphingolipid degradation (Kolter and Sandhoff 2005). The four saposins share lipid-binding and membrane-perturbing properties, but their mode of action, as well as their binding specificity, differ significantly. For example, saposin C is involved in glucosylceramide-β-glucosidase-mediated degradation of glucosylceramide by directly interacting with the enzyme and activating it in an allosteric manner. By contrast, saposin B interacts with a variety of sphingolipids and facilitates their digestion by specific lysosomal enzymes, such as α-galactosidase A, which is involved in processing of αGalGalCer, as discussed above (Kolter and Sandhoff 2005). Indeed, DCs derived from saposin-deficient mice are totally unable to present αGalGalCer to the invariant Vα14$^+$ NKT cells (Kang and Cresswell 2004; Zhou et al. 2004). Further, development of this T cell population is specifically impaired in these mutant mice, underscoring a critical role for saposins in CD1d-mediated antigen presentation (Zhou et al. 2004). It remains to be established whether saposins may be involved directly in the transfer of processed αGalCer to the CD1d antigen-binding groove, but such a lipid transfer function has been demonstrated for all the four saposins, which are capable of transferring phosphatidylserine, and for saposins A, B, and C, which transfer sulfatide to CD1d (Zhou et al. 2004). Saposin-dependent antigen processing and loading pathways have also been noted for human CD1b-presented glycolipid antigens of microbial origin (Fig. 1) (Winau et al. 2004).

Similar to saposins, the GM2 activator protein, capable of associating with β-hexosaminidase A and assisting GM2 degradation, functions as a lipid transfer protein involved in lipid loading onto CD1. Besides its ability to bind GM2, the GM2 activator protein can interact in vitro with the acidic trisialoganglioside GT1b bound to CD1d and remove it from the CD1d antigen-binding groove (Zhou et al. 2004). Further, a role for the GM2 activator protein to assist αGalCer loading onto CD1d has been suggested. It remains to be answered directly, however, whether the GM2 activator protein plays an essential role in NKT cell development, as has been shown for saposins. Together, these studies point to a key role for SAPs in lipid antigen processing and loading onto CD1 molecules in lysosomes.

7
Conclusion

It is now clear that CD1 molecules present antigens for recognition by the T cell antigen receptor. However, compared to MHC molecules, the unique nature of these integral membrane proteins and the lipid antigens they present utilize entirely different mechanisms of antigen delivery, trafficking, processing, and loading. The CD1 molecules survey the endosomal compartments of APCs by localizing preferentially in distinct endosomal subcompartments in order to intersect with a wide range of lipid antigens. Lipid antigens may be delivered to APCs in lipoprotein particles or bound to other lipid binding molecules and are then taken up by a range of cell-surface receptors including those receptors used in lipid metabolism such as LDL-R, scavenger receptors, and cell-surface lectins. Once internalized, lipid antigens traffic to different subcompartments of the endocytic system, with some localizing in the ERC and others in late endosomes and lysosomes. Studies on lipid antigens in lysosomes have revealed utilization of glycosidases as glycolipid processing enzymes and an accessory function for CD1e in that process as well as sphingolipid activator proteins as molecules that load lipids onto CD1. Together, a picture is emerging that reveals how the immune system has co-opted lipid transport, processing, and loading molecules that function in lipid metabolism also for the purpose of delivering, taking up, loading, and presenting lipid antigens bound to CD1 for recognition by T cells. The intersection of these processes with CD1 antigen-presenting molecules enables the universe of self and microbial lipid antigens to stimulate T cell immunity.

References

Amano M, Baumgarth N, Dick MD, Brossay L, Kronenberg M, Herzenberg LA, Strober S (1998) CD1 expression defines subsets of follicular and marginal zone B cells in the spleen: beta 2-microglobulin-dependent and independent forms. J Immunol 161:1710–1717

Angenieux C, Salamero J, Fricker D, Cazenave JP, Goud B, Hanau D, and de La Salle H (2000) Characterization of CD1e, a third type of CD1 molecule expressed in dendritic cells. J Biol Chem 275:37757–37764

Angenieux C, Fraisier V, Maitre B, Racine V, van der Wel N, Fricker D, Proamer F, Sachse M, Cazenave JP, Peters P, Goud B, Hanau D, Sibarita JB, Salamero J, and de la Salle H (2005) The cellular pathway of CD1e in immature and maturing dendritic cells. Traffic 6:286–302

Balk SP, Burke S, Polischuk JE, Frantz ME, Yang L, Porcelli S, Colgan SP, Blumberg RS (1994) Beta 2-microglobulin-independent MHC class Ib molecule expressed by human intestinal epithelium. Science 265:259–262

Barboni E, Coade S, Fiori A (2005) The binding of mycolic acids to galectin-3: a novel interaction between a host soluble lectin and trafficking mycobacterial lipids? FEBS Lett 579:6749–6755

Bonifacino JS (2004) Insights into the biogenesis of lysosome-related organelles from the study of the Hermansky-Pudlak syndrome. Ann N Y Acad Sci 1038:103–114

Briken V, Jackman RM, Dasgupta S, Hoening S, Porcelli SA (2002) Intracellular trafficking pathway of newly synthesized CD1b molecules. EMBO J 21:825–834

Brown MS, Goldstein JL (1983) Lipoprotein metabolism in the macrophage: implications for cholesterol deposition in atherosclerosis. Annu Rev Biochem 52:223–261

Brozovic S, Nagaishi T, Yoshida M, Betz S, Salas A, Chen D, Kaser A, Glickman J, Kuo T, Little A, Morrison J, Corazza N, Kim JY, Colgan SP, Young SG, Exley M, Blumberg RS (2004) CD1d function is regulated by microsomal triglyceride transfer protein. Nat Med 10:535–539

Cao X, Sugita M, Van Der Wel N, Lai J, Rogers RA, Peters PJ, Brenner MB (2002) CD1 molecules efficiently present antigen in immature dendritic cells and traffic independently of MHC class II during dendritic cell maturation. J Immunol 169:4770–4777

Caplan S, Dell'Angelica EC, Gahl WA, Bonifacino JS (2000) Trafficking of major histocompatibility complex class II molecules in human B-lymphoblasts deficient in the AP-3 adaptor complex. Immunol Lett 72:113–117

Cella M, Engering A, Pinet V, Pieters J, Lanzavecchia A (1997) Inflammatory stimuli induce accumulation of MHC class II complexes on dendritic cells. Nature 388:782–787

Cernadas M, Sugita M, van der Wel N, Cao X, Gumperz JE, Maltsev S, Besra GS, Behar SM, Peters PJ, Brenner MB (2003) Lysosomal localization of murine CD1d mediated by AP-3 is necessary for NK T cell development. J Immunol 171:4149–4155

Chiu YH, Park SH, Benlagha K, Forestier C, Jayawardena-Wolf J, Savage PB, Teyton L, Bendelac A (2002) Multiple defects in antigen presentation and T cell development by mice expressing cytoplasmic tail-truncated CD1d. Nat Immunol 3:55–60

Conner SD, Schmid SL (2003) Regulated portals of entry into the cell. Nature 422:37–44

De la Salle H, Mariotti S, Angenieux C, Gilleron M, Garcia-Alles LF, Malm D, Berg T, Paoletti S, Maitre B, Mourey L, Salamero J, Cazenave JP, Hanau D, Mori L, Puzo G, De Libero G (2005) Assistance of microbial glycolipid antigen processing by CD1e. Science 310:1321–1324

De Silva AD, Park JJ, Matsuki N, Stanic AK, Brutkiewicz RR, Medof ME, Joyce S (2002) Lipid protein interactions: the assembly of CD1d1 with cellular phospholipids occurs in the endoplasmic reticulum. J Immunol 168:723–733

Dell'Angelica EC, Shotelersuk V, Aguilar RC, Gahl WA, Bonifacino JS (1999) Altered trafficking of lysosomal proteins in Hermansky-Pudlak syndrome due to mutations in the beta 3A subunit of the AP-3 adaptor. Mol Cell 3:11–21

Diedrich G, Bangia N, Pan M, Cresswell P (2001) A role for calnexin in the assembly of the MHC class I loading complex in the endoplasmic reticulum. J Immunol 166:1703–1739

Dougan SK, Salas A, Rava P, Agyemang A, Kaser A, Morrison J, Khurana A, Kronenberg M, Johnson C, Exley M, Hussain MM, Blumberg RS (2005) Microsomal triglyceride transfer protein lipidation and control of CD1d on antigen-presenting cells. J Exp Med 202:529–539

Ehehalt R, Fullekrug J, Pohl J, Ring A, Herrmann T, Stremmel W (2006) Mol Cell Biochem Translocation of long chain fatty acids across the plasma membrane-lipid rafts and fatty acid transport proteins. 284:135–140

Elewaut D, Lawton AP, Nagarajan NA, Maverakis E, Khurana A, Honing S, Benedict CA, Sercarz E, Bakke O, Kronenberg M, Prigozy TI (2003) The adaptor protein AP-3 Is required for CD1d-mediated antigen presentation of glycosphingolipids and development of Valpha14i NKT cells. J Exp Med 198:1133–1146

Figdor CG, van Kooyk Y, Adema GJ (2002) C-type lectin receptors on dendritic cells and Langerhans cells. Nat Rev Immunol 2:77–84

Gagescu R, Demaurex N, Parton RG, Hunziker W, Huber LA, Gruenberg J (2000) The recycling endosome of Madin-Darby canine kidney cells is a mildly acidic compartment rich in raft components. Mol Biol Cell 11:2775–2791

Gordon DA, Jamil H (2000) Progress towards understanding the role of microsomal triglyceride transfer protein in apolipoprotein-B lipoprotein assembly. Biochim Biophys Acta 1486:72–83

Greaves DR, Gordon S (2005) Thematic review series: the immune system and atherogenesis. Recent insights into the biology of macrophage scavenger receptors. J Lipid Res 46:11–20

Herz J, Strickland DK (2001) LRP: a multifunctional scavenger and signaling receptor. J Clin Invest 108:779–784

Honey K, Benlagha K, Beers C, Forbush K, Teyton L, Kleijmeer MJ, Rudensky AY, Bendelac A (2002) Thymocyte expression of cathepsin L is essential for NKT cell development. Nat Immunol 3:1069–1074

Hughes EA, Cresswell P (1998) The thiol oxidoreductase ERp57 is a component of the MHC class I peptide-loading complex. Curr Biol 8:709–712

Hunger RE, Sieling PA, Ochoa MT, Sugaya M, Burdick AE, Rea TH, Brennan PJ, Belisle JT, Blauvelt A, Porcelli SA, Modlin RL (2004) Langerhans cells utilize CD1a and langerin to efficiently present nonpeptide antigens to T cells. J Clin Invest 113:701–708

Huttinger R, Staffler G, Majdic O, Stockinger H (1999) Analysis of the early biogenesis of CD1b: involvement of the chaperones calnexin and calreticulin, the proteasome and beta(2)-microglobulin. Int Immunol 11:1615–1623

Ikonen E (2001) Roles of lipid rafts in membrane transport. Curr Opin Cell Biol 13:470–477

Jackman RM, Stenger S, Lee A, Moody DB, Rogers RA, Niazi KR, Sugita M, Modlin RL, Peters PJ, Porcelli SA (1998) The tyrosine-containing cytoplasmic tail of CD1b is essential for its efficient presentation of bacterial lipid antigens. Immunity 8:341–351

Jamil H, Dickson JK Jr, Chu CH, Lago MW, Rinehart JK, Biller SA, Gregg RE, Wetterau JR (1995) Microsomal triglyceride transfer protein. Specificity of lipid binding and transport. J Biol Chem 270:6549–6554

Jayawardena-Wolf J, Benlagha K, Chiu YH, Mehr R, Bendelac A (2001) CD1d endosomal trafficking is independently regulated by an intrinsic CD1d-encoded tyrosine motif and by the invariant chain. Immunity 15:897–908

Joyce S, Woods AS, Yewdell JW, Bennink JR, De Silva AD, Boesteanu A, Balk SP, Cotter RJ, Brutkiewicz RR (1998) Natural ligand of mouse CD1d1: cellular glycosylphosphatidylinositol. Science 279:1541–1544

Kang SJ, Cresswell P (2002) Regulation of intracellular trafficking of human CD1d by association with MHC class II molecules. EMBO J 21:1650–1660

Kang SJ, Cresswell P (2004) Saposins facilitate CD1d-restricted presentation of an exogenous lipid antigen to T cells. Nat Immunol 5:175–181

Kim HS, Garcia J, Exley M, Johnson KW, Balk SP, Blumberg RS (1999) Biochemical characterization of CD1d expression in the absence of beta2-microglobulin. J Biol Chem 274:9289–9295

Kobayashi T, Gu F, Gruenberg J (1998a) Lipids, lipid domains and lipid-protein interactions in endocytic membrane traffic. Semin Cell Dev Biol 9:517–526

Kobayashi T, Stang E, Fang KS, de Moerloose P, Parton RG, Gruenberg J (1998b) A lipid associated with the antiphospholipid syndrome regulates endosome structure and function. Nature 392:193–197

Kolter T, Sandhoff K (2005) Principles of lysosomal membrane digestion: stimulation of sphingolipid degradation by sphingolipid activator proteins and anionic lysosomal lipids. Annu Rev Cell Dev Biol 21:81–103

Moody DB, Briken V, Cheng T-YRoura-Mir C, Guy MR, Geho DH, Tykocinski ML, Besra GS, Porcelli SA (2002) Lipid length controls antigen entry into endosomal and nonendosomal pathways for CD1b presentation. Nat Immunol 3:435–442

Morrice NA, Powis SJ (1998) A role for the thiol-dependent reductase ERp57 in the assembly of MHC class I molecules. Curr Biol 8:713–716

Mukherjee S, Maxfield FR (2000) Role of membrane organization and membrane domains in endocytic lipid trafficking. Traffic 1:203–211

Mukherjee S, Soe TT, Maxfield FR (1999) Endocytic sorting of lipid analogues differing solely in the chemistry of their hydrophobic tails. J Cell Biol 144:1271–1284

Nabi IR, Le PU (2003) Caveolae/raft-dependent endocytosis. J Cell Biol 161:673–677

Nijman HW, Kleijmeer MJ, Ossevoort MA, Oorschot VM, Vierboom MP, van de Keur M, Kenemans P, Kast WM, Geuze HJ, Melief CJ (1995) Antigen capture and major histocompatibility class II compartments of freshly isolated and cultured human blood dendritic cells. J Exp Med 182:163–174

Ortmann B, Androlewicz MJ, Cresswell P (1994) MHC class I/beta 2-microglobulin complexes associate with TAP transporters before peptide binding. Nature 368:864–867

Park JJ, Kang SJ, De Silva AD, Stanic AK, Casorati G, Hachey DL, Cresswell P, Joyce S (2004) Lipid-protein interactions: biosynthetic assembly of CD1 with lipids in the endoplasmic reticulum is evolutionarily conserved. Proc Natl Acad Sci U S A 101:1022–1026

Peden AA, Oorschot V, Hesser BA, Austin CD, Scheller RH, Klumperman J (2004) Localization of the AP-3 adaptor complex defines a novel endosomal exit site for lysosomal membrane proteins. J Cell Biol 164:1065–1076

Pierre P, Turley SJ, Gatti E, Hull M, Meltzer J, Mirza A, Inaba K, Steinman RM, Mellman I (1997) Developmental regulation of MHC class II transport in mouse dendritic cells. Nature 388:787–792

Prigozy TI, Naidenko O, Qasba P, Elewaut D, Brossay L, Khurana A, Natori T, Koezuka Y, Kulkarni A, Kronenberg M (2001) Glycolipid antigen processing for presentation by CD1d molecules. Science 291:664–667

Prigozy TI, Sieling PA, Clemens D, Stewart PL, Behar SM, Porcelli SA, Brenner MB, Modlin RL, Kronenberg M (1997) The mannose receptor delivers lipoglycan antigens to endosomes for presentation to T cells by CD1b molecules. Immunity 6:187–197

Raggers RJ, Pomorski T, Holthuis JC, Kalin N, and van Meer G (2000) Lipid traffic: the ABC of transbilayer movement. Traffic 1:226–234

Riese RJ, Shi GP, Villadangos J, Stetson D, Driessen C, Lennon-Dumenil AM, Chu CL, Naumov Y, Behar SM, Ploegh H, Locksley R, Chapman HA (2001) T cell selection and maturation by cathepsin S. Immunity 15:909–919

Sadasivan B, Lehner PJ, Ortmann B, Spies T, Cresswell P (1996) Roles for calreticulin and a novel glycoprotein, tapasin, in the interaction of MHC class I molecules with TAP. Immunity 5:103–114

Salamero J, Bausinger H, Mommaas AM, Lipsker D, Proamer F, Cazenave JP, Goud B, de la Salle H, Hanau D (2001) CD1a molecules traffic through the early recycling endosomal pathway in human Langerhans cells. J Invest Dermatol 116:401–408

Sallusto F, Cella M, Danieli C, Lanzavecchia A (1995) Dendritic cells use macropinocytosis and the mannose receptor to concentrate macromolecules in the major histocompatibility complex class II compartment: downregulation by cytokines and bacterial products. J Exp Med 182:389–400

Schaffer JE, Lodish HF (1994) Expression cloning and characterization of a novel adipocyte long chain fatty acid transport protein. Cell 79:427–436

Schaible UE, Winau F, Sieling PA, Fischer K, Collins HL, Hagens K, Modlin RL, Brinkmann V, Kaufmann SH (2003) Apoptosis facilitates antigen presentation to T lymphocytes through MHC-I and CD1 in tuberculosis. Nat Med 9:1039–1046

Sevilla LM, Richter SS, Miller J (2001) Intracellular transport of MHC class II and associated invariant chain in antigen presenting cells from AP-3-deficient mocha mice. Cell Immunol 210:143–53

Sugita M, Brenner MB (1994) An unstable beta 2-microglobulin: major histocompatibility complex class I heavy chain intermediate dissociates from calnexin and then is stabilized by binding peptide. J Exp Med 180:2163–2171

Sugita M, Porcelli SA, Brenner MB (1997) Assembly and retention of CD1b heavy chains in the endoplasmic reticulum. J Immunol 159:2358–2365

Sugita M, Grant EP, van Donselaar E, Hsu VW, Rogers RA, Peters PJ, Brenner MB (1999) Separate pathways for antigen presentation by CD1 molecules. Immunity 11:743–752

Sugita M, Jackman RM, van Donselaar E, Behar SM, Rogers RA, Peters PJ, Brenner MB, Porcelli SA (1996) Cytoplasmic tail-dependent localization of CD1b antigen-presenting molecules to MIICs. Science 273:349–352

Sugita M, van Der Wel N, Rogers RA, Peters PJ, Brenner MB (2000) CD1c molecules broadly survey the endocytic system. Proc Natl Acad Sci U S A 97:8445–8450

Sugita M, Cao X, Watts GF, Rogers RA, Bonifacino JS, Brenner MB (2002) Failure of trafficking and antigen presentation by CD1 in AP-3-deficient cells. Immunity 16:697–706

Van den Elzen P, Garg S, Leon L, Brigl M, Leadbetter EA, Gumperz JE, Dascher CC, Cheng TY, Sacks FM, Illarionov PA, Besra GS, Kent SC, Moody DB, Brenner MB (2005) Apolipoprotein-mediated pathways of lipid antigen presentation. Nature 437:906–910

Van der Wel NN, Sugita M, Fluitsma DM, Cao X, Schreibelt G, Brenner MB, Peters PJ (2003) CD1 and major histocompatibility complex II molecules follow a different course during dendritic cell maturation. Mol Biol Cell 14:3378–3388

Willnow TE, Nykjaer A, Herz J (1999) Lipoprotein receptors: new roles for ancient proteins. Nat Cell Biol 1:E157–E162

Winau F, Schwierzeck V, Hurwitz R, Remmel N, Sieling PA, Modlin RL, Porcelli SA, Brinkmann V, Sugita M, Sandhoff K, Kaufmann SH, Schaible UE (2004) Saposin C is required for lipid presentation by human CD1b. Nat Immunol 5:169–174

York IA, Rock KL (1996) Antigen processing and presentation by the class I major histocompatibility complex. Annu Rev Immunol 14:369–396

Zhou D, Cantu C 3rd, Sagiv Y, Schrantz N, Kulkarni AB, Qi X, Mahuran DJ, Morales CR, Grabowski GA, Benlagha K, Savage P, Bendelac A, Teyton L (2004) Editing of CD1d-bound lipid antigens by endosomal lipid transfer proteins. Science 303:523–527

CTMI (2007) 314:165–192

TCR-Mediated Recognition of Glycolipid CD1 Complexes

B. A. Sullivan · M. Kronenberg (✉)

La Jolla Institute for Allergy and Immunology, 9420 Athena Circle,
La Jolla, CA 92037, USA
mitch@liai.org

Abstract Populations of unconventional T lymphocytes that express αβ T cell antigen receptors (TCRs) have been characterized, including T cells reactive to glycolipids presented by CD1 molecules. The CD1 molecules have a structure broadly similar to major histocompatibility complex (MHC) class I and class II proteins, but because the antigens CD1 presents are so different from peptides, it is possible that glycolipid reactive TCRs have properties that distinguish them from TCRs expressed by conventional T cells. Consistent with this possibility, CD1-reactive T cells have an unrestrained pattern of co-receptor expression, as they include CD4$^+$, CD8$^+$, and double-negative cells. Furthermore, unlike peptide-reactive T cells, there are populations of glycolipid-reactive T cells with invariant α chain TCRs that are conserved across species. There are also glycolipid reactive populations with more variable TCRs, however, suggesting that it may be difficult to make categorical generalizations about glycolipid reactive TCRs. Among the glycolipid reactive TCRs, the invariant TCR expressed by CD1d reactive NKT cells has been by far the most thoroughly studied, and in this article we emphasize the unique features of this antigen recognition system, including repertoire formation, fine specificity, TCR affinity, and TCR structure.

Abbreviations

αGalCer	α-Galactosylceramide
αGluCer	α-Glucosylceramide
αManCer	α-Mannosylceramide
C	Constant
CDR	Complementarity determining region
DN	Double negative
DP	Double positive
i	Invariant
iGb3	Isoglobotrihexosylceramide
Hex	Hexosaminidase
MHC	Major histocompatibility complex
p	Peptide
NK	Natural killer
PIM$_4$	Phosphatidylinositol tetramannoside
TCR	T cell antigen receptor
V	Variable

1
Introduction to glycolipid reactive T cells

T lymphocytes that recognize lipids belong to a diverse group of unconventional T cells that express αβ T cell antigen receptors (TCRs). This group also includes various types of T lymphocytes that do not recognize lipids, including major histocompatibility complex (MHC) class I-reactive T cells that co-express natural killer (NK) cell receptors such as NK1.1, and the T cells reactive with nonclassical class I or class Ib molecules. Some properties of these different populations are compared in Fig. 1. TCR αβ intraepithelial lymphocytes that express CD8αα homodimers, but which lack expression of one of the known TCR co-receptors, CD4 or CD8αβ, certainly are also unconventional (Gangadharan and Cheroutre 2004), but they are omitted from the table because although they may react to a variety of self antigens (Leishman et al. 2002), their specificity remains unknown.

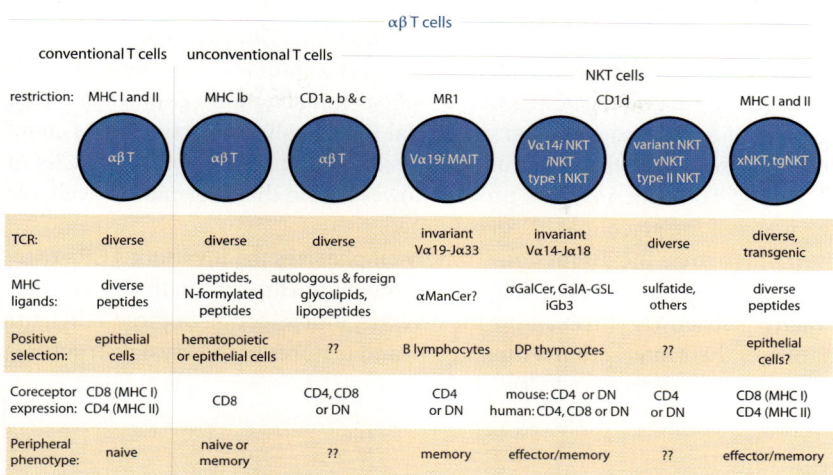

Fig. 1 Features of unconventional αβ T cell subsets. Unconventional αβ T cells share unusual features such as positive selection by hematopoietic cells in many cases, unrestricted co-receptor expression, and a peripheral memory phenotype in the absence of deliberate immunization

Are there any features that distinguish the TCRs of glycolipid reactive T cells? A major population of mouse T cells reactive to glycolipids presented by CD1d expresses a semi-invariant TCR. This is composed of an invariant TCR α chain (Vα14i) and only one or a few predominant Vβ segments (Bendelac et al. 1997), although there is great variability in the CDR3 regions of the β chain (Gui et al. 2001; Matsuda et al. 2001; Ronet et al. 2001). Mucosal invariant T cells (MAIT) have a different invariant α chain (Vα19i) (Treiner et al. 2005), and recently it was reported that they respond to glycolipids presented by the class Ib protein MR1 (Okamoto et al. 2005). It would be misleading, however, to conclude that all glycolipid reactive T cells have invariant TCRs. There are T cells reactive with CD1d that do not express the invariant TCR α chain (Cardell et al. 1995; Jahng et al. 2004), and moreover, the T cells reactive with human CD1a, CD1b, and CD1c molecules have diverse TCRs (Brigl and Brenner 2004; Grant et al. 1999).

One property that does seem to distinguish the glycolipid reactive T cells, however, is their pattern of co-receptor expression. In general, T cells reactive to a particular CD1 molecule can express either CD4, CD8 or they can be double negative (DN) (Porcelli and Modlin 1999), although the mouse T cells that express the Vα14i TCR constitute an exception in that they never are CD8⁺ (Bendelac et al. 1994). These data, particularly the relatively large percentage of CD1 reactive T cells that are DN, suggest that the TCRs of glycolipid reactive T cells are co-receptor independent. As the co-receptors enhance both the TCR avidity (Garcia et al. 1996) as well as signal transduction (Zamoyska 1998), these data further suggest that in general the glycolipid reactive TCRs could have different properties, including possibly an increased avidity or altered signaling. This remains to be proven, however, and the information available for many of the glycolipid TCRs is limited.

In this article the discussion strongly emphasizes the invariant TCRs reactive to CD1d, because there is by far the most information on this glycolipid-reactive subset. We will examine the diversity and selection of these TCRs, the nature of their interaction with antigen, and features of the crystal structures of human CD1d-reactive TCRs.

2
Background on Vα14*i* NKT Cells

NKT cells are a diverse population of T lymphocytes defined operationally by the co-expression of NK receptors such as NK1.1 and an αβ TCR (Fig. 1). The majority of NKT cells in the mouse express a TCR with an invariant Vα14-Jα18 rearrangement (Lantz and Bendelac 1994). These cells have been variously called Vα14*i* NKT cells, the term we use here, invariant NK T cells (*i*NKT), or type I NKT cells (Godfrey et al. 2004). The invariant TCR α chain pairs with a limited set of Vβ segments, with Vβ8.2 being the most predominant followed in frequency by Vβ7 and Vβ2. The TCR of Vα14*i* NKT cells specifically recognizes glycolipid antigens presented by CD1d, a nonpolymorphic class I-like antigen-presenting molecule. A potent glycolipid, α-galactosyl ceramide (αGalCer), has been used in numerous studies to activate Vα14*i* NKT cells and to identify them by staining with fluorescent αGalCer/CD1d multimers. In humans, a homologous population of NKT cells, which expresses TCR α chains using the Vα24-gene segment (Vα24*i* NKT), exists that is reactive to αGalCer presented by human CD1d (hCD1d). The structures of αGalCer and some other glycolipid antigens recognized by *i*NKT cells are depicted in Fig. 2. The nomenclature for the Vα*i* TCR genes is summarized in Table1. Here we employ the widely used colloquial nomenclature, as outlined above.

Vα14*i* NKT cells play an important role in numerous mouse models of human diseases. They are a naturally occurring memory-like population with the capacity to produce both pro- and anti-inflammatory cytokines rapidly after TCR engagement. Vα14*i* NKT cells are regulatory in the traditional sense – they are able to alter the initiation of an adaptive immune response by augmenting or dampening the early immune response or by diverting it

Table 1 Vα14*i* and Vα24*i* NKT TCR nomenclature. T cell receptor gene nomenclature is not always intuitive. Here is a quick reference guide for *i*NKT biologists

Mouse	Human
Protein name: Vα14	Protein name: Vα24
Gene name: **TRAV11*01** and **TRAV11*02**	Genename: **TRAV10** or **TCRAV10S1**
(**T cell receptor alpha chain variable gene 11 allele*01**)	(**T cell receptor alpha chain variable gene 10 segment 1**)
Also TRAV11D*01 and*02 (from the Vα cluster duplication)	
Formerly known as TRAV14 or AV14S2	Formerly known as TRAV24S1
Gene ID: 547422	Gene ID: 28676
Genbank ID	Genbank ID: AE000659
TRAV11*01: AY158221, AY158220	Protein ID: AAB69005
TRAV11*02: AY158218	
Invariant Vα14-Jα18 arrangement	
Genbank ID	
TRAV11*01: M14506, AF093872	
TRAV11*02: S75451	
Protein name: Vβ8.2	Protein name: Vβ11
Gene name: **TRBV8S2** or **Tcrb-V8.2**	Gene name: **TRBV11-1**
(**T cell receptor beta chain variable gene 8 segment 2**)	
Gene ID: 21607	Gene ID: 28582
Genbank ID: L37869	Genbank ID: NG_001333

in either a T helper type 1 or T helper type 2 direction. Studies of the role of Vα14*i* NKT cells in immune regulation most commonly use mice that are selectively deficient in these cells as they lack the Jα segment required to form the invariant TCR ($J\alpha18^{-/-}$). In other studies, the larger population of CD1d-restricted T cells are deleted by removing the antigen-presenting molecule required for their selection ($CD1d^{-/-}$). Some CD1d-restricted T cells do not express the invariant TCR and therefore these two knockout strategies do not always produce the same outcome in vivo. Because this invariant population is conserved across numerous mammalian species (Brossay and Kronenberg 1999) and because of their pivotal position in the immune system, understanding the mechanism of activation and antagonism is essential for the production of therapeutics designed to target these cells.

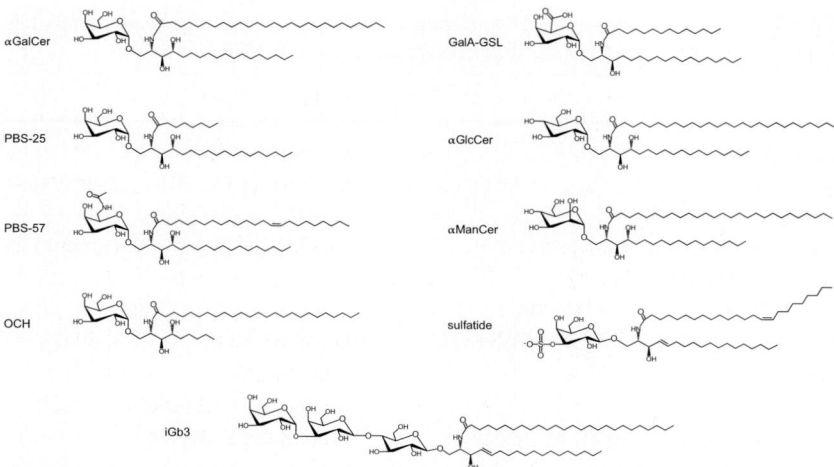

Fig. 2 Structure of some glycolipid compounds recognized by *i*NKT cells

3
Selection of Vα14*i* NKT Cells

The antigen receptor repertoire of naïve αβ T cells within an individual is highly diverse in order to identify pathogen-derived antigens to protect the host from disease (Nikolich-Zugich et al. 2004). TCR diversity is acquired during development in the thymic organs. The recent description of a second thymus in the neck, the cervical thymus, requires new experiments to examine both conventional and unconventional T cell development in this organ (Terszowski et al. 2006). For simplicity, the term "thymus" will be used to describe studies of the thoracic thymus. In the thymus, T cell precursors recombine genes of their TCR β and α loci and test the paired chains against the pool of self-MHC–antigen complexes expressed predominantly by epithelial cells for positive selection and dendritic cells, among others, for negative selection. T cell precursors with high-affinity αβTCRs are deleted, those with intermediate affinity mature, and low-affinity T cell precursors succumb to "death by neglect."

Vα14*i* NKT cell development in the thymus shares features with the development of conventional CD4[+] and CD8[+] T cells. There are, however, major differences. Genes required for Vα14*i* NKT cell differentiation that are dispensable for conventional T cells include genes required for the presentation or recognition of the selecting antigen such as *CD1d*, *TCR Jα18*, *prosaposin*, *hexosaminidase B* (*Hexb*), *ap3* and perhaps *cathepsin L* (Kronenberg and

Gapin 2002; Matsuda and Gapin 2005). Furthermore, there is a set of signaling molecules and transcription factors also required for Vα14*i* NKT cell differentiation, including *fyn*, *SLAM-associated-protein* (*SAP*), *DOCK2*, *T-bet*, and members of the ets and NF-κB families, although the reasons for the requirement for these diverse elements are not known (Elewaut et al. 2003; Kronenberg and Gapin 2002; Kunisaki et al. 2006; Matsuda and Gapin 2005). For positive selection of Vα14*i* NKT cells, CD1d expressed exclusively on $CD4^+CD8^+$ (double positive or DP) thymocytes, driven by the lck proximal promoter, is sufficient (Wei et al. 2005). Selection by hematopoietic cells is a feature that Vα14*i* NKT cells share with some other T cells restricted by class Ib and class I-like proteins, such as those restricted to MR1, Qa-1, and H2-M3 (Sullivan et al. 2002; Treiner et al. 2003; Urdahl et al. 2002). Expression of human CD1d on DP thymocytes in transgenic mice also leads to the selection of Vα14*i* NKT cells (Schumann et al. 2005), highlighting the remarkable cross-reactivity and conservation of *i*NKT cell specificity. Surprisingly, however, alleles of the rat Vα14*i* TCR exhibit a high degree of specificity for αGalCer presented by rat CD1d, with little or no reactivity for the mouse CD1d ortholog (Pry et al. 2006).

TCR β and α gene rearrangement and pairing of the Vα14*i* NKT TCR appear to conform to the standards of conventional αβ selection. Difference in selection the DP stage. DP Vα14*i* NKT cell precursors interact with other DPs that express antigenic CD1d/glycolipid complexes. Those cells that receive an appropriate signal are positively selected. DP Vα14*i* NKT cell precursors express high levels of heat-stable antigen (HSA or CD24). Selected Vα14*i* NKT cell precursors become $CD4^+$ or double negative (DN) and HSA^{low}. Finally, the cells expand and express activation and memory markers, such as CD44, and NK cell lineage markers, such as NK1.1 (Benlagha et al. 2002; Matsuda and Gapin 2005; Pellicci et al. 2002; Wei et al. 2005). The positive selection signal for Vα14*i* NKT cells is thought to be agonistic, as suggested by recent studies of isoglobotrihexosylceramide (iGb3), a glycolipid that activates the mature cells, and studies of mice that cannot form iGb3/CD1d complexes (Zhou et al. 2004). These mice, $Hexb^{-/-}$, completely lack Vα14*i* NKT cells.

4
Diversity and Selection of the Invariant α Chains

For all TCR αβ+ T cells, recombination of both the α and β gene segments results in highly variable TCRs. Germ line variability in the V region genes is encoded primarily in the complementarity determining regions (CDRs) 1 and 2. The CDR3 region, by contrast, is generated by rearrangement. CDR3β is defined by the rearrangement of three segments, Vβ, Dβ, and Jβ, while CDR3α is defined by Vα-Jα rearrangement. Additional diversity is added with the inclusion of hairpin nucleotides and nongermline encoded nucleotides by terminal deoxynucleotidyl transferase. This acquisition of diversity is a hallmark of adaptive immune receptors and is also used by developing B cells to generate antibodies.

In the case of mouse Vα14i and human Vα24i NKT cells, there is essentially no amino acid sequence diversity in the rearranged α genes (Dellabona et al. 1994; Lantz and Bendelac 1994; Makino et al. 1995; Porcelli et al. 1993), and moreover, the CDR3α sequences are very closely related (10/13 amino acids identical) when the two species are compared, providing further evidence for the high degree of evolutionary conservation of the iNKT cell specificity. In humans, the Vα24i rearrangement is most often formed by a Vα–Jα joining in which there are no N region nucleotide additions or nucleotide deletions from the Vα24 segment, and two nucleotides are deleted from the germline Jα18 segment. In both humans and mice, however, the invariant α gene rearrangement can be formed in some iNKT cells with different patterns of nucleotide deletion as well as N region additions (Lantz and Bendelac 1994). These data provide evidence for the selection of the invariant α chain at the protein level, as opposed to a mechanism based on preferential gene rearrangement. Consistent with the absence of a preferential rearrangement mechanism, analysis of Vα14i NKT cell hybridomas indicated random rearrangements of the α gene on the silent allele (Lantz and Bendelac 1994; Shimamura et al. 1997). In contrast to the strong selection for a conserved CDR3α sequence, allelic polymorphisms in Vα14 in mice and rats affecting CDR2 do not strongly alter the recognition of CD1d/glycolipid complexes (Pry et al. 2006; Sim et al. 2003). It should be noted, however, that some human T cells bind αGalCer/hCD1d tetramers without expressing Vα24 (Gadola et al. 2006), and these constitute an average of 22% of the αGalCer/hCD1d tetramer binding cells in human peripheral blood (Brigl et al. 2006). A similar population has not been reported in mice. This difference may reflect the predominant analysis of populations of Vα14i NKT cells in mice as opposed to cultured lines and expanded Vα24i clones in humans. It is also possible that human TCRs capable of recognizing αGalCer presented by CD1d contain a somewhat more diverse repertoire of α chains. Interestingly, the cells with noncanonical TCR α chains reactive with αGalCer presented by CD1d express Vβ11 and they rearrange several different Vα segments to Jα18, most notably Vα3.1 and Vα10.1 (Brigl et al. 2006; Gadola et al. 2006).

5
The Role of the TCR β Chain

The Vα14*i* TCR pairs with a restricted set of mouse Vβ chains, with Vβ8.2 most frequent and constituting at least 50% of invariant NKT cells, followed by Vβ7 and then Vβ2. It was found that Vβ6, Vβ10, and Vβ14 are also expressed in this population, but at lower frequencies (Matsuda et al. 2001). In contrast to the CDR3 region of the α chain, the CDR3 regions of the β chains of Vα14*i* NKT cells from the thymus, liver, and spleen are highly diverse in composition and length (Matsuda et al. 2001; Gui et al. 2001; Ronet et al. 2001). Consistent with a lack of stringent selection on CDR3β, the capacity to bind αGalCer/CD1d tetramers is not limited to Vβ genes selected in developing Vα14*i* NKT cells. Therefore, Vα14 can pair with Vβ8.2 chains from several TCR transgenic mice obtained from TCRs selected for other specificities, and the resulting TCRs bind αGalCer/CD1d tetramers (Cantu et al. 2003; Matsuda et al. 2001; Wingender et al. 2006). In human Vα24*i* NKT cells, Vα24 pairs almost exclusively with Vβ11, the ortholog of mouse Vβ8. The CDR3β regions of the β chains expressed by Vα24*i* NKT cells have also been reported to be quite diverse (Exley et al. 1997; Porcelli et al. 1993), although this was not the case in one study (Dellabona et al. 1994).

CD1d tetramers loaded with αGalCer are extremely useful for the identification and analysis of primary Vα14*i* NKT cells. Soluble divalent mouse or human CD1d–IgG1 fusion proteins can also be loaded with glycolipids and are available commercially. To assess the influence of the TCR β chain on glycolipid–CD1d complex binding, the binding of αGalCer/mouse CD1d (mCD1d) tetramers (higher avidity), αGalCer/hCD1d-IgG1 dimers (intermediate avidity), and αGalCer/mCD1d-IgG1 dimers (low avidity) to populations of mouse Vα14*i* NKT cells has been compared (Schumann et al. 2003). Vβ8.2 containing TCRs have the highest avidity for this synthetic ligand, but this may not necessarily be the case for endogenous or natural antigens. To test the role of different β chains in the recognition of endogenous ligands and the positive selection of Vα14*i* NKT cells, *CD1d*$^{+/-}$ mice, which express approximately half the normal level of CD1d, were analyzed. Although the numbers of preselection DP Vα14*i* NKT cell precursors were the same in these heterozygotes, the number of mature thymic Vβ7$^+$ Vα14*i* NKT cells increased, while the numbers of Vβ8.2$^+$ Vα14*i* NKT cells remained unchanged. This suggests that Vβ7 has a higher avidity and is better able to compete for limited ligand–CD1d complexes. If this is true, then overexpression of CD1d might lead to the selective deletion of Vβ7$^+$ Vα14*i* NKT cells. Transgenic expression of CD1d under the control of the K^b promoter significantly increased CD1d levels on hematopoietic and epithelial cells in the thymus (Chun et al. 2003). These mice have fewer Vα14*i* NKT cells in the thymus, liver and spleen, with a approximately 50% reduction Vβ7$^+$ and Vβ8$^+$ cells and an increase in the frequency of Vβ2$^+$ cells. This study demonstrated that Vβ2$^+$ Vα14*i* NKT cells are likely to have a lower avidity for endogenous ligands, and overall, considering the influence of endogenous antigen(s), the data are consistent with an affinity hierarchy for Vα14*i* NKT cells of Vβ7 greater than Vβ8.2 greater than Vβ2.

The restriction in Vβ use in Vα14*i* NKT cells could be due to constraints in pairing, such as the possibility that only certain Vβ genes form stable heterodimers with the Vα14*i* TCR. Alternatively, the disfavored Vβ genes could be eliminated either by negative selection or by a failure of positive selection. Mice expressing a Vα14*i* α chain transgene were crossed to the *CD1d$^{-/-}$* background to provide a glimpse of the unselected TCR β chain repertoire of Vα14*i* expressing T lymphocytes (Wei et al. 2006). This analysis provided little evidence for a strong β chain pairing bias for the Vα14*i* α chain. Moreover, the double-negative spleen cells in these mice had cells that could bind αGalCer/CD1d tetramers that expressed diverse Vβ segments, including those such as Vβ9 and Vβ10 that are rarely found among mature Vα14*i* NKT cells. By various criteria, however, including their activation after intrathymic injection, tetramer binding cells expressing these rarely used Vβ segments have lower-affinity TCRs. According to these functional studies, Vβ7 TCRs have the highest affinity. Therefore, the restricted Vβ repertoire of Vα14*i* NKT cells may reflect primarily the imprint of the positively selecting ligand as opposed to negative selection of thymocytes expressing unusual pairs such as Vβ9/Vα14*i*.

6
Methods for assuming TCR Avidity and Affinity

For conventional αβ T cells, antigenic potency has been correlated in different studies with TCR affinity or avidity, the kinetics of TCR engagement, or the heat capacity of TCR binding. Much of the data relies on surface plasmon resonance (SPR) assays that measure the binding of soluble TCRs and peptide–MHC (pMHC) complexes in real time. Based on this method, in several studies the *off*-rate of TCR binding to pMHC was shown to correlate best with biologic outcome (Kersh et al. 1998; Matsui et al. 1994). For example, pMHC complexes that bound to TCRs with a long half-life ($t_{1/2}$) led to complete activation (agonist peptides) and those with shorter half-lives led to weaker activation (weak agonist peptides) or activation of one but not all of the T cell's effector functions (partial agonist peptides). Measurements of equilibrium tetramer binding and decay of tetramer binding have also been used, although this provides only an avidity measurement, because of the multimeric nature of the ligand. Tetramer-binding methods have the advantage, however, of assessing the binding of molecules expressed by living cells, and they are useful for the analysis of populations of lymphocytes. Similar methods have been employed for the analysis of the TCRs expressed by $V\alpha14i$ and $V\alpha24i$ NKT cells.

7
Measurements of CD1d Glycolipid Binding

Any analysis of the biochemical interactions of the semi-invariant TCRs expressed by iNKT cells must also concern the formation of the TCR ligand, which is a complex of glycolipid plus CD1d. A problem in the analysis of TCR binding to CD1d is the difficulty in achieving reliable and quantitative measurements of glycolipid binding to CD1d molecules. Methods that have been used to measure CD1d binding to glycolipids include direct binding assays using surface plasmon resonance (SPR), isothermal titration calorimetry (ITC) or isoelectric focusing (IEF), as well as indirect assays based on T cell activation as a readout of CD1d glycolipid binding. Using these methods, the equilibrium binding constant of αGalCer for CD1d was calculated to be in the 0.2- to 2.6-μM range (Cantu et al. 2003; Sidobre et al. 2002), but for the SPR and ITC methods, there were problems in verifying the specificity of the binding, although the binding could be competed with gangliosides, which are glycosphingolipids like αGalCer. Moreover, at least for the SPR measurements, the $t_{1/2}$ of the interaction was artificially low. In the functional assay, lipids were loaded onto CD1d-coated plates for various times before culture with $V\alpha14i$ NKT cell hybridomas. Alternatively, the excess glycolipid was washed out, and the plates incubated for various times and rewashed before culture with cells, in order to measure decay of lipid binding to CD1d. This type of *off*-rate assay may be more reliable than binding assays when lipid antigens are concerned, as lipids may form micelles or require lipid transfer proteins for efficient loading in solution. The results revealed the high degree of stability of the glycolipid–CD1d interaction, as it took more than 24 h to lose only 25% of the bound compound (Cantu et al. 2003; Stanic et al. 2003). PBS-25 is a glycolipid ligand closely related to αGalCer, but with a shorter acyl chain. PBS-25 bound CD1d more rapidly than αGalCer, and when bound, the interaction with CD1d was as stable as the αGalCer–CD1d interaction, with little dissociation after 24 h (Zajonc et al. 2005a). Another glycolipid ligand related to αGalCer, OCH, has a shorter sphingosine base and it exhibits some properties of an altered glycolipid ligand, by analogy with altered peptide ligands, in that it stimulated an increased ratio of IL-4 to IFNγ synthesis (Oki et al.

2004). It shares this property with several other αGalCer analogs with shorter aliphatic chains or unsaturated bonds in the acyl chain (Goff et al. 2004; Yu et al. 2005). Interestingly, OCH dissociated more quickly from plate-bound CD1d than αGalCer, with approximately 40% fewer antigenic complexes after 24 h (Oki et al. 2004; Stanic et al. 2003). Regardless, these data indicate that CD1d complexes with different glycosphingolipids have a relatively long $t_{1/2}$, sufficient to permit measurements of TCR binding.

CD1d molecules probably are never empty, and the soluble molecules produced in insect tissue culture cells are loaded predominantly with phosphatidylcholine (PC) (Giabbai et al. 2005). When glycolipids with acyl chains shorter than αGalCer, such as the *Sphingomonas* bacterial antigen GalA-GSL, bind CD1d, part of the binding groove is filled with a palmitic acid spacer lipid (Wu et al. 2006). Despite being loaded with glycolipid, the soluble CD1d molecules from insect cells appear to efficiently exchange PC for glycosphingolipids in vitro. The glycolipid most commonly used in the production of tetramers for the detection or stimulation of *i*NKT cells is the very potent agonist αGalCer, but a newly synthesized and closely related variant, PBS-57, which contains an amino modification of the galactose sugar, loads onto CD1d as well as αGalCer, and has been chosen for tetramer production by the tetramer core facility at the National Institutes of Health (Liu et al. 2006). Tetramers loaded with αGalCer and PBS-57 identify the same population of Vα14*i* NKT cells in vivo and can be used interchangeably. Other glycolipid ligands have been loaded into CD1d to produce tetramers, including GalA-GSL (Kinjo et al. 2005; Mattner et al. 2005; Sriram et al. 2005) and sulfatide (Jahng et al. 2004). Efficient CD1d loading does not occur spontaneously in solution for all antigens, however, and there has been difficulty in producing tetramers of the self antigen iGb3 (Zhou et al. 2004).

Crystal structures of mouse and human CD1d glycolipid complexes have been recently described and will be analyzed in greater detail elsewhere in this volume. However, certain features of glycolipid binding to CD1d are of particular interest, in that they almost certainly affect TCR recognition. Positions R79 and D80 on the CD1d α helix hydrogen bind to the hydroxyls of the sphingosine base of PBS-25, and on the α2 helix D153 hydrogen bonds with positions 2′ and 3′ of the galactose and T156 forms hydrogen bonds with the 1′-O glycosidic bond and the nitrogen linked to the acyl chain. Conserved amino acids in hCD1d form similar hydrogen bonds with αGalCer (R79, D151 and T154) (Koch et al. 2005). Interestingly, in both structures, the galactose lies nearly flat, held in place by hydrogen bonds slightly above the α1 and α2 helices. The structure of a natural *Sphingomonas* glycolipid bound to mCD1d reveals a similar mode of antigen binding (Wu et al. 2006). Studies of the antigen-presenting function of CD1d molecules bearing point mutations identified several upward-pointing amino acids that do not bind αGalCer, but that are likely to be involved in TCR recognition because they altered the Vα14i NKT cell response. These include E83 (Kamada et al. 2001) and S76 (Burdin et al. 2000).

8
Measurements of Vα14 TCR:CD1d Affinity

To better understand the biochemistry and biophysics of the interaction of the Vαi TCR with complexes of αGalCer bound to CD1d, several groups have produced soluble mouse or human TCRs for use in SPR studies (Cantu et al. 2003; Gadola et al. 2006; Kjer-Nielsen et al. 2006; Sidobre et al. 2002). The mouse Vα14i NKT cell TCR was shown to have a relatively high affinity for αGalCer–CD1d complexes, ranging from 31 to 350 nM in the four Vα14i TCRs tested (Cantu et al. 2003; Sidobre et al. 2002). For most of the peptide-reactive TCRs that have been measured, the affinity is in the micromolar range, although there are some exceptional TCRs that have a stronger binding interaction (Davis et al. 1998). The most extraordinary difference compared to the TCRs expressed by conventional T cells, however, was the long $t_{1/2}$ of the interaction, approximately 3 min compared to the 1–10 s that is typical for peptide-reactive TCRs measured under similar conditions. Two compounds with identical lipids but with different sugars, α-glucosylceramide (αGluCer) and α-mannosylceramide (αManCer) were found to be less potent agonists than αGalCer. They exhibited reduced K_Ds of 3.8 µM (αGluCer) and 13.23 µM (αManCer), as well as reduced $t_{1/2}$s of 57 and 17 s, respectively (Sidobre et al. 2004). Therefore, the measurements of both affinity and $t_{1/2}$ correlated with antigenic potency using this small set of compounds. The study of αManCer, however, is complicated by the fact that in the crystal structures of glycolipid–CD1d complexes, CD1d forms a hydrogen bond with the equatorial 2′OH of galactose. In αManCer, however, this OH group is in the axial position, and therefore αManCer may not bind CD1d as well as αGalCer, thereby affecting TCR affinity and avidity measurements. This is a general issue for these types of studies and controls demonstrating that glycolipid binding to CD1d is more stable than TCR binding to the CD1d–glycolipid complex would be useful.

Vα14i TCR binding to αGalCer–CD1d complexes was not found to be temperature-dependent (Cantu et al. 2003; Sidobre et al. 2004), suggesting that this TCR does not make significant conformational changes in the recognition of αGalCer–CD1d complexes. Conventional αβTCRs, by contrast, make such accommodations in binding to pMHC complexes and they show a temperature dependence of binding (Wu et al. 2002). This is in accordance with the hypothesis that the $V\alpha14i$ TCR binds to a rigid galactose structure together with the CD1d α helices.

Surprisingly, the TCRs of human T cells that recognize αGalCer bound to hCD1d had a K_D ranging between 4.2 and 16.8 µM (Gadola et al. 2006; Kjer-Nielsen et al. 2006), exhibiting an approximately 50-fold reduction in binding strength compared to their mouse counterparts. Moreover, the $t_{1/2}$ of the interaction was on the order of seconds, comparable to TCRs from conventional T cells. The significance of this difference is uncertain, because αGalCer is not a natural antigen, and the affinities of the same mouse and human TCRs for the natural endogenous glycolipids or for exogenous bacterial glycolipids presented by CD1d could be similar. The degree of selection on different portions of the TCR clearly is also different if the mouse and human αGalCer-reactive TCRs are compared. In human, the repertoire of αGalCer-reactive TCRs exhibits more selection for a single Vβ (Vβ11) and a lesser degree of selection for a single Vα chain (Vα24). Substitution of the CDR3β region with three alanines had little effect on the TCR affinity, although a complete swap replacing CDR3 and the Jβ from a peptide-reactive TCR did reduce the binding interaction (Kjer-Nielsen et al. 2006). Therefore, CDR3β amino acids are not critical for the human $V\alpha24i$ TCR, similar to the mouse, although they can exert an influence. There was no difference in αGalCer–hCD1d binding when $V\alpha24i$-positive and -negative TCRs were compared (Gadola et al. 2006), but cells lacking the canonical TCR α chain did not respond either to αGlcCer or iGb3, raising the possibility that there are additional self antigens in humans (Brigl et al. 2006).

9
Avidity Measurement: Analyzing Multimeric Interactions

The relatively high avidity of binding and long $t_{1/2}$ of the interaction were verified by measuring tetramer binding at equilibrium and the decay of tetramer staining of hybridomas and $V\alpha14i$ NKT cells in the thymus (Sidobre et al. 2002; Sim et al. 2003; Stanic et al. 2003). To calculate the avidity of αGalCer/CD1d complexes, cells were incubated with a dose range of the tetramers until equilibrium binding has been achieved, washed and analyzed by flow cytometry for the mean fluorescence intensity of the tetramer. Avidity (K_D) measurements for equilibrium binding of αGalCer/CD1d tetramers ranged from 0.49 to 17.6 nM, stronger binding than has been observed for peptide reactive T cells, despite conventional T cell expression of co-receptors that could increase the avidity of tetramer binding (Garcia et al. 1996). However in two studies, CD4 did not increase the binding to class II tetramers (Crawford et al. 1998; Hamad et al. 1998). Binding of tetrameric complexes of CD1d with additional glycolipids, including αGlcCer, OCH, 4-deoxy (Sidobre et al. 2004; Stanic et al. 2003), and the bacterial ligand GalA-GSL (Wu et al. 2006), to Vα14i NKT cells have also been measured. When loaded into CD1d, all of these compounds have lower avidity interactions than αGalCer–CD1d complexes, corresponding well with the rank order of antigenic potency of the different compounds as well as their TCR affinity measurements.

An intriguing experiment conducted with αGalCer–CD1d tetramers was to measure Hill coefficients to determine if tetramers bound to cells in a cooperative manner (Benlagha et al. 2000; Stanic et al. 2003). Cooperative binding may allow for small concentrations of agonistic glycolipids to sensitively trigger the Vα14i NKT TCR and might help to explain the rapid activity of Vα14i NKT cells after exposure to antigen in vivo. Hill coefficients greater than 1 indicate positive cooperativity, and those with high values (>5) allow the system to exhibit nearly switch-like responsiveness, with maximal responses to very low amounts of activating ligand (Germain 2001). Benlagha et al. observed a Hill coefficient of 4.5 for αGalCer–CD1d tetramer binding to one hybridoma. Stanic et al. obtained Hill coefficients of thymic, splenic, and two-hybridoma NKT cells for αGalCer–CD1d tetramers from 2.09 to 3.17. Thus αGalCer–CD1d tetrameric complexes appear to bind to the TCR on Vα14i NKT cells with moderate cooperativity, more so than for MHC-restricted $CD8^+$ T cells. It would be interesting to determine if the cooperative engagement of the Vα14i TCR with αGalCer–CD1d complexes were influenced by the presence of endogenous glycolipid–CD1d complexes that may be continuously activating Vα14i NKT cells in vivo. Vα14i NKT cells transferred into $CD1d^{-/-}$ mice have been shown to survive (Matsuda et al. 2002; McNab et al. 2005), making this experiment feasible.

A decay of tetramer binding assay has been used to measure the *off*-rate of TCR binding for conventional T cells (Savage et al. 1999; Wang and Altman 2003). To do this for Vα14i NKT cells, αGalCer–CD1d tetramers were incubated with cells until saturation, washed, and the decay of tetramer staining over time was determined by flow cytometry. Two groups measured *off*-rates in this manner, although one group added a blocking CD1d monoclonal antibody to the culture to prevent rebinding of the tetramer to the TCR during the decay period (Sidobre et al. 2002), while the other group added sodium azide to prevent internalization of the TCR with the fluorescent CD1d tetramer complexes, but did not adding a blocking reagent (Stanic et al. 2003). Each method has advantages. Tetramers might rebind to the TCR in the absence of a blocking reagent. Consistent with this hypothesis, in optimizing the tetramer decay assay for $CD8^+$ T cells, it was observed that adding a blocking reagent was essential for the calculation of *off*-rates (Wang and Altman

2003). It is possible, however, that an anti-CD1d antibody might cross-link the tetramers to the $V\alpha 14i$ NKT cells that also express CD1d, thereby resulting in an artificially long $t_{1/2}$. With the inclusion of blocking CD1d antibodies, αGalCer–CD1d complexes did not decay at $4°$C and exhibited a $t_{1/2}$ of 300 min at $37°$C using a hybridoma or thymocytes (Sidobre et al. 2002). Conventional $\alpha\beta$ T cells have relatively fast tetramer *off*-rates that are typically measured at $4°$C (Wang and Altman 2003), with $t_{1/2}$s of 21 and 240 min for 5C.C7 and 2B4 TCR transgenic T cells, respectively (Savage et al. 1999). In the absence of blocking antibody, a shorter $t_{1/2}$ of 16.4–42.1 min for binding to $V\alpha 14i$ NKT hybridomas was observed at $37°$C. The $t_{1/2}$ of peptide/K^b tetramers specific for CTL clones measured in parallel was 2.1–9.4 min. The data suggest that the absence of blocking antibody may not artificially prolong the $t_{1/2}$ due to tetramer rebinding, but it is not possible to directly compare these two sets of results, as they were performed in different laboratories using different $V\alpha 14i$ NKT hybridomas. Regardless of these differences in methodology, the data from both studies are consistent with a higher avidity interaction for the $V\alpha 14i$ TCR compared to conventional T cells.

10
TCR Crystal Structures

Crystal structures of several human TCRs that bind αGalCer–hCD1d tetramers recently have been solved, providing a breakthrough in the understanding of glycolipid antigen recognition. The structures solved include several $V\alpha 24i$ TCRs and two $V\beta 11$ TCRs with noncanonical $V\alpha$ segments, either $V\alpha 3.1$ or $V\alpha 10.1$, rearranged to $J\alpha 18$ (Gadola et al. 2006; Kjer-Nielsen et al. 2006). One of the $V\alpha 24i$ TCRs (NKT12) (Kjer-Nielsen et al. 2006) is depicted in Fig. 3, with a view from the side and from the perspective of CD1d. Each TCR had an architecture similar to conventional TCRs, with two immunoglobulin (Ig)-like V domains ($V\alpha$ and $V\beta$) and two constant ($C\alpha$ and $C\beta$) domains. The glycolipid–CD1d-specific binding surface of the TCR contains a significantly electropositive, 120 $Å^3$ pocket formed by CDR1α, CDR3α, CDR1β, and CDR3β. Certain amino acids found only in a few TCR $V\alpha$ genes, including human $V\alpha 24$ and mouse $V\alpha 14$, and in human and mouse $J\alpha 18$ help to form this pocket. Overall, this pocket is similar regardless of presence of $V\alpha 24$ (Gadola et al. 2006). It has been proposed that this preformed cavity is the appropriate size for binding a small polar moiety, such as a galactose ring, that might protrude from the CD1d-binding groove. Kjer-Nielsen and colleagues predict that the volume of this pocket is flexible and would be influenced by the sequence of CDR3β (Kjer-Nielsen et al.

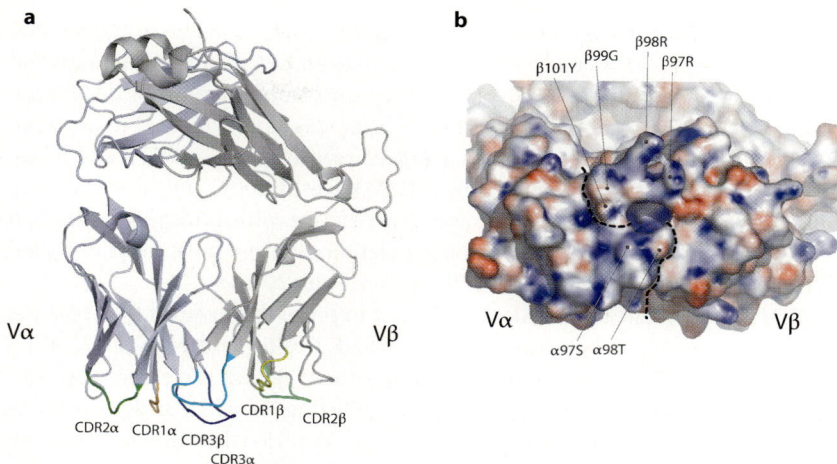

Fig. 3a, b View of a Vα24*i* TCR from the side and from the CD1d perspective. **a** Side view of the NKT12 Vα24*i*/Vβ11 human αβ NKT TCR. The α chain (*lavender*) and β chain (*grey*) are labeled along with the CDRs: CDR1α (*dark green*), CDR2α (*orange*), CDR3α (*dark blue*), CDR1β (*yellow*), CDR2β (*light green*), and CDR3β (*light blue*). **b** Looking down at the electrostatic potential of the NKT12 Vα24*i*/Vβ11 human αβ NKT TCR. The 120 Å³ pocket is visible in the *center*: the amino acids of the CDR regions that form the pocket are labeled and a *dashed line* shows the α/β boundary. (The figure is based on the coordinates published originally in Kjer-Nielsen et al. 2006)

2006). Models of TCR docking in a diagonal mode have been constructed, and these suggest the invariant CDR3α loop is biased to bind the ligand as well as CD1d. The data are consistent with a conformational change of the CDR3 loops of the human NKT cell TCR to the glycolipid ligand, which was not predicted from the biophysical data on mouse Vα14*i* TCR binding, but it is not certain if this reflects a species difference. Furthermore, it remains unknown how large glycolipids, such as iGb3, will interact with the Vα24*i* TCR, but the Vα24*i* TCR might accommodate this trisaccharide antigen by altering the conformation of CDR3β. Perhaps the suboptimal recognition of endogenous ligands such as iGb3 causes the natural, low-level autoreactivity that characterizes Vα24*i* and Vα14*i* NKT cells.

11
Diversity in the CD1d-Reactive TCR Repertoire

Although nearly all Vα14*i* NKT cells are αGalCer-reactive (Gui et al. 2001), there are subspecificities that provide some diversity in the antigen reactivity;

presumably this heterogeneity is due to β chain diversity. Approximately 25% of splenic Vα14i NKT cells were reported to bind to CD1d tetramers loaded with a mycobacterial glycolipid, phosphatidylinositol tetramannoside (PIM$_4$), although the PIM$_4$-reactive proportion in liver was closer to 1% (Fischer et al. 2004). Moreover, a small subset of αGalCer-reactive Vα14i NKT cells cross-reacts with the autologous ganglioside GD3 (Wu et al. 2003) and several mouse and human αGalCer clones that are also reactive with phospholipids such as phosphatidylinositol and phosphatidylethanolamine have been reported (Brigl et al. 2006; Gumperz et al. 2000; Rauch et al. 2003).

CD1d-dependent NKT cells that do not express the invariant Vα14-Jα18 rearrangement are sometimes called type II NKT cells (Godfrey et al. 2004). It has not been possible to precisely enumerate these cells in mixed populations, although they were detected initially by analyzing T cell hybridomas made from the residual CD4$^+$ population in MHC class II-deficient mice (Cardell et al. 1995; Park et al. 2001), but they have been found in several other contexts (Behar et al. 1999; Jahng et al. 2004). For example, peripheral T cell clones stimulated by CD1d transfectants of the mouse T cell lymphoma RMAS, cells which are deficient for the transporter associated with antigen processing, predominantly expressed Vβ8 paired with Vα22, Vα11, Vα14, Vα10, or Vα17 (Behar et al. 1999). Those Vα14/Vβ8 expressing T cells did not use the canonical Vα14-Jα18 junction and they were reactive against CD1d-transfected RMAS without the addition of an exogenous glycolipid antigen. Although these CD1d-dependent cells that do not express a Vα14i TCR unquestionably have more variable TCRs, in one study a Vα3.2–Jα9 rearrangement was most common in this subpopulation (Park et al. 2001). If the Vα3.2-Jα9 TCR were characteristic of a significant non-Vα14i but CD1d-restricted T cell population, then they should be easier to detect in mice deficient in Jα18$^{-/-}$ mice that lack Vα14i NKT cells. Likewise, mice with a limited Vα14i NKT repertoire, such as the HexB$^{-/-}$ mice, could be informative to examine for the presence of non-Vα14i CD1d-restricted T cells.

Vα14i NKT cells are dependent on the ability of CD1d to traffic to endosomes for their selection (Chiu et al. 2002) and autoreactivity (Chiu et al. 1999). Type II NKT cells, which have more diverse TCRs and which therefore do not usually express a Vα14i TCR, are not dependent on the ability of CD1d to traffic to endosomes for their autoreactivity (Chiu et al. 1999). The functional capability of type II NKT cells is best revealed by comparing CD1d$^{-/-}$ mice to Jα18$^{-/-}$ mice, which lack only the type I NKT cells. The results from studies of the hepatitis virus response (Baron et al. 2002) and the suppression of tumor rejection (Terabe et al. 2006) suggested that the type II cells with more diverse TCRs are functionally distinct from their type I NKT cell counterparts. The analysis of CD1d-reactive clones from human bone marrow suggests that T lymphocytes expressing the invariant TCR may be less abundant than those with more variable TCRs (Exley et al. 2001).

The CD1d-reactive T cells with diverse TCRs are likely to recognize diverse antigens. This was inferred initially from the requirement for different types of APC by hybridomas from this population (Cardell et al. 1995). A population of non-Vα14i expressing T cells is specific for sulfatide–CD1d complexes. Sulfatide is β–galactosylceramide, with the galactose ring sulfated at the 3 position (Fig. 2). These cells are enriched in the central nervous system (CNS) during experimental autoimmune encephalomyelitis (EAE), a rodent model for multiple sclerosis, and they have been reported to be important in the prevention of EAE after in vivo stimulation with sulfatide (Jahng et al. 2004). Tetramers of sulfatide bound to CD1d detect approximately 5% the number of αGalCer–CD1d-reactive cells, and the two glycolipid-reactive T cell populations do not overlap, as shown by several criteria including dual αGalCer–CD1d and sulfatide–CD1d tetramer staining, as well as the detection of sulfatide reactive T cells in $J\alpha18^{-/-}$ mice. There is little information on the TCR repertoire of these lymphocytes, although a panel of $V\alpha3.2^+$ NKT cell hybridomas did not respond to sulfatide–CD1d complexes. CD1a molecules can present lipopeptides (Moody et al. 2004; Zajonc et al. 2005b), providing a precedent for the recognition of nonpeptidic antigens other than glycolipids. Therefore the antigens recognized by CD1d reactive cells need not be confined to glycolipids. In fact, a human T cell clone with a noncanonical $V\alpha2/V\beta21$ TCR was found to be specific for a nonlipidic, sulfonate-containing molecule presented by CD1d (Van Rhijn et al. 2004).

12
TCRs Reactive with Group I CD1 Molecules

As discussed elsewhere in this volume, the T cells reactive with group I CD1 molecules recognize diverse antigens including mycolic acids, phospholipids, glycosphingolipids, polyisoprenol glycolipids, diacylated sulfoglycolipids, and lipopeptides (Brigl and Brenner 2004). The concept has emerged that the different human CD1 isoforms—CD1a, CD1b, and CD1c—survey different endosomal compartments (Sugita et al. 1999). Moreover, the crystal structures indicate that the capacity for binding lipid antigens varies, with CD1b having the biggest groove and capable of binding lipids that are more than 80 carbons long (Gadola et al. 2002), while CD1a has a much smaller antigen-binding groove (Zajonc et al. 2003). Consistent with the functional and structural diversity of the CD1 isoforms, the group I CD1-reactive T cells are a diverse set of lymphocytes. They can express either CD4 or CD8 or they are double negative, they can be reactive to self antigen, foreign antigen, or both (Vincent et al. 2005). Although an αβ TCR is most frequently expressed, some γδ T cells expressing Vδ1 are reactive to CD1c (Spada et al. 2000) and αβ T cells restricted to the CD1a, CD1b, or CD1c are highly diverse, with junctional diversity in both the α and β chains and N nucleotide additions (Grant et al. 1999; Vincent et al. 2005). Like CD1d, CD1a, CD1b, and CD1c present autologous and foreign glycolipid antigens to αβ T cells, and CD1-mediated antigen recognition occurs during the natural course of bacterial infection in humans (Gilleron et al. 2004; Moody et al. 2000a, 2000b; Ulrichs et al. 2003). The antigens presented by group I CD1 molecules to reactive T cells include foreign antigens from the mycobacterial cell wall and from plant pollen (Agea et al. 2005) and autologous glycosphingolipids (Shamshiev et al. 1999; Shamshiev et al. 2000).

13
Mucosal Invariant T Cells

Mucosal invariant T cells (MAIT) are a second population of invariant NKT cells found in mice and humans. In mice, they express an invariant Vα19-Jα33 rearranged TCR, with a highly similar Vα7.2–Jα33 rearrangement in humans, and they are reactive to MR1, a nonpolymorphic MHC class I-like antigen-presenting molecule. Interestingly, CD1d and MR1 are encoded in the same region of chromosome 1 in a locus paralogous to the MHC (Shiina et al. 2001). MR1 is highly conserved, with more than 89% sequence identity at the protein level in the α1 and α2 domains when mice and humans are compared (Treiner et al. 2005). Mouse CD1d, by contrast, is only approximately 61% identical at the protein level for the α1 and α2 domains compared to its human ortholog (Brossay et al. 1998). Although the study of Vα19i MAIT cells is less advanced compared to CD1d-reactive Vα14i NKT cells, Vα19i MAIT cells share a number of features in common with their CD1d-reactive counterparts. For example, in mice the majority of these cells are NK1.1$^+$ and DN, although some express CD4, they express a restricted set of Vβ regions including Vβ8.2 and Vβ6, they are selected by hematopoietic cells in the thymus, and they rapidly produce effector cytokines such as IL-4 after TCR activation (Kawachi et al. 2006; Treiner et al. 2005). Despite these similarities, Vα19i MAIT cells clearly are functionally distinct from Vα14i NKT cells, as Vα19i MAIT cells are uniquely dependent upon B lymphocytes and the gut flora for their normal accumulation in the periphery, and they are enriched in the intestinal lamina propria (Kawachi et al. 2006; Treiner et al. 2005). Recent papers suggest that Vα19i MAIT cells are reactive to mannose-containing glycolipids, including αManCer, when presented by MR1 (Okamoto et al. 2005; Shimamura et al. 2006), but this requires further confirmation.

14
Implications and Unresolved Questions

Although our understanding of glycolipid antigen recognition has progressed rapidly, important questions remain unanswered. A primary issue is the extent to which the invariant TCRs have to be considered separately from the more variable TCRs. The significance of the cooperative binding phenomenon remains to be determined and it is unknown how the glycolipid-reactive TCRs act independently of the known co-receptors in DN cells. It is also not known why CDR3α tends to be conserved and not CDR3β, and we do not know how oligosaccharides such as iGb3 are accommodated by the TCR. Human Vα24i TCRs have a reduced affinity for αGalCer presented by CD1d, but it is not known if this is also true for the response to natural autologous or foreign glycolipid antigens. The resolution of a trimolecular structures of TCR bound to the complex of glycolipid plus CD1 constitutes the next likely breakthrough, and combined with other findings, an intense pace of continued progress will expand knowledge of glycolipid antigen recognition.

Acknowledgements This review was funded by National Institutes of Health grants AI45053 (to M.K.) and AI062015 (to B.A.S.). We gratefully acknowledge the help of Dirk Zajonc in constructing Fig. 3. This is manuscript number 775 from the La Jolla Institute for Allergy and Immunology.

Notes added in proof   Three manuscripts have been published since the submission of this review that pertain dreirectly to the topics addressed; here we have summarized these recent findings. These include the first identification of a novel class of CD1d-binding Vα14i/Vα24i NKT cell antigens, those of the diacylglycerol family from *Borrelia burgdorferi* bacteria . Secondly, an analysis of several mouse models of lysosomal glycosphingolipid storage diseases revealed, in each mouse model, an impaired development of Vα14i NKT cells. This suggests that the paucity of Vα14i NKT cells in Hexosaminidase B deficient mice could be due to a problem in CD1d trafficking and/or a more general defect in glycolipid antigen acquisition, rather than the inability to synthesize the self antigen iGb3 . Finally, a new study of the MR1-restricted Vα19i MAIT cells suggested that TCR transgenic Vα19i MAIT cells could inhibit the induction and progression of experimental autoimmune encephalomyelitis (EAE) , which is a mouse model of multiple sclerosis.

References

Agea E, Russano A, Bistoni O, Mannucci R, Nicoletti I, Corazzi L, Postle AD, De Libero G, Porcelli SA, Spinozzi F (2005) Human CD1-restricted T cell recognition of lipids from pollens. J Exp Med 202:295–308

Baron JL, Gardiner L, Nishimura S, Shinkai K, Locksley R, Ganem D (2002) Activation of a nonclassical NKT cell subset in a transgenic mouse model of hepatitis B virus infection. Immunity 16:583–594

Behar SM, Podrebarac TA, Roy CJ, Wang CR, Brenner MB (1999) Diverse TCRs recognize murine CD1. J Immunol 162:161–167

Bendelac A, Killeen N, Littman DR, Schwartz RH (1994) A subset of CD4+ thymocytes selected by MHC class I molecules. Science 263:1774–1778

Bendelac A, Rivera MN, Park SH, Roark JH (1997) Mouse CD1-specific NK1 T cells: development, specificity, and function. Annu Rev Immunol 15:535–562

Benlagha K, Weiss A, Beavis A, Teyton L, Bendelac A (2000) In vivo identification of glycolipid antigen-specific T cells using fluorescent CD1d tetramers. J Exp Med 191:1895–1903

Benlagha K, Kyin T, Beavis A, Teyton L, Bendelac A (2002) A thymic precursor to the NK T cell lineage. Science 296:553–555

Brigl M, Brenner MB (2004) CD1: antigen presentation and T cell function. Annu Rev Immunol 22:817–890

Brigl M, van den Elzen P, Chen X, Meyers JH, Wu D, Wong CH, Reddington F, Illarianov PA, Besra GS, Brenner MB, Gumperz JE (2006) Conserved and heterogeneous lipid antigen specificities of CD1d-restricted NKT cell receptors. J Immunol 176:3625–3634

Brossay L, Kronenberg M (1999) Highly conserved antigen-presenting function of CD1d molecules. Immunogenetics 50:146–151

Brossay L, Chioda M, Burdin N, Koezuka Y, Casorati G, Dellabona P, Kronenberg M (1998) CD1d-mediated recognition of an alpha-galactosylceramide by natural killer T cells is highly conserved through mammalian evolution. J Exp Med 188:1521–1528

Burdin N, Brossay L, Degano M, Iijima H, Gui M, Wilson IA, Kronenberg M (2000) Structural requirements for antigen presentation by mouse CD1. Proc Natl Acad Sci U S A 97:10156–10561

Cantu C 3rd, Benlagha K, Savage PB, Bendelac A, Teyton L (2003) The paradox of immune molecular recognition of alpha-galactosylceramide: low affinity, low specificity for CD1d, high affinity for alpha beta TCRs. J Immunol 170:4673–4682

Cardell S, Tangri S, Chan S, Kronenberg M, Benoist C, Mathis D (1995) CD1-restricted CD4+ T cells in major histocompatibility complex class II-deficient mice. J Exp Med 182:993–1004

Chiu YH, Jayawardena J, Weiss A, Lee D, Park SH, Dautry-Varsat A, Bendelac A (1999) Distinct subsets of CD1d-restricted T cells recognize self-antigens loaded in different cellular compartments. J Exp Med 189:103–110

Chiu YH, Park SH, Benlagha K, Forestier C, Jayawardena-Wolf J, Savage PB, Teyton L, Bendelac A (2002) Multiple defects in antigen presentation and T cell development by mice expressing cytoplasmic tail-truncated CD1d. Nat Immunol 3:55–60

Chun T, Page MJ, Gapin L, Matsuda JL, Xu H, Nguyen H, Kang HS, Stanic AK, Joyce S, Koltun WA, Chorney MJ, Kronenberg M, Wang CR (2003) CD1d-expressing dendritic cells but not thymic epithelial cells can mediate negative selection of NKT cells. J Exp Med 197:907–918

Crawford F, Kozono H, White J, Marrack P, Kappler J (1998) Detection of antigen-specific T cells with multivalent soluble class II MHC covalent peptide complexes. Immunity 8:675–682

Davis MM, Boniface JJ, Reich Z, Lyons D, Hampl J, Arden B, Chien Y (1998) Ligand recognition by alpha beta T cell receptors. Annu Rev Immunol 16:523–544

Dellabona P, Padovan E, Casorati G, Brockhaus M, Lanzavecchia A (1994) An invariant V alpha 24-J alpha Q/V beta 11 T cell receptor is expressed in all individuals by clonally expanded CD4⁻8⁻ T cells. J Exp Med 180:1171–1176

Elewaut D, Lawton AP, Nagarajan NA, Maverakis E, Khurana A, Honing S, Benedict CA, Sercarz E, Bakke O, Kronenberg M, Prigozy TI (2003) The adaptor protein AP-3 is required for CD1d-mediated antigen presentation of glycosphingolipids and development of Valpha14i NKT cells. J Exp Med 198:1133–1146

Exley M, Garcia J, Balk SP, Porcelli S (1997) Requirements for CD1d recognition by human invariant Valpha24⁺ CD4⁻CD8⁻ T cells. J Exp Med 186:109–120

Exley MA, Tahir SM, Cheng O, Shaulov A, Joyce R, Avigan D, Sackstein R, Balk SP (2001) A major fraction of human bone marrow lymphocytes are Th2-like CD1d-reactive T cells that can suppress mixed lymphocyte responses. J Immunol 167:5531–5534

Fischer K, Scotet E, Niemeyer M, Koebernick H, Zerrahn J, Maillet S, Hurwitz R, Kursar M, Bonneville M, Kaufmann SH, Schaible UE (2004) Mycobacterial phosphatidylinositol mannoside is a natural antigen for CD1d-restricted T cells. Proc Natl Acad Sci U S A 101:10685–10690

Gadola SD, Zaccai NR, Harlos K, Shepherd D, Castro-Palomino JC, Ritter G, Schmidt RR, Jones EY, Cerundolo V (2002) Structure of human CD1b with bound ligands at 2.3 A, a maze for alkyl chains. Nat Immunol 3:721–726

Gadola SD, Koch M, Marles-Wright J, Lissin NM, Shepherd D, Matulis G, Harlos K, Villiger PM, Stuart DI, Jakobsen BK, Cerundolo V, Jones EY (2006) Structure and binding kinetics of three different human CD1d-alpha-galactosylceramide-specific T cell receptors. J Exp Med 203:699–710

Gangadharan D, Cheroutre H (2004) The CD8 isoform CD8alphaalpha is not a functional homologue of the TCR co-receptor CD8alphabeta. Curr Opin Immunol 16:264–270

Garcia KC, Scott CA, Brunmark A, Carbone FR, Peterson PA, Wilson IA, Teyton L (1996) CD8 enhances formation of stable T-cell receptor/MHC class I molecule complexes. Nature 384:577–81

Germain RN (2001) The art of the probable: system control in the adaptive immune system. Science 293:240–245

Giabbai B, Sidobre S, Crispin MD, Sanchez-Ruiz Y, Bachi A, Kronenberg M, Wilson IA, Degano M (2005) Crystal structure of mouse CD1d bound to the self ligand phosphatidylcholine: a molecular basis for NKT cell activation. J Immunol 175:977–984

Gilleron M, Stenger S, Mazorra Z, Wittke F, Mariotti S, Bohmer G, Prandi J, Mori L, Puzo G, De Libero G (2004) Diacylated sulfoglycolipids are novel mycobacterial antigens stimulating CD1-restricted T cells during infection with *Mycobacterium tuberculosis*. J Exp Med 199:649–659

Godfrey DI, MacDonald HR, Kronenberg M, Smyth MJ, Van Kaer L (2004) NKT cells: what's in a name? Nat Rev Immunol 4:231–237

Goff RD, Gao Y, Mattner J, Zhou D, Yin N, Cantu C 3rd, Teyton L, Bendelac A, Savage PB (2004) Effects of lipid chain lengths in alpha-galactosylceramides on cytokine release by natural killer T cells. J Am Chem Soc 126:13602–13603

Grant EP, Degano M, Rosat JP, Stenger S, Modlin RL, Wilson IA, Porcelli SA, Brenner MB (1999) Molecular recognition of lipid antigens by T cell receptors. J Exp Med 189:195–205

Gui M, Li J, Wen LJ, Hardy RR, Hayakawa K (2001) TCR beta chain influences but does not solely control autoreactivity of V alpha 14J281T cells. J Immunol 167:6239–6246

Gumperz JE, Roy C, Makowska A, Lum D, Sugita M, Podrebarac T, Koezuka Y, Porcelli SA, Cardell S, Brenner MB, Behar SM (2000) Murine CD1d-restricted T cell recognition of cellular lipids. Immunity 12:211–221

Hamad AR, O'Herrin SM, Lebowitz MS, Srikrishnan A, Bieler J, Schneck J, Pardoll D (1998) Potent T cell activation with dimeric peptide-major histocompatibility complex class II ligand: the role of CD4 coreceptor. J Exp Med 188:1633–1640

Jahng A, Maricic I, Aguilera C, Cardell S, Halder RC, Kumar V (2004) Prevention of autoimmunity by targeting a distinct, noninvariant CD1d-reactive T cell population reactive to sulfatide. J Exp Med 199:947–957

Kamada N, Iijima H, Kimura K, Harada M, Shimizu E, Motohashi S, Kawano T, Shinkai H, Nakayama T, Sakai T, Brossay L, Kronenberg M, Taniguchi M (2001) Crucial amino acid residues of mouse CD1d for glycolipid ligand presentation to V(alpha)14 NKT cells. Int Immunol 13:853–861

Kawachi I, Maldonado J, Strader C, Gilfillan S (2006) MR1-restricted V alpha 19i mucosal-associated invariant T cells are innate T cells in the gut lamina propria that provide a rapid and diverse cytokine response. J Immunol 176:1618–1627

Kersh GJ, Kersh EN, Fremont DH, Allen PM (1998) High- and low-potency ligands with similar affinities for the TCR: the importance of kinetics in TCR signaling. Immunity 9:817–826

Kinjo Y, Wu D, Kim G, Xing GW, Poles MA, Ho DD, Tsuji M, Kawahara K, Wong CH, Kronenberg M (2005) Recognition of bacterial glycosphingolipids by natural killer T cells. Nature 434:520–525

Kjer-Nielsen L, Borg NA, Pellicci DG, Beddoe T, Kostenko L, Clements CS, Williamson NA, Smyth MJ, Besra GS, Reid HH, Bharadwaj M, Godfrey DI, Rossjohn J, McCluskey J (2006) A structural basis for selection and cross-species reactivity of the semi-invariant NKT cell receptor in CD1d/glycolipid recognition. J Exp Med 203:661–673

Koch M, Stronge VS, Shepherd D, Gadola SD, Mathew B, Ritter G, Fersht AR, Besra GS, Schmidt RR, Jones EY, Cerundolo V (2005) The crystal structure of human CD1d with and without alpha-galactosylceramide. Nat Immunol 6:819–826

Kronenberg M, Gapin L (2002) The unconventional lifestyle of NKT cells. Nat Rev Immunol 2:557–568

Kunisaki Y, Tanaka Y, Sanui T, Inayoshi A, Noda M, Nakayama T, Harada M, Taniguchi M, Sasazuki T, Fukui Y (2006) DOCK2 is required in T cell precursors for development of Valpha14 NK T cells. J Immunol 176:4640–4645

Lantz O, Bendelac A (1994) An invariant T cell receptor alpha chain is used by a unique subset of major histocompatibility complex class I-specific CD4+ and CD4−8− T cells in mice and humans. J Exp Med 180:1097–1106

Leishman AJ, Gapin L, Capone M, Palmer E, MacDonald HR, Kronenberg M, Cheroutre H (2002) Precursors of functional MHC class I- or class II-restricted CD8alphaalpha(+) T cells are positively selected in the thymus by agonist self-peptides. Immunity 16:355–364

Liu Y, Goff RD, Zhou D, Mattner J, Sullivan BA, Khurana A, Cantu C 3rd, Ravkov EV, Ibegbu CC, Altman JD, Teyton L, Bendelac A, Savage PB (2006) A modified alpha-galactosyl ceramide for staining and stimulating natural killer T cells. J Immunol Methods 312:34–39

Makino Y, Kanno R, Ito T, Higashino K, Taniguchi M (1995) Predominant expression of invariant V alpha 14+ TCR alpha chain in NK1.1+ T cell populations. Int Immunol 7:1157–1161

Matsuda JL, Gapin L (2005) Developmental program of mouse Valpha14i NKT cells. Curr Opin Immunol 17:122–130

Matsuda JL, Gapin L, Fazilleau N, Warren K, Naidenko OV, Kronenberg M (2001) Natural killer T cells reactive to a single glycolipid exhibit a highly diverse T cell receptor beta repertoire and small clone size. Proc Natl Acad Sci U S A 98:12636–12641

Matsuda JL, Gapin L, Sidobre S, Kieper WC, Tan JT, Ceredig R, Surh CD, Kronenberg M (2002) Homeostasis of V alpha 14i NKT cells. Nat Immunol 3:966–974

Matsui K, Boniface JJ, Steffner P, Reay PA, Davis MM (1994) Kinetics of T-cell receptor binding to peptide/I-Ek complexes: correlation of the dissociation rate with T-cell responsiveness. Proc Natl Acad Sci U S A 91:12862–12866

Mattner J, Debord KL, Ismail N, Goff RD, Cantu C 3rd, Zhou D, Saint-Mezard P, Wang V, Gao Y, Yin N, Hoebe K, Schneewind O, Walker D, Beutler B, Teyton L, Savage PB, Bendelac A (2005) Exogenous and endogenous glycolipid antigens activate NKT cells during microbial infections. Nature 434:525–529

McNab FW, Berzins SP, Pellicci DG, Kyparissoudis K, Field K, Smyth MJ, Godfrey DI (2005) The influence of CD1d in postselection NKT cell maturation and homeostasis. J Immunol 175:3762–3768

Moody DB, Guy MR, Grant E, Cheng TY, Brenner MB, Besra GS, Porcelli SA (2000a) CD1b-mediated T cell recognition of a glycolipid antigen generated from mycobacterial lipid and host carbohydrate during infection. J Exp Med 192:965–976

Moody DB, Ulrichs T, Muhlecker W, Young DC, Gurcha SS, Grant E, Rosat JP, Brenner MB, Costello CE, Besra GS, Porcelli SA (2000b) CD1c-mediated T-cell recognition of isoprenoid glycolipids in *Mycobacterium tuberculosis* infection. Nature 404:884–888

Moody DB, Young DC, Cheng TY, Rosat JP, Roura-Mir C, O'Connor PB, Zajonc DM, Walz A, Miller MJ, Levery SB, Wilson IA, Costello CE, Brenner MB (2004) T cell activation by lipopeptide antigens. Science 303:527–531

Nikolich-Zugich J, Slifka MK, Messaoudi I (2004) The many important facets of T-cell repertoire diversity. Nat Rev Immunol 4:123–132

Okamoto N, Kanie O, Huang YY, Fujii R, Watanabe H, Shimamura M (2005) Synthetic alpha-mannosyl ceramide as a potent stimulant for an NKT cell repertoire bearing the invariant Valpha19-Jalpha26 TCR alpha chain. Chem Biol 12:677–683

Oki S, Chiba A, Yamamura T, Miyake S (2004) The clinical implication and molecular mechanism of preferential IL-4 production by modified glycolipid-stimulated NKT cells. J Clin Invest 113:1631–1640

Park SH, Weiss A, Benlagha K, Kyin T, Teyton L, Bendelac A (2001) The mouse CD1d-restricted repertoire is dominated by a few autoreactive T cell receptor families. J Exp Med 193:893–904

Pellicci DG, Hammond KJ, Uldrich AP, Baxter AG, Smyth MJ, Godfrey DI (2002) A natural killer T (NKT) cell developmental pathway involving a thymus-dependent NK1.1(–)CD4(+) CD1d-dependent precursor stage. J Exp Med 195:835–844

Porcelli S, Yockey CE, Brenner MB, Balk SP (1993) Analysis of T cell antigen receptor (TCR) expression by human peripheral blood CD4⁻8⁻ alpha/beta T cells demonstrates preferential use of several V beta genes and an invariant TCR alpha chain. J Exp Med 178:1–16

Porcelli SA, Modlin RL (1999) The CD1 system: antigen-presenting molecules for T cell recognition of lipids and glycolipids. Annu Rev Immunol 17:297–329

Pry E, Naidenko O, Miyake S, Yamamura T, Berberich I, Cardell S, Kronenberg M, Herrmann T (2006) The complementarity determining region 2 of BV8S2 (Vb8.2) contributes to antigen recognition by rat invariant NK T cell TCR. J Immunol 176:7447–7455

Rauch J, Gumperz J, Robinson C, Skold M, Roy C, Young DC, Lafleur M, Moody DB, Brenner MB, Costello CE, Behar SM (2003) Structural features of the acyl chain determine self-phospholipid antigen recognition by a CD1d-restricted invariant NKT (iNKT) cell. J Biol Chem 278:47508–47515

Ronet C, Mempel M, Thieblemont N, Lehuen A, Kourilsky P, Gachelin G (2001) Role of the complementarity-determining region 3 (CDR3) of the TCR-beta chains associated with the V alpha 14 semi-invariant TCR alpha-chain in the selection of CD4+ NK T Cells. J Immunol 166:1755–1762

Savage PA, Boniface JJ, Davis MM (1999) A kinetic basis for T cell receptor repertoire selection during an immune response. Immunity 10:485–492

Schumann J, Voyle RB, Wei BY, MacDonald HR (2003) Cutting edge: influence of the TCR V beta domain on the avidity of CD1d:alpha-galactosylceramide binding by invariant V alpha 14 NKT cells. J Immunol 170:5815–5819

Schumann J, Pittoni P, Tonti E, Macdonald HR, Dellabona P, Casorati G (2005) Targeted expression of human CD1d in transgenic mice reveals independent roles for thymocytes and thymic APCs in positive and negative selection of Valpha14i NKT cells. J Immunol 175:7303–7310

Shamshiev A, Donda A, Carena I, Mori L, Kappos L, De Libero G (1999) Self glycolipids as T-cell autoantigens. Eur J Immunol 29:1667–1675

Shamshiev A, Donda A, Prigozy TI, Mori L, Chigorno V, Benedict CA, Kappos L, Sonnino S, Kronenberg M, De Libero G (2000) The alphabeta T cell response to self-glycolipids shows a novel mechanism of CD1b loading and a requirement for complex oligosaccharides. Immunity 13:255–264

Shiina T, Ando A, Suto Y, Kasai F, Shigenari A, Takishima N, Kikkawa E, Iwata K, Kuwano Y, Kitamura Y, Matsuzawa Y, Sano K, Nogami M, Kawata H, Li S, Fukuzumi Y, Yamazaki M, Tashiro H, Tamiya G, Kohda A, Okumura K, Ikemura T, Soeda E, Mizuki N, Kimura M, Bahram S, Inoko H (2001) Genomic anatomy of a premier major histocompatibility complex paralogous region on chromosome 1q21-q22. Genome Res 11:789–802

Shimamura M, Ohteki T, Beutner U, MacDonald HR (1997) Lack of directed V alpha 14-J alpha 281 rearrangements in NK1+ T cells. Eur J Immunol 27:1576–1579

Shimamura M, Okamoto N, Huang YY, Yasuoka J, Morita K, Nishiyama A, Amano Y, Mishina T (2006) Induction of promotive rather than suppressive immune responses from a novel NKT cell repertoire Valpha19 NKT cell with alpha-mannosyl ceramide analogues consisting of the immunosuppressant ISP-I as the sphingosine unit. Eur J Med Chem 41:569–576

Sidobre S, Naidenko OV, Sim BC, Gascoigne NR, Garcia KC, Kronenberg M (2002) The V alpha 14 NKT cell TCR exhibits high-affinity binding to a glycolipid/CD1d complex. J Immunol 169:1340–1348

Sidobre S, Hammond KJ, Benazet-Sidobre L, Maltsev SD, Richardson SK, Ndonye RM, Howell AR, Sakai T, Besra GS, Porcelli SA, Kronenberg M (2004) The T cell antigen receptor expressed by Valpha14i NKT cells has a unique mode of glycosphingolipid antigen recognition. Proc Natl Acad Sci U S A 101:12254–12259

Sim BC, Holmberg K, Sidobre S, Naidenko O, Niederberger N, Marine SD, Kronenberg M, Gascoigne NR (2003) Surprisingly minor influence of TRAV11 (Valpha14) polymorphism on NK T-receptor mCD1/alpha-galactosylceramide binding kinetics. Immunogenetics 54:874–883

Spada FM, Grant EP, Peters PJ, Sugita M, Melian A, Leslie DS, Lee HK, van Donselaar E, Hanson DA, Krensky AM, Majdic O, Porcelli SA, Morita CT, Brenner MB (2000) Self-recognition of CD1 by gamma/delta T cells: implications for innate immunity. J Exp Med 191:937–948

Sriram V, Du W, Gervay-Hague J, Brutkiewicz RR (2005) Cell wall glycosphingolipids of Sphingomonas paucimobilis are CD1d-specific ligands for NKT cells. Eur J Immunol 35:1692–1701

Stanic AK, Shashidharamurthy R, Bezbradica JS, Matsuki N, Yoshimura Y, Miyake S, Choi EY, Schell TD, Van Kaer L, Tevethia SS, Roopenian DC, Yamamura T, Joyce S (2003) Another view of T cell antigen recognition: cooperative engagement of glycolipid antigens by Va14Ja18 natural T(iNKT) cell receptor [corrected]. J Immunol 171:4539–4551

Sugita M, Grant EP, van Donselaar E, Hsu VW, Rogers RA, Peters PJ, Brenner MB (1999) Separate pathways for antigen presentation by CD1 molecules. Immunity 11:743–752

Sullivan BA, Kraj P, Weber DA, Ignatowicz L, Jensen PE (2002) Positive selection of a Qa-1-restricted T cell receptor with specificity for insulin. Immunity 17:95–105

Terabe M, Khanna C, Bose S, Melchionda F, Mendoza A, Mackall CL, Helman LJ, Berzofsky JA (2006) CD1d-restricted natural killer T cells can down-regulate tumor immunosurveillance independent of interleukin-4 receptor-signal transducer and activator of transcription 6 or transforming growth factor-beta. Cancer Res 66:3869–3875

Terszowski G, Muller SM, Bleul CC, Blum C, Schirmbeck R, Reimann J, Pasquier LD, Amagai T, Boehm T, Rodewald HR (2006) Evidence for a functional second thymus in mice. Science 312:284–287

Treiner E, Duban L, Bahram S, Radosavljevic M, Wanner V, Tilloy F, Affaticati P, Gilfillan S, Lantz O (2003) Selection of evolutionarily conserved mucosal-associated invariant T cells by MR1. Nature 422:164–169

Treiner E, Duban L, Moura IC, Hansen T, Gilfillan S, Lantz O (2005) Mucosal-associated invariant T (MAIT) cells: an evolutionarily conserved T cell subset. Microbes Infect 7:552–559

Ulrichs T, Moody DB, Grant E, Kaufmann SH, Porcelli SA (2003) T-cell responses to CD1-presented lipid antigens in humans with *Mycobacterium tuberculosis* infection. Infect Immun 71:3076–3087

Urdahl KB, Sun JC, Bevan MJ (2002) Positive selection of MHC class Ib-restricted CD8(+) T cells on hematopoietic cells. Nat Immunol 3:772–779

Van Rhijn I, Young DC, Im JS, Levery SB, Illarionov PA, Besra GS, Porcelli SA, Gumperz J, Cheng TY, Moody DB (2004) CD1d-restricted T cell activation by nonlipidic small molecules. Proc Natl Acad Sci U S A 101:13578–13583

Vincent MS, Xiong X, Grant EP, Peng W, Brenner MB (2005) CD1a-, b-, and c-restricted TCRs recognize both self and foreign antigens. J Immunol 175:6344–6351

Wang XL, Altman JD (2003) Caveats in the design of MHC class I tetramer/antigen-specific T lymphocytes dissociation assays. J Immunol Methods 280:25–35

Wei DG, Lee H, Park SH, Beaudoin L, Teyton L, Lehuen A, Bendelac A (2005) Expansion and long-range differentiation of the NKT cell lineage in mice expressing CD1d exclusively on cortical thymocytes. J Exp Med 202:239–248

Wei DG, Curran SA, Savage PB, Teyton L, Bendelac A (2006) Mechanisms imposing the Vbeta bias of Valpha14 natural killer T cells and consequences for microbial glycolipid recognition. J Exp Med 203:1197–1207

Wingender G, Berg M, Jungerkes F, Diehl L, Sullivan BA, Kronenberg M, Limmer A, Knolle PA (2006) Immediate antigen-specific effector functions by TCR-transgenic CD8+ NKT cells. Eur J Immunol 36:570–582

Wu D, Zajonc DM, Fujio M, Sullivan BA, Kinjo Y, Kronenberg M, Wilson IA, Wong CH (2006) Design of natural killer T cell activators: structure and function of a microbial glycosphingolipid bound to mouse CD1d. Proc Natl Acad Sci U S A 103:3972–1397

Wu DY, Segal NH, Sidobre S, Kronenberg M, Chapman PB (2003) Cross-presentation of disialoganglioside GD3 to natural killer T cells. J Exp Med 198:173–181

Wu LC, Tuot DS, Lyons DS, Garcia KC, Davis MM (2002) Two-step binding mechanism for T-cell receptor recognition of peptide MHC. Nature 418:552–556

Yu KO, Im JS, Molano A, Dutronc Y, Illarionov PA, Forestier C, Fujiwara N, Arias I, Miyake S, Yamamura T, Chang YT, Besra GS, Porcelli SA (2005) Modulation of CD1d-restricted NKT cell responses by using N-acyl variants of alpha-galactosylceramides. Proc Natl Acad Sci U S A 102:3383–3388

Zajonc DM, Elsliger MA, Teyton L, Wilson IA (2003) Crystal structure of CD1a in complex with a sulfatide self antigen at a resolution of 2.15 A. Nat Immunol 4:808–815

Zajonc DM, Cantu C 3rd, Mattner J, Zhou D, Savage PB, Bendelac A, Wilson IA, Teyton L (2005a) Structure and function of a potent agonist for the semi-invariant natural killer T cell receptor. Nat Immunol 6:810–818

Zajonc DM, Crispin MD, Bowden TA, Young DC, Cheng TY, Hu J, Costello CE, Rudd PM, Dwek RA, Miller MJ, Brenner MB, Moody DB, Wilson IA (2005b) Molecular mechanism of lipopeptide presentation by CD1a. Immunity 22:209–219

Zamoyska R (1998) CD4 and CD8: modulators of T-cell receptor recognition of antigen and of immune responses? Curr Opin Immunol 10:82–87

Zeng Z, Castano AR, Segelke BW, Stura EA, Peterson PA, Wilson IA (1997) Crystal structure of mouse CD1: an MHC-like fold with a large hydrophobic binding groove. Science 277:339–345

Zhou D, Mattner J, Cantu C 3rd, Schrantz N, Yin N, Gao Y, Sagiv Y, Hudspeth K, Wu YP, Yamashita T, Teneberg S, Wang D, Proia RL, Levery SB, Savage PB, Teyton L, Bendelac A (2004) Lysosomal glycosphingolipid recognition by NKT cells. Science 306:1786–1789

CTMI (2007) 314:195–210
© Springer-Verlag Berlin Heidelberg 2007

Development and Selection of Vα14i NKT Cells

H. R. MacDonald (✉) · M. P. Mycko

Ludwig Institute for Cancer Research, Lausanne Branch, University of Lausanne,
1066 Epalinges, Switzerland
hughrobson.macdonald@isrec.unil.ch

Abstract Vα14 invariant natural killer T (Vα14i NKT) cells are a unique lineage of mouse T cells that share properties with both NK cells and memory T cells. Vα14i NKT cells recognize CD1d-associated glycolipids via a semi-invariant T cell receptor (TCR) composed of an invariant Vα14-Jα18 chain paired preferentially with a restricted set of TCRβ chains. During development in the thymus, rare CD4⁺ CD8⁺ (DP) cortical thymocytes that successfully rearrange the semi-invariant TCR are directed to the Vα14i NKT cell lineage via interactions with CD1d-associated endogenous glycolipids expressed by other DP thymocytes. As they mature, Vα14i NKT lineage cells upregulate activation markers such as CD44 and subsequently express NK-related molecules such as NK1.1 and members of the Ly-49 inhibitory receptor family. The developmental program of Vα14i NKT cells is critically regulated by a number of signaling cues that have little or no effect on conventional T cell development, such as the Fyn/SAP/SLAM pathway, NFκB and T-bet transcription factors, and the cytokine IL-15. The unique developmental requirements of Vα14i NKT cells may represent a paradigm for other unconventional T cell subsets that are positively selected by agonist ligands expressed on hematopoietic cells.

Abbreviations

αGalCer	α-Galactosylceramide
DN	CD4⁻ CD8⁻
DP	CD4⁺ CD8⁺
iGb3	Isoglobotrihexosylceramide
MAIT	Mucosa-associated invariant T
MHC	Major histocompatibility complex
NF-κB	Nuclear factor κB
NIK	NF-κB inducing kinase
NKT	Natural killer T
PKCθ	Protein kinase Cθ
SAP	SLAM-associated protein
SLAM	Signaling lymphocytic activation molecule
TCR	T cell receptor
Vα14i	Vα14 invariant

1
Introduction

Natural killer T (NKT) cells are a subset of unconventional T cells that play an immunoregulatory role in microbial and tumor immunity and have been implicated in the pathogenesis of autoimmunity and allergy. As suggested by their name, NKT cells are a hybrid lineage between T and NK cells, expressing a CD3-associated αβ T cell receptor (TCR) as well as NK-related markers such as NK1.1 and members of the Ly-49 inhibitory receptor family. In contrast to conventional T cells that recognize peptides presented by highly polymorphic major histocompatibility complex (MHC) class I and class II molecules, a large proportion of NKT cells recognize glycolipids associated with the monomorphic CD1d molecule. In mice, the TCR responsible for CD1d and glycolipid recognition by NKT cells is composed of an invariant Vα14-Jα18 chain paired with a restricted subset of TCRβ chains using primarily Vβ8.2, Vβ7 and Vβ2. For simplicity, the subset of NKT cells expressing this TCR will subsequently be referred to as Vα14 invariant (Vα14i) NKT cells. Importantly Vα14i NKT cells can be directly identified by virtue of the fact that their semi-invariant TCR binds tetramers of CD1d complexed with the synthetic glycolipid α-galactosylceramide (αGalCer) [5, 32]. Humans possess an apparently equivalent population utilizing a Vα24-Jα18 chain, which likewise pairs with limited TCR β chains and responds to αGalCer.

Several unusual features of Vα14i NKT cells indicate that they belong to a unique T cell lineage. In addition to their semi-invariant TCR, Vα14i NKT cells constitutively express activation markers such as CD44 and CD69, which are not expressed by naïve conventional T cells. Furthermore, the requirements for the development and selection of Vα14i NKT cells differ markedly from those of conventional T cells. This latter aspect of Vα14i NKT cells will provide the focus for this review.

2
Developmental Pathway of Vα14i NKT Cells

2.1
Thymic Origin of Vα14i NKT Cells

Initially there was considerable controversy surrounding the role of the thymus in the development of Vα14i NKT cells. Since the liver is a major anatomical site for the accumulation of Vα14i NKT cells in the mouse [38] it was postulated that liver Vα14i NKT cells arise in situ [30]. However subsequent experiments provided compelling evidence that most if not all Vα14i NKT cells in the liver and in peripheral lymphoid tissues are thymus-derived since they are essentially absent in athymic nude mice [12, 56].

2.2
Precommitment or Instruction?

The developmental pathway of Vα14i NKT cells in the thymus has been controversial. Given their unique semi-invariant TCR, two distinct models for Vα14i NKT cell development have been proposed [28]. By analogy with certain other unconventional T cell subsets bearing highly restricted TCR, such as Vγ3 cells in the epidermis, it was initially postulated that Vα14i NKT cells arose from precommitted precursors that had undergone directed Vα14-Jα18 rearrangement at the TCRα locus [45]. However subsequent analysis of the "silent" TCRα allele in Vα14i NKT cell hybridomas revealed no evidence for such directed rearrangements [50]. Rather it is now generally agreed that random TCRα (and TCRβ) rearrangements followed by stringent selection by CD1d is the driving force that shapes the semi-invariant TCR repertoire expressed by Vα14i NKT cells.

One obvious corollary of this instructional model is that Vα14i NKT cell precursors expressing CD1d-reactive TCR must be extremely rare, perhaps of the order of 1 in 10^5, thereby posing serious problems for their definitive identification (see Sect. 2.3). A second implication is that Vα14i NKT cell precursors do not form a distinct lineage prior to TCR rearrangement. Indeed the simplest model, which is now widely accepted, is that the existing pool of CD4$^+$ CD8$^+$ double-positive (DP) thymocytes provides precursors for both the Vα14i NKT and conventional T cell lineages.

2.3
The Elusive DP Vα14i NKT Precursor

Rearranged TCR α chains first appear on DP thymocytes. Therefore, the instructive model of Vα14i NKT cell development implies that CD1d-reactive DP thymocytes expressing the semi-invariant TCR would serve as precursors for mature Vα14i NKT cells. Nevertheless direct identification of such putative DP Vα14i NKT precursor cells has been controversial, most likely because of their extremely low frequency. Several groups have shown that purified DP thymocytes contain a detectable frequency of in-frame Vα14-Jα18 rearrangements [13, 21]. These rearrangements can even be detected in DP thymocytes from CD1d$^{-/-}$ mice [21], suggesting the presence of unselected DP Vα14i NKT precursors. Attempts to directly identify DP Vα14i NKT precursors with CD1d–αGalCer tetramers have met with varying results, leading to controversy. Although it is generally agreed that no cells staining with CD1d tetramers can be detected among conventional DP thymocytes expressing high levels of both CD4 and CD8, several groups have identified rare CD1d tetramer-stained cells in a DP "dull" subset of cells, which could represent post-selection Vα14i NKT precursors that have partially downregulated CD4 and CD8 [4, 19, 21]. However DP dull tetramer-staining cells were not observed in another study [41] and were in fact only observed when tetramer-based enrichment procedures were utilized. Moreover, there are major discrepancies in the phenotype of DP dull tetramer$^+$ cells described by different groups [4, 19, 21], raising the possibility that the enrichment procedure may have led to an altered phenotype.

Despite the lack of definitive evidence for DP Vα14i NKT precursors that express a semi-invariant TCR, a number of other observations support the hypothesis that mature Vα14i NKT cells are indeed derived from DP precursors. First, intrathymic transfer of purified DP thymocytes derived from wild type or CD1d$^{-/-}$ mice into recipient mice that are unable to make the canonical Vα14-Jα18 rearrangement (Jα18$^{-/-}$) led to the development of mature Vα14i NKT cells [21]. Second Vα14i NKT cell development is completely dependent upon the retinoic acid-related orphan receptor, RORγt. This transcription factor is selectively expressed in DP thymocytes and is required to promote their survival via bcl-X$_L$, so that distal Vα to Jα rearrangements, including Vα14–Jα18, can occur [6, 15]. Significantly, Vα14i NKT cell development is rescued in RORγt$^{-/-}$ mice in the presence of either a bcl-X$_L$ transgene or a rearranged Vα14–Jα18 transgene [6, 15], suggesting that Vα14–Jα18 rearrangements at the DP thymocyte stage are necessary for subsequent Vα14i NKT cell development. Finally a fate mapping strategy in which thymocytes were selectively marked with enhanced green fluorescent protein (EGFP) at the DP stage using a RORγt-driven Cre recombinase provided compelling evidence that Vα14i NKT cells are the progeny of DP thymocytes [15].

2.4
Phenotypic Stages of Intrathymic Vα14i NKT Cell Development

Following rearrangement of the semi-invariant TCR at the DP thymocyte stage, Vα14i NKT cell precursors undergo a differentiation program that is driven by engagement of CD1d. This differentiation pathway can be subdivided into at least four sequential stages based upon the expression of a variety of phenotypic markers [3, 4, 19, 41] (Fig. 1). The earliest post-DP Vα14i NKT stage is CD4$^+$ and is characterized by high expression of heat stable antigen (HSA or CD24), a phenotype consistent with developmental immaturity. This CD4$^+$ CD24^{high} subset has a CD44^{low} NK1.1$^-$ phenotype indicative of its immature status. Interestingly, CD4$^+$ CD24^{high} Vα14i NKT cells are not yet cycling but already display a marked bias for expression of Vβ8, indicating that Vβ repertoire selection by CD1d precedes cell expansion in this lineage. Furthermore, most CD4$^+$ CD24^{high} Vα14i NKT cells express the early activation marker CD69, suggesting that they may represent cells that have recently undergone positive selection.

The second well-defined stage of intrathymic Vα14i NKT cell development is characterized by downregulation of CD24 and CD69. At this stage, the developing Vα14i NKT cells remain CD44^{low} and do not express NK1.1. Importantly, CD4$^+$ CD24^{low} CD44^{low} NK1.1$^-$ Vα14i NKT cells are rapidly cycling, as determined by their large size and ability to incorporate 5-bromo-2-deoxyuridine (BrdU) in short-term in vivo labeling studies. A third stage of Vα14i NKT cell development is defined by upregulation of CD44. CD4$^+$ CD24^{low} CD44^{high} Vα14i NKT cells do not yet express NK1.1 or other NK-related markers such as the Ly-49 family of inhibitory receptors but continue to undergo rapid proliferation. Stage 4 marks an important late step in Vα14i NKT cell development distinguished by the acquisition of NK1.1 and Ly-49 inhibitory receptors. Microarray analysis indicates a coordinate expression of multiple NK-related markers at this stage [33]. Significantly, stage 4 Vα14i NKT cells cease to cycle, consistent with their entering a terminal stage of differentiation.

Phenotype

Signaling cues

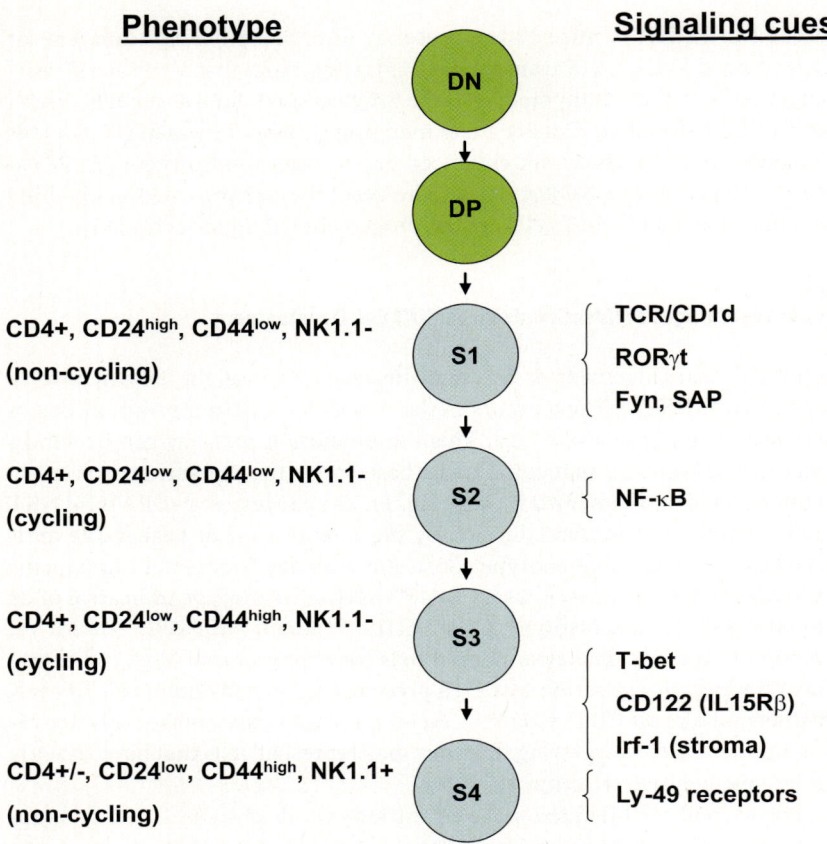

CD4+, CD24^{high}, CD44^{low}, NK1.1- (non-cycling)

CD4+, CD24^{low}, CD44^{low}, NK1.1- (cycling)

CD4+, CD24^{low}, CD44^{high}, NK1.1- (cycling)

CD4+/-, CD24^{low}, CD44^{high}, NK1.1+ (non-cycling)

Fig. 1 Stages of intrathymic development of Vα14i NKT cells. Like conventional T cells, Vα14i NKT cells arise from CD4⁻ CD8⁻ (*DN*) immature precursors and proceed to the CD4⁺ CD8⁺ (*DP*) stage. Following rearrangement of the semi-invariant TCR and interaction with CD1d on neighboring DP thymocytes, Vα14i NKT cells undergo differentiation and maturation through at least four defined stages (*S1–S4*). Phenotypic characteristics and signaling cues associated with each developmental stage are indicated. See text for details

2.5
Late Origin of CD4⁻ CD8⁻ Vα14i NKT Cells

The four sequential phenotypic stages of Vα14i NKT cell development described above have all been characterized as expressing CD4. Nevertheless, it is clear that an important subset of Vα14i NKT cells, which can constitute 30–40% of CD1d tetramer-staining cells in the thymus of the adult mouse, have a CD4⁻ CD8⁻ (double negative, or DN) phenotype. DN Vα14i NKT cells appear to be mature cells since they express NK cell markers such as NK1.1 and Ly-49 family members. Using intrathymic cell transfers of purified Vα14i NKT cell subsets, several groups have demonstrated that DN Vα14i NKT cells are in fact derived from immature CD4⁺ (stage 2 or 3) precursors [3, 19, 41]. However, the mechanism responsible for downregulation of CD4 expression during this maturation step remains obscure.

2.6
Mysterious Absence of CD8⁺ Vα14i NKT Cells

Although selection of DP precursors by CD1d results in the appearance of CD4⁺ and DN Vα14i NKT cells, no CD8⁺ Vα14i NKT cells are generated. The mysterious absence of CD8 lineage Vα14i NKT cells, which contrasts with the large number of CD8⁺ cells among conventional T cells, has been attributed to negative selection imposed by a putative interaction between CD1d and CD8, since mice constitutively expressing transgenic CD8 are depleted of Vα14i NKT cells [2]. Nevertheless there is no direct evidence to support such a co-receptor function for CD8 on Vα14i NKT cells, and transgenic CD8 over-expression may interfere indirectly with Vα14i NKT cell development, for example by sequestration of src kinases. Alternatively, the exclusive CD4 phenotype of post-selection Vα14i NKT cells may be an inescapable consequence of the kinetic signaling model of CD4:CD8 lineage commitment [52]. According to this scenario, DP thymocyte precursors expressing a semi-invariant TCR with high affinity for CD1d would be directed automatically to the CD4 lineage, as is the case for DP precursors of conventional T cells with high affinity TCR for MHC class II. If true, this model would predict that CD8⁺ Vα14i NKT cells could develop if TCR affinity for CD1d was somehow reduced. Interestingly CD8⁺ NKT cells expressing the homologous human Vα24i TCR have been reported [22, 43], although no direct relationship between this phenotype and TCR affinity for CD1d has been examined.

2.7
Signaling Cues for Vα14i NKT Cell Development

Like other hematopoietic lineages, Vα14i NKT cell development is regulated by a combination of cytokines, transcription factors and other signaling molecules. A comprehensive list of factors influencing Vα14i NKT cell development at different developmental stages has been published recently [31]. This review concentrates on a few key signaling cues that have been well characterized.

2.7.1
The Fyn/SAP/SLAM Pathway

One signaling molecule that acts very early during Vα14i NKT cell development is the src family kinase Fyn. It has been known for some time that Fyn is required for Vα14i NKT cell development but largely dispensable for T or NK cell development [14, 18]. More recently, it was demonstrated that the requirement for Fyn in Vα14i NKT cell development could be completely rescued by the introduction of a transgenic rearranged Vα14–Jα18 chain [20]. This surprising finding suggests that Fyn is acting upstream of expression of the semi-invariant TCR in Vα14i NKT cell precursors. By analogy with the phenotype of RORγt$^{-/-}$ mice, where Vα14i NKT cells fail to develop because of a failure to rearrange distal Vα–Jα pairs such as Vα14–Jα18 at the DP thymocyte stage, it is tempting to speculate that Fyn deficiency shortens the time window available for DP thymocytes to undergo Vα–Jα rearrangements, thus reducing the probability that DP Vα14i NKT precursors expressing the semi-invariant TCR will be generated. Extending DP survival in Fyn$^{-/-}$ mice via the introduction of a bcl-2 or bcl-X$_L$ transgene would be one means of testing this interesting hypothesis.

Several mechanistic explanations for the selective role of Fyn in Vα14i NKT cell development can be entertained. First since Fyn, like Lck, can associate with intracellular TCR components to promote signaling in lymphocytes, it is possible that reduced agonist signaling via the semi-invariant TCR is responsible for the block in Vα14i NKT cell development in Fyn$^{-/-}$ mice. However, if the requirement for Fyn in the Vα14i NKT cell lineage is actually upstream of Vα14–Jα18 rearrangement [20], this hypothesis is unlikely.

A second important role of Fyn in the immune system is to mediate signaling via surface receptors of the signaling lymphocytic activation molecule (SLAM) family. In this pathway, homotypic interactions between SLAM family members on different cell types lead to activation of Fyn signaling via SLAM-associated protein (SAP), an adaptor molecule linking the SLAM cytoplasmic domain to Fyn. Importantly, mutations in SAP in humans lead to an X-linked immunodeficiency (XLP) characterized by defective Vα24i NKT cell development [11, 36, 40] in addition to functional defects in mature T and B cells. Moreover, mice deficient in SAP have very few Vα14i NKT cells, although development of other lymphocyte subsets is relatively normal [11, 36, 40]. Taken together, these data have led to speculation that the Fyn/SAP/SLAM pathway controls Vα14i NKT cell development at a very early stage, perhaps by regulating survival and hence rearrangement of the semi-invariant TCR in DP Vα14i NKT thymocyte precursors [29]. Nevertheless, the putative SLAM family member involved in Vα14i NKT cell development remains to be identified, and recent studies indicate that SAP can function independently of Fyn in some cases, for example in regulating cytokine production by mature CD4$^+$ T cells [9]. Analysis of Vα14i NKT cell development in knockin mice expressing a mutant form of SAP that cannot interact with Fyn [9] would be informative in this respect.

2.7.2
The NF-κB Connection

A second important signaling pathway implicated in Vα14i NKT cell development is the nuclear factor (NF)-κB pathway. The role of NF-κB signaling in Vα14i NKT cell development is complex since it involves independent effects on stromal cells (see Sect. 2.8) as well as Vα14i NKT cells. The effects of blocking NF-κB signaling via deficiencies in several components of the classical NF-κB pathway have been tested. Deletion of NF-κB1 and IκB kinase (IKK-2), as well as expression of a non-degradable mutant form of the IκBα molecule in the Vα14i NKT lineage using the T cell-specific lck proximal promoter, led to a severe and selective reduction in Vα14i NKT cells [16, 46, 53, 54]. Interestingly, the few remaining Vα14i NKT lineage cells in these latter mutant mice did not express mature NK markers, such as NK1.1 and Ly-49 inhibitory receptors, and displayed a predominantly CD4$^+$ CD44^{low} phenotype [54]. A proportion of these CD4$^+$ NK1.1$^-$ CD44^{low} Vα14i NKT cells also expressed high levels of CD24, suggesting that they were blocked in stage 1 (Fig. 1). This block at the immature Vα14i NKT cell stage could be completely rescued by overexpression of a bcl-X$_L$ transgene, suggesting that the main function of NF-κB in early Vα14i NKT cell development is to promote survival [54].

In considering the possible role of NF-κB signaling during Vα14i NKT cell development, it is noteworthy that the NF-κB pathway is also potentially linked to the Fyn/SAP/SLAM pathway via the protein kinase PKCθ [8]. Interestingly, deficiency of PKCθ also leads to a severe reduction in thymic Vα14i NKT cells [46, 55]. Although the reduced numbers of Vα14i NKT cells in PKCθ$^{-/-}$ mice has been attributed to the well-characterized role of PKCθ in TCR signaling [55], this interpretation is not consistent with the fact that thymic Vα14i NKT cell development is unaffected in mice deficient for the bcl-10 adapter protein [46], which is also required for downstream NF-κB-dependent TCR signaling. Thus PKCθ-mediated NF-κB signaling in Vα14i NKT cells may actually be downstream of the Fyn/SAP/SLAM pathway rather than the TCR [7]. This hypothesis predicts that the similar Vα14i NKT cell defects observed in mice deficient for Fyn, SAP and various components of the NF-κB pathway are the result of a single signaling cascade.

2.7.3
T-bet

Another transcription factor that plays a key role in Vα14i NKT cell development is T-bet. Initially identified as critical for the development of the Th1 subset of mature CD4$^+$ T cells, T-bet was subsequently found to influence both NK and Vα14i NKT cell development [57]. Vα14i NKT cells deficient in T-bet are selectively blocked at a relatively late stage of development (S3 in Fig. 1). Thus, T-bet$^{-/-}$ Vα14i NKT cells do not express NK1.1 or other NK-related markers such as members of the Ly-49 inhibitory receptor family [57]. Of particular interest is the fact that T-bet$^{-/-}$ Vα14i NKT cells express very low levels of CD122, the common β-chain of the IL-2R and IL-15R [57]. Given the strong dependence of Vα14i NKT cell development on IL-15 (see Sect. 2.7.4) these data raise the possibility that T-bet may specifically control IL-15 responsiveness of developing Vα14i NKT cells via regulation of CD122 expression. Nevertheless, it should be noted that T-bet controls multiple genes involved in migration, survival and effector function of Vα14i NKT cells [33], suggesting that its role in Vα14i NKT cell development may be relatively complex.

2.7.4
IL-15

Like many other hematopoietic cells, Vα14i NKT cells are critically dependent upon cytokines for their development. Since Vα14i NKT cells initially develop along the same pathway as conventional T cells up to the DP thymocyte stage, it is not surprising that IL-7 is required for their early development [60]. Once the specific Vα14i NKT cell developmental pathway is initiated, however, IL-15 is the key cytokine involved in their subsequent differentiation and maturation. Thus mice deficient for either IL-15 [23] or for the IL-15Rα [26] or CD122 [37] chains are severely depleted of Vα14i NKT cells, whereas conventional T cell development proceeds normally. In addition, mice lacking Irf-1, a transcription factor that controls IL-15 production by stromal cells, are selectively deficient in Vα14i NKT cells [39]. IL-15 deficiency selectively affects late stages of Vα14i NKT cell development (stage 4 in Fig. 1), consistent with the fact that CD122 is upregulated at this time point. The failure to rescue Vα14i NKT cell deficiency in CD122$^{-/-}$ mice by expression of a bcl-2 transgene [34] would seem to argue against a simple survival function of IL-15 during Vα14i NKT cell development. However, it should be remembered that only bcl-X$_L$, but not bcl-2, is able to restore Vα14i NKT cell development in other contexts, such as the absence of NF-κB signaling [54].

2.7.5
Inhibitory and Activating NK Receptors

A striking feature of Vα14i NKT cells is their expression of NK markers such as NK1.1 and members of the Ly-49 receptor family. In contrast to NK cells, which express both activating and inhibitory Ly-49 receptors, Vα14i NKT cells express only inhibitory family members [25]. The absence of activating Ly-49 receptors on Vα14i NKT cells appears to be necessary to avoid excessive ITAM signaling during development, since transgenic expression of the Ly-49D activating receptor in the presence of its MHC class I ligand H-2D^d seriously impairs Vα14i NKT cell development [61]. On the other hand, the role of inhibitory Ly-49 receptors in Vα14i NKT cell development is less clear. By analogy with NK cells, engagement of inhibitory Ly-49 receptors on Vα14i NKT cells by MHC class I ligands is widely believed to be necessary to dampen signaling via activating receptors (in this case the semi-invariant TCR) and thus prevent autoreactivity [27]. This interpretation is consistent with the fact that inhibitory Ly-49 receptors are only expressed by mature Vα14i NKT cells (stage 4 in Fig. 1). Moreover, forced ligation of a transgenic Ly-49A inhibitory receptor on immature Vα14i NKT cells significantly perturbs their development in the thymus [44], as might be expected if TCR signaling were inhibited.

2.8
Enigmatic Role of Stromal Cells

A generally under-appreciated aspect of Vα14i NKT cell development is that it is dependent upon stromal cells. This fact was first demonstrated in the spontaneous mouse mutant aly (alymphoplasia). Homozygous aly/aly mice have a small thymus but a relatively normal distribution of conventional T cell subsets. However, aly/aly mice are selectively deficient in Vα14i NKT cells [35], and the basis of this deficiency was mapped to stromal cells in radiation bone marrow chimeras [24]. With the subsequent identification of the aly gene as NF-κB-inducing kinase (NIK) [51], it became apparent that the NF-κB pathway plays a dual role in NKT cell development. On the one hand NF-κB signaling in Vα14i NKT cell precursors is essential for their early survival (see Sect. 2.7.2), whereas a second, less well-defined function of the NF-κB pathway in stromal cells promotes Vα14i NKT cell development. More recent studies have identified Rel B as the specific NF-κB family member that is required in stromal cells for Vα14i NKT cell development [16, 53]. Activation of Rel B requires NIK [16, 53], thus explaining the reduced numbers of Vα14i NKT cells in NIK-deficient aly/aly mice.

3
Selection of NKT Cells

3.1
Positive Selection

In contrast to conventional T cells, which are positively selected by peptide–MHC complexes expressed by thymic cortical epithelial cells, Vα14i NKT cells are positively selected by glycolipid–CD1d complexes expressed by hematopoietic cells [2, 38]. A number of experiments using bone marrow chimeras have identified DP thymocytes as being important for Vα14i NKT cell positive selection [1, 12]; however, this approach did not exclude the possibility that other thymic CD1d-expressing hematopoietic subsets might also be involved. Recently tissue-specific transgenic expression of CD1d has been used by several groups to more precisely identify hematopoietic subsets responsible for positive selection of Vα14i NKT cells. Using the proximal lck promoter to restrict expression of mouse [63, 65] or human [48] CD1d to DP thymocytes, it has been clearly demonstrated that CD1d-expressing DP thymocytes are sufficient to elicit positive selection of Vα14i NKT cells.

How homotypic interactions between DP Vα14i NKT precursors and other DP CD1d-expressing thymocytes can induce the unique developmental program of Vα14i NKT cells remains an enigma. In this regard, it could be speculated that specialized signaling pathways, such as the Fyn /SAP/SLAM pathway, may provide unique signals that favor Vα14i NKT cell development. In addition, it should be remembered that the intrinsic affinity of the semi-invariant TCR on NKT cells for CD1d–glycolipid complexes is probably significantly higher than typical TCR–peptide–MHC interactions. Thus strong signaling via the TCR and/or additional surface molecules may act in concert to initiate Vα14i NKT cell development upon interaction of DP precursors with other DP thymocytes expressing CD1d. Importantly, this interaction is sufficient to drive the complete developmental program of Vα14i NKT cells, as evidenced by the mature phenotype and functional competence of Vα14i NKT cells in mice that express CD1d uniquely on DP thymocytes [48, 63, 65]. Whatever the mechanism, positive selection on hematopoietic cells is not a unique property of Vα14i NKT cells, since other nonconventional T cell subsets such as H-2M-restricted CD8[+] T cells and mucosa-associated invariant T (MAIT) cells share this characteristic [58, 59].

A longstanding issue in Vα14i NKT cell biology has been the nature of the endogenous CD1d-binding glycolipid ligand that is responsible for positive selection. Until recently, the only well-characterized CD1d-binding glycolipid was the marine sponge-derived αGalCer, which obviously cannot participate in physiological Vα14i NKT cell selection. This question appears to have been at least partly resolved with the recent demonstration that isoglobotri-hexosylceramide (iGb3), an endogenous glycolipid resident in the lysosomal compartment, is able to bind CD1d and activate both human and mouse Vα14i NKT cells [64]. Importantly, Vα14i NKT cell development is severely impaired in mutant mice lacking hexB [64], a lysosomal enzyme that is required for iGb3 synthesis. Based on these results it has been proposed that iGb3 is the principal endogenous glycolipid involved in positive selection of Vα14i NKT cells [64], although a more general disruption of endosomal function in hexB-deficient mice cannot be excluded [17]. Whether other endogenous CD1d-binding glycolipids are able to participate in positive selection of Vα14i NKT cells remains to be investigated. In this regard it is interesting that iGb3 preferentially selects a subset of Vα14i NKT cells expressing Vβ7 [47, 62], raising the possibility that other glycolipids may be necessary to select a complete Vα14i NKT TCR repertoire.

3.2
Negative Selection

Although the mechanistic basis for positive selection of Vα14i NKT cells is gradually being clarified, the question of how or even whether Vα14i NKT cells are negatively selected remains controversial. The fact that Vα14i NKT cells are potentially susceptible to negative selection was first demonstrated by experiments in which αGalCer was added to fetal thymus organ cultures, resulting in a reduced generation of Vα14i NKT cells [42]. Nevertheless, since αGalCer is an artificial ligand for the semi-invariant TCR, these studies do not address the question of whether Vα14i NKT cells can be negatively selected under physiological conditions. More recent studies have examined negative selection of Vα14i NKT cells in transgenic mice with restricted expression of CD1d driven by the MHC class I [10] or CD11c [48] promoters. In both cases, it was concluded that dendritic cells expressing CD1d were able to mediate negative selection of Vα14i NKT cells; however, the extremely high levels of CD1d overexpression induced by the transgenes again precluded extrapolation of the results to the physiological situation. In one study, restricted expression of relatively physiological levels of human CD1d on DP thymocytes, using the proximal lck promoter, led to significant negative selection of developing Vα14i NKT cells, suggesting that both positive and negative selection can be induced by the same (DP) thymocyte subset [48]. This interpretation is, however, subject to the caveat that the subset of Vβ8.2$^+$ Vα14i NKT cells negatively selected by DP thymocytes in this model appears to bind human CD1d with unusually high avidity [49], again raising the issue of physiological relevance.

4
Concluding Remarks

During the past few years, it has become increasingly clear that Vα14i
NKT cells differ remarkably from conventional αβ T cells in terms of their
requirements for development and selection. Indeed, as outlined in this article, Vα14i NKT cells require specific ligands (CD1d–glycolipid complexes)
and specialized antigen-presenting cells (DP thymocytes) as well as particular signaling pathways (Fyn/SAP/SLAM, NF-κB, and T-bet) and cytokines
(IL-15) in order to complete their differentiation program. Although there is
a common tendency to consider Vα14i NKT cells as a unique lineage with
peculiar developmental requirements, the possibility should be considered
that this view is largely conditioned by comparison with the much better
studied conventional T cell development. In reality there are increasing numbers of unconventional T cell subsets that share at least some of the unusual
developmental properties of Vα14i NKT cells, such as their selection by ligands associated with monomorphic MHC class Ib molecules expressed on
hematopoietic cells [58, 59]. Thus Vα14i NKT cells may prove to be a useful
paradigm for a broad class of T cell subsets that are selected by high-affinity
(agonist) TCR interactions.

References

1. Bendelac A (1995) Positive selection of mouse NK1+ T cells by CD1-expressing
    cortical thymocytes. J Exp Med 182:2091–2096
2. Bendelac A, Killeen N, Littman DR, Schwartz RH (1994) A subset of CD4+ thy-
    mocytes selected by MHC class I molecules. Science 263:1774–1778
3. Benlagha K, Kyin T, Beavis A, Teyton L, Bendelac A (2002) A thymic precursor to
    the NKT cell lineage. Science 296:553–555
4. Benlagha K, Wei DG, Veiga J, Teyton L, Bendelac A (2005) Characterization of the
    early stages of thymic NKT cell development. J Exp Med 202:485–492
5. Benlagha K, Weiss A, Beavis A, Teyton L, Bendelac A (2000) In vivo identification
    of glycolipid antigen-specific T cells using fluorescent CD1d tetramers. J Exp Med
    191:1895–1903
6. Bezbradica JS, Hill T, Stanic AK, Van Kaer L, Joyce S (2005) Commitment toward
    the natural T (iNKT) cell lineage occurs at the CD4+8+ stage of thymic ontogeny.
    Proc Natl Acad Sci U S A 102:5114–119
7. Borowski C, Bendelac A (2005) Signaling for NKT cell development: the SAP-FynT
    connection. J Exp Med 201:833–836
8. Cannons JL, Yu LJ, Hill B, Mijares LA, Dombroski D, Nichols KE, Antonellis A,
    Koretzky GA, Gardner K, Schwartzberg PL (2004) SAP regulates T(H)2 differenti-
    ation and PKC-theta-mediated activation of NF-kappaB1. Immunity 21:693–706

9. Cannons JL, Yu LJ, Jankovic D, Crotty S, Horai R, Kirby M, Anderson S, Cheever AW, Sher A, Schwartzberg PL (2006) SAP regulates T cell-mediated help for humoral immunity by a mechanism distinct from cytokine regulation. J Exp Med 203:1551–165

10. Chun T, Page MJ, Gapin L, Matsuda JL, Xu H, Nguyen H, Kang HS, Stanic AK, Joyce S, Koltun WA, Chorney MJ, Kronenberg M, Wang CR (2003) CD1d-expressing dendritic cells but not thymic epithelial cells can mediate negative selection of NKT cells. J Exp Med 197:907–918

11. Chung B, Aoukaty A, Dutz J, Terhorst C, Tan R (2005) Signaling lymphocytic activation molecule-associated protein controls NKT cell functions. J Immunol 174:3153–3157

12. Coles MC, Raulet DH (2000) NK1.1+ T cells in the liver arise in the thymus and are selected by interactions with class I molecules on CD4+CD8+ cells. J Immunol 164:2412–2418

13. Dao T, Guo D, Ploss A, Stolzer A, Saylor C, Boursalian TE, Im JS, Sant'Angelo DB (2004) Development of CD1d-restricted NKT cells in the mouse thymus. Eur J Immunol 34:3542–3552

14. Eberl G, Lowin-Kropf B, MacDonald HR (1999) Cutting edge: NKT cell development is selectively impaired in Fyn- deficient mice. J Immunol 163:4091–4094

15. Egawa T, Eberl G, Taniuchi I, Benlagha K, Geissmann F, Hennighausen L, Bendelac A, Littman DR (2005) Genetic evidence supporting selection of the Valpha14i NKT cell lineage from double-positive thymocyte precursors. Immunity 22:705–716

16. Elewaut D, Shaikh RB, Hammond KJ, De Winter H, Leishman AJ, Sidobre S, Turovskaya O, Prigozy TI, Ma L, Banks TA, Lo D, Ware CF, Cheroutre H, Kronenberg M (2003) NIK-dependent RelB activation defines a unique signaling pathway for the development of V alpha 14i NKT cells. J Exp Med 197:1623–1633

17. Gadola SD, Silk JD, Jeans A, Illarionov PA, Salio M, Besra GS, Dwek R, Butters TD, Platt FM, Cerundolo V (2006) Impaired selection of invariant natural killer T cells in diverse mouse models of glycosphingolipid lysosomal storage diseases. J Exp Med 203:2293–2303

18. Gadue P, Morton N, Stein PL (1999) The Src family tyrosine kinase Fyn regulates natural killer T cell development. J Exp Med 190:1189–1196

19. Gadue P, Stein PL (2002) NKT cell precursors exhibit differential cytokine regulation and require Itk for efficient maturation. J Immunol 169:2397–2406

20. Gadue P, Yin L, Jain S, Stein PL (2004) Restoration of NKT cell development in fyn-mutant mice by a TCR reveals a requirement for Fyn during early NKT cell ontogeny. J Immunol 172:6093–6100

21. Gapin L, Matsuda JL, Surh CD, Kronenberg M (2001) NKT cells derive from double-positive thymocytes that are positively selected by CD1d. Nat Immunol 2:971–978

22. Gumperz JE, Miyake S, Yamamura T, Brenner MB (2002) Functionally distinct subsets of CD1d-restricted natural killer T cells revealed by CD1d tetramer staining. J Exp Med 195:625–636

23. Kennedy MK, Glaccum M, Brown SN, Butz EA, Viney JL, Embers M, Matsuki N, Charrier K, Sedger L, Willis CR, Brasel K, Morrissey PJ, Stocking K, Schuh JC, Joyce S, Peschon JJ (2000) Reversible defects in natural killer and memory CD8. T cell lineages in interleukin 15-deficient mice. J Exp Med 191:771–780

24. Konishi J, Iwabuchi K, Iwabuchi C, Ato M, Nagata JI, Onoe K, Nakagawa KI, Kasai M, Ogasawara K, Kawakami K (2000) Thymic epithelial cells responsible for impaired generation of NK-T thymocytes in Alymphoplasia mutant mice. Cell Immunol 206:26–35

25. Lees RK, Ferrero I, MacDonald HR (2001) Tissue-specific segregation of TCRgamma delta+ NKT cells according to phenotype TCR repertoire and activation status: parallels with TCR alphabeta+ NKT cells. Eur J Immunol 31:2901–2909

26. Lodolce JP, Boone DL, Chai S, Swain RE, Dassopoulos T, Trettin S, Ma A (1998) IL-15 receptor maintains lymphoid homeostasis by supporting lymphocyte homing and proliferation. Immunity 9:669–676

27. MacDonald HR (2002) Immunology. T before NK. Science 296:481–482

28. MacDonald HR (2002) Development and selection of NKT cells. Curr Opin Immunol 14:250–254

29. MacDonald HR, Schumann J (2005) The need for natural killer T cells. Nat Med 11:256–257

30. Makino Y, Yamagata N, Sasho T, Adachi Y, Kanno R, Koseki H, Kanno M, Taniguchi M (1993) Extrathymic development of V alpha 14-positive T cells. J Exp Med 177:1399–1408

31. Matsuda JL, Gapin L (2005) Developmental program of mouse Valpha14i NKT cells. Curr Opin Immunol 17:122–130

32. Matsuda JL, Naidenko OV, Gapin L, Nakayama T, Taniguchi M, Wang CR, Koezuka Y, Kronenberg M (2000) Tracking the response of natural killer T cells to a glycolipid antigen using CD1d tetramers. J Exp Med 192:741–754

33. Matsuda JL, Zhang Q, Ndonye R, Richardson SK, Howell AR, Gapin L (2006) T-bet concomitantly controls migration, survival, and effector functions during the development of Valpha14i NKT cells. Blood 107:2797–2805

34. Minagawa M, Watanabe H, Miyaji C, Tomiyama K, Shimura H, Ito A, Ito M, Domen J, Weissman IL, Kawai K (2002) Enforced expression of Bcl-2 restores the number of NK cells, but does not rescue the impaired development of NKT cells or intraepithelial lymphocytes, in IL-2/IL-15 receptor beta-chain-deficient mice. J Immunol 169:4153–4160

35. Nakagawa K, Iwabuchi K, Ogasawara K, Ato M, Kajiwara M, Nishihori H, Iwabuchi C, Ishikura H, Good RA, Onoe K (1997) Generation of NK1.1+ T cell antigen receptor alpha/beta+ thymocytes associated with intact thymic structure. Proc Natl Acad Sci U S A 94:2472–2477

36. Nichols KE, Hom J, Gong SY, Ganguly A, Ma CS, Cannons JL, Tangye SG, Schwartzberg PL, Koretzky GA, Stein PL (2005) Regulation of NKT cell development by SAP, the protein defective in XLP. Nat Med 11:340–345

37. Ohteki T, Ho S, Suzuki H, Mak TW, Ohashi PS (1997) Role for IL-15/IL-15 receptor beta-chain in natural killer 1.1+ T cell receptor-alpha beta+ cell development. J Immunol 159:5931–5935

38. Ohteki T, MacDonald HR (1994) Major histocompatibility complex class I related molecules control the development of CD4$^+$8$^-$ and CD4$^-$8$^-$ subsets of natural killer 1.1$^+$ T cell receptor-alpha/beta$^+$ cells in the liver of mice. J Exp Med 180:699–704

39. Ohteki T, Yoshida H, Matsuyama T, Duncan GS, Mak TW, Ohashi PS (1998) The transcription factor interferon regulatory factor 1 (IRF-1) is important during the maturation of natural killer 1.1+ T cell receptor-alpha/beta+ (NK1+ T) cells, natural killer cells, and intestinal intraepithelial T cells. J Exp Med 187:967–972

40. Pasquier B, Yin L, Fondaneche MC, Relouzat F, Bloch-Queyrat C, Lambert N, Fischer A, de Saint-Basile G, Latour S (2005) Defective NKT cell development in mice and humans lacking the adapter SAP, the X-linked lymphoproliferative syndrome gene product. J Exp Med 201:695–701

41. Pellicci DG, Hammond KJ, Uldrich AP, Baxter AG, Smyth MJ, Godfrey DI (2002) A natural killer T (NKT) cell developmental pathway involving a thymus-dependent NK1.1(-)CD4(+) CD1d-dependent precursor stage. J Exp Med 195:835–844

42. Pellicci DG, Uldrich AP, Kyparissoudis K, Crowe NY, Brooks AG, Hammond KJ, Sidobre S, Kronenberg M, Smyth MJ, Godfrey DI (2003) Intrathymic NKT cell development is blocked by the presence of alpha-galactosylceramide. Eur J Immunol 33:1816–1823

43. Prussin C, Foster B (1997) TCRV alpha 24 and V beta 11 coexpression defines a human NK1. T cell analog containing a unique Th0 subpopulation. J Immunol 159:5862–5870

44. Robson MacDonald H, Lees RK, Held W (1998) Developmentally regulated extinction of Ly-49 receptor expression permits maturation and selection of NK1.1+ T cells. J Exp Med 187:2109–2114

45. Sato H, Nakayama T, Tanaka Y, Yamashita M, Shibata Y, Kondo E, Saito Y, Taniguchi M (1999) Induction of differentiation of pre-NKT cells to mature Valpha14. NKT cells by granulocyte/macrophage colony-stimulating factor. Proc Natl Acad Sci U S A 96:7439–7444

46. Schmidt-Supprian M, Tian J, Grant EP, Pasparakis M, Maehr R, Ovaa H, Ploegh HL, Coyle AJ, Rajewsky K (2004) Differential dependence of CD4+CD25+ regulatory and natural killer-like T cells on signals leading to NF-kappaB activation. Proc Natl Acad Sci U S A 101:4566–4571

47. Schumann J, Mycko MP, Dellabona P, Casorati G, MacDonald HR (2006) Cutting edge: influence of the TCRVbeta domain on the selection of semi-invariant NKT cells by endogenous ligands. J Immunol 176:2064–2068

48. Schumann J, Pittoni P, Tonti E, Macdonald HR, Dellabona P, Casorati G (2005) Targeted expression of human CD1d in transgenic mice reveals independent roles for thymocytes and thymic APCs in positive and negative selection of Valpha14i NKT cells. J Immunol 175:7303–7310

49. Schumann J, Voyle RB, Wei BY, MacDonald HR (2003) Cutting edge: influence of the TCRV beta domain on the avidity of CD1d:alpha-galactosylceramide binding by invariant V alpha 14. NKT cells. J Immunol 170:5815–5819

50. Shimamura M, Ohteki T, Beutner U, MacDonald HR (1997) Lack of directed V alpha 14-J alpha 281 rearrangements in NK1+ T cells. Eur J Immunol 27:1576–1579

51. Shinkura R, Kitada K, Matsuda F, Tashiro K, Ikuta K, Suzuki M, Kogishi K, Serikawa T, Honjo T (1999) Alymphoplasia is caused by a point mutation in the mouse gene encoding Nf-kappa b-inducing kinase. Nat Genet 22:74–77

52. Singer A (2002) New perspectives on a developmental dilemma: the kinetic signaling model and the importance of signal duration for the CD4/CD8 lineage decision. Curr Opin Immunol 14:207–215

53. Sivakumar V, Hammond KJ, Howells N, Pfeffer K, Weih F (2003) Differential requirement for Rel/nuclear factor kappa B family members in natural killer T cell development. J Exp Med 197:1613–1621

54. Stanic AK, Bezbradica JS, Park JJ, Matsuki N, Mora AL, Van Kaer L, Boothby MR, Joyce S (2004) NF-kappa B controls cell fate specification, survival, and molecular differentiation of immunoregulatory natural T lymphocytes. J Immunol 172:2265–2273

55. Stanic AK, Bezbradica JS, Park JJ, Van Kaer L, Boothby MR, Joyce S (2004) Cutting edge: the ontogeny and function of Va14Ja18 natural T lymphocytes require signal processing by protein kinase C theta and NF-kappa B. J Immunol 172:4667–4671

56. Tilloy F, Di Santo JP, Bendelac A, Lantz O (1999) Thymic dependence of invariant V alpha 14+ natural killer-T cell development. Eur J Immunol 29:3313–3318

57. Townsend MJ, Weinmann AS, Matsuda JL, Salomon R, Farnham PJ, Biron CA, Gapin L, Glimcher LH (2004) T-bet regulates the terminal maturation and homeostasis of NK and Valpha14i NKT cells. Immunity 20:477–494

58. Treiner E, Duban L, Bahram S, Radosavljevic M, Wanner V, Tilloy F, Affaticati P, Gilfillan S, Lantz O (2003) Selection of evolutionarily conserved mucosal-associated invariant T cells by MR1. Nature 422:164–169

59. Urdahl KB, Sun JC, Bevan MJ (2002) Positive selection of MHC class Ib-restricted CD8(+) T cells on hematopoietic cells. Nat Immunol 3:772–779

60. Vicari AP, Herbelin A, Leite-de-Moraes MC, Von Freeden-Jeffry U, Murray R, Zlotnik A (1996) NK1.1+ T cells from IL-7-deficient mice have a normal distribution and selection but exhibit impaired cytokine production. Int Immunol 8:1759–1766

61. Voyle RB, Beermann F, Lees RK, Schumann J, Zimmer J, Held W, MacDonald HR (2003) Ligand-dependent inhibition of CD1d-restricted NKT cell development in mice transgenic for the activating receptor Ly49D. J Exp Med 197:919–925

62. Wei DG, Curran SA, Savage PB, Teyton L, Bendelac A (2006) Mechanisms imposing the Vbeta bias of Valpha14 natural killer T cells and consequences for microbial glycolipid recognition. J Exp Med 203:1197–1207

63. Wei DG, Lee H, Park SH, Beaudoin L, Teyton L, Lehuen A, Bendelac A (2005) Expansion and long-range differentiation of the NKT cell lineage in mice expressing CD1d exclusively on cortical thymocytes. J Exp Med 202:239–248

64. Zhou D, Mattner J, Cantu C 3rd, Schrantz N, Yin N, Gao Y, Sagiv Y, Hudspeth K, Wu YP, Yamashita T, Teneberg S, Wang D, Proia RL, Levery SB, Savage PB, Teyton L, Bendelac A (2004) Lysosomal glycosphingolipid recognition by NKT cells. Science 306:1786–1789

65. Zimmer MI, Colmone A, Felio K, Xu H, Ma A, Wang CR (2006) A cell-type specific CD1d expression program modulates invariant NKT cell development and function. J Immunol 176:1421–1430

Section III
Disease

CTMI (2007) 314:215–248
© Springer-Verlag Berlin Heidelberg 2007

CD1-Restricted T Cells in Host Defense to Infectious Diseases

S. M. Behar[1] · S. A. Porcelli[2] (✉)

[1]Division of Rheumatology, Immunology and Allergy, Brigham and Women's
Hospital, Smith Building Room 518, One Jimmy Fund Way, Boston, MA 02115, USA

[2]Department of Microbiology and Immunology, Albert Einstein College of Medicine,
Room 416 Forchheimer Building, 1300 Morris Park Avenue, Bronx, NY 10461, USA
porcelli@aecom.yu.edu

Abstract CD1 has been clearly shown to function as a microbial recognition system for activation of T cell responses, but its importance for mammalian protective responses against infections is still uncertain. The function of the group 1 CD1 isoforms, including human CD1a, CD1b, and CD1c, seems closely linked to adaptive immunity. These CD1 molecules control the responses of T cells that are highly specific for particular lipid antigens, the best known of which are abundantly expressed by pathogenic mycobacteria such as *Mycobacterium tuberculosis* and *Mycobacterium leprae*. Studies done mainly on human circulating T cells ex vivo support a significant role for group I CD1-restricted T cells in protective immunity to mycobacteria and potentially other pathogens, although supportive data from animal models is currently limited. In contrast, group 2 CD1 molecules, which include human CD1d and its orthologs, have been predominantly associated with the activation of CD1d-restricted NKT cells, which appear to be more appropriately viewed as a facet of the innate immune system. Whereas the recognition of certain self-lipid ligands by CD1d-restricted NKT cells is well accepted, the importance of these T cells in mediating adaptive immune recognition of specific microbial lipid antigens remains controversial. Despite continuing uncertainty about the role of CD1d-restricted NKT cells in natural infections, studies in mouse models demonstrate the potential of these T cells to exert various effects on a wide spectrum of infectious diseases, most likely by serving as a bridge between innate and adaptive immune responses.

1
Introduction

The essential function of CD1 molecules in the presentation of lipid antigens to T cells is well established, but their precise roles in the overall function of the immune system are still largely matters of conjecture. Clearly, CD1 molecules have the potential to function as a key component of a microbial recognition system that alerts the immune system to the presence of pathogens harboring relevant lipid targets as part of their essential structure. Detailed structural studies of CD1 molecules confirm their basic lipid-binding and -presentation function, and T cell responses to microbial lipids that depend on CD1 presentation have been repeatedly demonstrated. All lines of investigation point clearly to the conclusion that CD1 evolved as a family of proteins with the primary function of serving as a microbial recognition system. Nevertheless, major questions remain regarding the importance of this system in adaptive and innate immune responses. In this chapter, we attempt to summarize the considerable body of information that has accumulated on the involvement of CD1 and CD1-restricted T cells in host immunity to infectious agents.

2
Group 1 Versus Group 2 CD1: Separate Roles in Antimicrobial Immunity?

One of the problems in attempting to resolve the question of in vivo relevance of CD1-restricted T cell responses in infectious diseases has been the extensive reliance of immunologists on rodent models for this purpose. As is now well-recognized, mice and rats appear to be endowed with a smaller number of CD1 isoforms than most other mammals, and completely lack orthologs of a major set of CD1 isoforms known as group 1 CD1 molecules (CD1a, CD1b, and CD1c). These are believed to perform important roles in immune responses in humans and many other species that are known to express group 1 CD1 proteins [1, 2]. Thus, mice have substantial limitations as a model species for studies of the human CD1 system, and only partially reflect the full potential of human CD1-restricted T cell responses. Extensive reliance on the mouse as a model for human immune responses represents a serious obstacle for research on human CD1 that has yet to be overcome.

While there is a reasonable concern that a major part of the story of CD1-restricted T cells is missing from studies that rely only on mouse models, a great deal of valuable information can be gained from mice on the function of the CD1d protein, which has been found to be expressed in all mouse strains examined to date. CD1d is classified as group 2 CD1 because it shows significant divergence from the group 1 CD1 molecules in terms of its structure, expression, and apparent immunological functions [1, 3]. There is little doubt that the group 2 CD1 system plays a significant role in modulating immune responses to many infections through the activities of CD1d-restricted natural killer T cells (NKT cells) and potentially other distinct T cell subsets [4]. CD1d-restricted T cells have thus far been predominantly linked to more innate-like than adaptive functions in anti-microbial immune responses. These responses appear innate in that they generally do not require priming by prior pathogen exposure, are rapidly triggered upon infection, and may not exhibit the characteristic memory of classical antigen-specific, adaptive T cell responses [5].

In contrast to mice, humans and most other mammals have a larger family of CD1 isoforms, which includes group 1 CD1 molecules consisting of CD1a, CD1b, and CD1c isoforms. The fifth isoform, CD1e, is difficult to classify and may deserve its own designation as group 3 [1, 4]. Unlike CD1d, the group 1 CD1 molecules have been mainly associated with the responses of T cells that exist at low precursor frequencies and appear to constitute adaptive responses to specific microbial challenges. Thus, the impression from currently available data is that the group 1 CD1 system functions primarily as a component of antigen-specific adaptive immunity and provides immunological memory to previously encountered pathogens in a manner analogous to conventional major histocompatibility complex (MHC)-restricted T cells.

For clarity, the current review has been organized largely around the distinction between group 1 and group 2 CD1 molecules, and their respective involvement mainly in adaptive vs innate immune responses during infection. However, the extent to which this apparent dichotomy in CD1-restricted immune responses represents a full and accurate view of how the two different types of CD1 molecules function, as opposed to biases inherent in the available experimental systems, remains to be fully evaluated.

3
Expression of Group 1 CD1 and Its Modulation by Infection

A striking feature of group 1 CD1 molecules is their restricted pattern of expression on relatively few cell types. Other than the strong expression of all CD1 proteins on cortical thymocytes, only myeloid dendritic cells and a few other cell types express group 1 CD1 proteins at readily detectable levels [1, 6]. In humans, CD1a and CD1b have been found exclusively on dendritic cells in vivo and in vitro. CD1c may be slightly more widely distributed, with clear expression on a subset of B cells and low levels occasionally detected on monocytes [7, 8]. So far, this restriction of group 1 CD1 proteins mainly to dendritic cells seems to hold up for other mammalian species, with the exception of the much more prominent expression of one or more CD1b isoforms on virtually all B cells that has been observed in guinea pigs [9]. This restricted expression on dendritic cells and very few other cell types suggests that CD1-restricted T cells may function in infections similarly to class II MHC-restricted T cells, which also recognize antigens on a fairly restricted range of host cells. Thus, functions such as cytokine secretion, activation of dendritic cells and B cells might be among the crucial functions of group 1 CD1-restricted T cells in immune responses to infections.

Several studies have evaluated the modulation of group 1 CD1 expression on myeloid lineage dendritic cells following exposure to infectious microbes or components of microorganisms. This has been analyzed using in vitro mycobacterial infection of monocyte-derived cells, and conflicting results have been obtained. An initial report found that infection of CD1-expressing, monocyte-derived dendritic cells with a virulent strain of *Mycobacterium tu-*

berculosis led to a rapid decrease in cell surface CD1a, -b, and -c expression that was essentially complete by 48 h [10]. This correlated with the disappearance of CD1 transcripts from the cells. Not surprisingly, this loss of CD1 expression by *M. tuberculosis*-infected cells led to their inability to stimulate a CD1-restricted T cell line specific for the bacterium. These findings were interpreted as possible evidence of an immune evasion mechanism used by *M. tuberculosis* to avoid recognition through presentation of its antigens by CD1. Subsequent studies examining the effects of *M. bovis* BCG on the ability of CD1b to be induced on monocytes by exposure to GM-CSF also found evidence for inhibition of CD1 expression by live mycobacterial infection [11, 12]. A similar downmodulation of group 1 CD1 expression and blockade of CD1 induction by GM-CSF has been shown to occur with infection of human monocyte-derived dendritic cells in vitro with the intracellular protozoan *Leishmania donovani* [13].

In contrast to these results, a recent study showed that infection of freshly isolated monocytes with an avirulent strain of *M. tuberculosis* (H37Ra) actually stimulated significant induction of CD1a, CD1b, and CD1c molecules over a period of 72 h [14]. Group 1 CD1 induction in these experiments was associated with increased transcript levels and new protein synthesis. This was shown to be triggered by ligands of toll-like receptor-2 (TLR-2), including polar lipids from the mycobacterium that are known to signal through this receptor. The cells that were induced to express group 1 CD1 molecules by infection had a phenotype more characteristic of dendritic cells than macrophages, suggesting that infection can drive differentiation of monocytes to become more potent antigen-presenting cells. Interestingly, the upregulation of group 1 CD1 on monocytes by stimulation with mycobacterial lipids was also associated with a concurrent reduction in expression of CD1d, emphasizing further the apparent differences in the way that group 1 and group 2 CD1 molecules interact with infections.

Taken together, these in vitro studies support the idea that infections of myeloid cells may either positively or negatively modulate the expression of group 1 CD1 molecules, with the final outcome depending on several factors such as the particular pathogen involved, the differentiated state of the cell at the time of infection, or other features of the local microenvironment. Evidence for modulation of group 1 CD1 expression on myeloid lineage cells during infections in vivo is currently extremely limited and is an area in need of further investigation. One study using immunohistochemistry to analyze group 1 CD1 expression in human cutaneous leprosy lesions demonstrated the prominent expression of CD1a, -b, and -c on dendritic cells localizing to dermal granulomas that are sites of active *M. leprae* infection [15]. The expression of CD1b in leprosy lesions was confirmed in a study that linked this to the development of increased local immunity to *M. leprae*, and suggested that toll-like receptor signaling could induce monocytes to differentiate into these group 1 CD1$^+$ dendritic cells [16]. Recent progress in defining group 1 CD1 molecules in a variety of other mammalian species, such as guinea pigs [9, 17, 18], rabbits [19], cows [20], and nonhuman primates [21], may allow the development of more advanced studies on the modulation of group 1 CD1 molecules by infection in vivo.

4
Identification of Group 1 CD1-Restricted T Cells in Infectious Diseases

Nearly all descriptions of group 1 CD1-restricted T cell responses against infectious agents have been focused on mycobacterial pathogens, primarily *M. tuberculosis* and *M. leprae*. In part, this may reflect the historical fact that CD1-restriction of T cell responses was discovered by using mycobacterial antigen preparations to elicit human T cell responses in vitro [22]. In addition, mycobacteria are extremely lipid-rich and harbor a broad array of known and potential CD1-presented antigens [23]. As described in detail in other chapters of this volume, a number of specific lipid and glycolipid components of mycobacteria that are recognized by group 1 CD1-restricted T cells have been isolated and fully characterized.

4.1
Mycobacteria-Reactive, CD1-Restricted T Cell Responses in Humans

CD1-restricted T cells were initially identified in cultures of human leukocytes stimulated ex vivo with CD1-expressing, monocyte-derived dendritic cells plus crude extracts of *M. tuberculosis*. This led to the identification of CD4$^-$CD8$^-$ TCR$\alpha\beta^+$ T cell lines (often referred to as double negative, or DN T cells) that proliferated and secreted interferon-γ in response to *M. tuberculosis* extracts [22, 24–27]. In follow-up studies, similar T cell lines were isolated from the CD8$^+$ and CD4$^+$ circulating pools [28, 29]. Most of these T cell lines showed cytotoxic activity against infected or antigen-pulsed target cells, which was mediated by either FasL- or perforin-dependent mechanisms [30]. Examples of mycobacteria-specific T cells restricted by each of the three group 1 CD1 proteins have been reported. All of these have been shown to respond to different lipid or glycolipid antigens unique to mycobacteria and other closely related bacterial species. The T cell antigen receptor (TCR) α and β chains expressed by these T cells appear highly diverse, and no repeating or canonical features of group 1 CD1-restricted TCRs have yet been found [31].

Several studies have attempted to quantitate levels of circulating CD1-restricted T cell reactivity against mycobacterial antigens in humans. One of the goals of these studies was to determine whether increased levels of such T cell responses could be correlated with prior infection with the pathogen, which would be indicative of sustained memory responses characteristic of true adaptive immunity. Four published reports currently indicate that this is indeed the case. Thus, group 1 CD1-restricted T cells specific for either whole lipid extracts or fully characterized glucose monomycolate or acylated sulfotrehalose antigens of *M. tuberculosis* were generally detectable only in humans with positive tuberculin skin tests, which are indicative of previous infection with *M. tuberculosis* [32, 33]. A similar observation was documented for CD1c-restricted T cells specific for a synthetic analog of an *M. tuberculosis* mannosyl-phosphomycoketide antigen [34], and a study of *M. bovis* BCG-vaccinated subjects found that a majority of the CD8+ T cells responsive to live BCG-infected dendritic cells in vitro was restricted by group 1 CD1 molecules [35].The precursor frequencies of lipid-reactive T cells in *M. tuberculosis*-immune human subjects were measured by interferon-γ enzyme-linked immunospot (ELISPOT) assays in one study and were reported to have median values of 46 per 100,000 circulating mononuclear cells for responses to a crude mycobacterial lipid extract, and 43 per 100,000 for responses to the purified glucose monomycolate antigen [32]. Assuming that these represent frequencies of circulating CD1-restricted memory T cells, these values are not insignificant, as they are only slightly lower than values reported for some of the more well-studied immunodominant *M. tuberculosis* protein antigens in similar patients. Lipid antigen-reactive T cells have been detected by ELISPOT in both the CD4+ and CD8+ fractions of circulating lymphocytes from *M. tuberculosis*-immune donors, with a two- to threefold higher median frequency observed in the CD4+ fraction [32].

An interesting feature of human CD1-restricted T cells specific for mycobacteria that has recently been reported is the strong tendency of these T cells to cross-react between different species of mycobacteria [36]. This property of CD1-restricted T cells appears to contrast sharply with class II MHC-restricted peptide antigen-reactive T cells, as the latter tend, in the majority of cases, to distinguish between closely related mycobacterial species such as *M. leprae* and *M. tuberculosis*. This high level of cross-reactivity for related pathogens among CD1-restricted T cells may reflect the relatively high level of conservation of the structures of CD1-presented lipid and glycolipid antigens, and also the almost complete lack of significant allelic polymorphism of the CD1 molecules themselves. This apparent fundamental difference between the specificities of the MHC-restricted and CD1-restricted T cell repertoires suggest that these two classes of T cells play distinct roles in the host response. In particular, it has been suggested that the more cross-reactive CD1-restricted subset may have a greater ability to respond to pathogens that have not been previously encountered, and thus provide a way of bridging innate and adaptive immunity.

4.2
Animal Models of CD1-Restricted Immunity to Mycobacteria

Now that many fundamental features of CD1-restricted antigen presentation have been well studied, it is clear that there is a pressing need for the development of practical animal models to evaluate the importance of this component of immunity to infection and vaccination in vivo. Unfortunately, progress in meeting this challenge has been relatively slow. As mentioned earlier, mice, rats, and presumably other small rodents do not provide an opportunity for modeling group 1 CD1-restricted responses because they lack orthologs of CD1a, CD1b, CD1c, and CD1e molecules. However, a variety of other animals may ultimately prove useful in this regard, particularly guinea pigs, rabbits, cows, and nonhuman primates. Given the fact that cows are a natural host of *M. bovis*, another human pathogen that causes a tuberculosis-like disease, it is possible that these animals may ultimately prove to be extremely useful for gaining insights into the in vivo function of the group 1 CD1 antigen-presenting system [20].

However, so far only the guinea pig has been studied in any detail with respect to the immunological functions of the group 1 CD1 molecules during infection or vaccination in vivo. Initial studies of this animal showed that it has at least seven functional CD1 genes, including multiple orthologs of human CD1b and CD1c [17]. It may be possible to induce CD1-restricted T cell responses in guinea pigs via immunization with purified *M. tuberculosis* lipids [18]. Furthermore, guinea pigs immunized with *M. tuberculosis* lipids, using a regimen that induced CD1-restricted T cell responses, showed significant protection against a subsequent aerosol challenge with virulent *M. tuberculosis* organisms [37]. The level of protective immunity achieved in the lungs of guinea pigs immunized with *M. tuberculosis* lipids was actually similar to that seen in animals that had been immunized with standard BCG vaccination. These studies provide further evidence that group 1 CD1-restricted T cell responses constitute a significant form of T cell memory, which can be potentially exploited for development of novel vaccination strategies against *M. tuberculosis* and possibly other organisms that contain relevant lipid antigens.

4.3
Group 1 CD1-Restricted Responses to Pathogens Other Than Mycobacteria

In contrast to the copious data on responses to mycobacteria, strikingly little data have been reported on group 1 CD1-restricted responses to other types of pathogens. One early study reported isolation of CD1b- and CD1c-restricted T cell lines specific for a protease resistant fraction of *Haemophilus influenzae* type B [38]. These findings have not yet been replicated in further reports, and it remains unclear whether Gram-negative bacteria such as *Haemophilus* species actually harbor lipids that are presented by group 1 CD1 and what the immunological consequences of this would be. Although most bacteria and other more complex pathogens would appear to contain lipids and glycolipids that could be presented by group 1 CD1 molecules to generate adaptive T cell responses, this has yet to be demonstrated. It remains at present unclear whether this reflects a lack of effort in seeking such responses, or alternatively, if the group 1 CD1 system is effective mainly or exclusively in the presentation of lipid antigens associated with mycobacteria and a few other related genera of bacteria.

5
Mechanisms of Group 2 CD1-Restricted T Cell Responses in Infectious Diseases

As discussed above, human T cells that recognize microbial lipid antigens presented by group 1 CD1 are elicited following infection and express antimicrobial effector functions. Group 2 CD1-restricted T cells are also thought to contribute to immunity against infection. Mice have been used extensively to determine the role of CD1d-restricted T cells in immunity to microbial pathogens. Murine CD1d-restricted T cells frequently express cell surface proteins encoded by the NK locus, and the NK1.1 antigen (CD161) has been used to identify CD1d-restricted T cells in mice. However, as previously noted, NK1.1 and other NK cell markers are induced on conventional MHC-restricted T cells following activation, particularly during infection, and therefore, NK1.1^{+} T cells are not synonymous with CD1d-restricted T cells. One major subset of CD1d-restricted T cells is distinguished by their use of a semi-invariant TCR [39]. These T cells have a canonical rearrangement of Vα14 and Jα18, and this invariant TCRα chain pairs with a limited number of TCRβ chains, which come predominantly from the Vβ2, Vβ7, and Vβ8 families. These CD1d-restricted T cells are sometimes referred to as type 1 NKT cells, or invariant NKT cells. They uniformly recognize the synthetic antigen α-galactosylceramide (αGalCer), a molecule based on the structure of lipids identified in marine sponges, which were found to activate the immune system. While the biological or evolutionary links between marine sponge lipids and CD1 are unclear, treatment with αGalCer induces protection from certain types of tumors [40]. The capacity of invariant NKT cells to recognize αGalCer is useful experimentally as CD1d tetramers loaded with αGalCer can bind to the invariant TCR and can be used to identify these T cells by flow cytometry [41]. A second population of CD1d-restricted T cells also expresses NK markers, but in contrast to invariant NKT cells, this second population uses a more diverse TCR repertoire [42]. In general, diverse (or type 2) NKT cells do not recognize αGalCer and there are no known markers that specifically identify this population of cells. However, they can be identified largely based on their functional characterization. Additional T cell populations exist that express NK1.1 or other NK cell-associated markers and are not CD1d-restricted but are sometimes referred to as NKT cells in the literature [43]. These constitute a poorly characterized and apparently heterogeneous group of T cells, and we will thus limit our discussion to invariant NKT cells (i.e., type 1 NKT cells) and to CD1d-restricted T cells that express a diverse TCR repertoire (i.e., type 2 NKT cells) [43].

The capacity of αGalCer treatment to improve the outcome of infection is an important indication that invariant NKT cells have the potential to enhance immunity against microbial pathogens [44–46]. While pharmacological activation of invariant NKT cells demonstrates their antimicrobial potential, and raises the possibility that αGalCer could have a role in the therapy of certain infectious diseases, the ability of αGalCer to ameliorate infectious disease does not prove a physiological role for invariant NKT cells in microbial immunity. For example, αGalCer-induced invariant NKT cell activation enhances host resistance to tuberculosis; however, the absence of CD1d or invariant NKT cells does not impair host susceptibility to *M. tuberculosis* infection [47–49]. Since pharmacologically activated invariant NKT cells modulate host immunity by multiple mechanisms, the finding that CD1d and/or invariant NKT cells are dispensable in certain infection models raises the question of whether CD1d-restricted T cells truly play a physiological role in immunity to infectious agents. To present a clear analysis of the physiological role that CD1d-restricted T cells play in immunity to infection, the following section focuses on studies in which CD1d or invariant NKT cell TCRs have been deleted, rather than studies of αGalCer treatment of animals, a topic that has been addressed in several recent reviews [49, 50].

Certain infectious processes are exacerbated in the absence of CD1d-restricted T cells, which suggests that CD1d-restricted T cells serve a protective role against microbial pathogens. However, the severity of disease caused by other microbial pathogens is lessened in the absence of CD1d-restricted

T cells, which indicates that NKT cells can also have a detrimental effect on the outcome of infection. This detrimental effect may result mainly or exclusively from immune-mediated tissue damage. Importantly, both of these findings imply that NKT cells are physiologically activated during infection, and raise the interesting question of how diverse pathogens lead to NKT cell activation. Group 1 CD1-restricted T cells appear to share many similarities with conventional MHC-restricted T cells, particularly with respect to their diverse TCR repertoire, fine specificity for antigens, and requirement for co-stimulation and accessory signals. Analogous to the paradigm established for conventional MHC-restricted T cells, activation of group 1 CD1-restricted T cells requires their clonotypic TCR to bind to a microbial lipid antigen presented by CD1. Activation of CD1d-restricted T cells during infection may be triggered by a similar sequence of events; alternatively, recent data suggest that microbial pathogens may activate NKT cells indirectly by inducing host factors that provide co-stimulation to weakly autoreactive CD1d-restricted T cells. These possible modes of activation are discussed below.

5.1
Direct Recognition of Pathogen-Derived Lipid Antigens by CD1d-Restricted T Cells

Since many microbial lipids differ structurally from mammalian lipids, it was anticipated that lipid-antigen presentation by CD1 would play a role in host immunity against infection. This is true for group 1 CD1, as CD1a-, CD1b-, and CD1c-restricted T cells recognize *M. tuberculosis*-infected cells. Although studies in animal models have established that CD1d-restricted T cells participate in the host response to infection, only a limited number of microbial lipid antigens have been identified that are recognized by CD1d-restricted T cells. This is surprising since the intracellular trafficking patterns and the structure of murine CD1d resemble human CD1b, which clearly binds and presents mycobacterial lipids [51]. Microbial lipids that bind to murine CD1d include *Escherichia coli* phosphatidylethanolamine, *M. tuberculosis* lipoarabinomannan, and *Trypanosoma cruzi* glycophosphatidylinositol. However, it is uncertain whether CD1d-restricted T cells that recognize these antigens are elicited during infection [52–54]. Other microbial lipid antigens have been identified that are presented by CD1d and activate NKT cells. These include monoglycosylceramides from sphingomonas species [55, 56] phosphatidylinositolmannosides from *M. tuberculosis*, and lipophosphoglycan from *Leishmania donovani* [57, 58].

The paucity of microbial lipid antigens has made it difficult to characterize antigen-specific CD1d-restricted NKT cell responses following infection. However, the examples that exist are important ones as they show that, like human group 1 CD1, CD1d-restricted NKT cells can recognize microbial lipid antigens. The power of the mouse model can now be exploited to determine the exact role of CD1d-restricted T cells in immunity to infection by these pathogens. In particular, there is widespread interest in determining whether vaccination with lipid antigens will induce protective immunity and whether specific activation of CD1d-restricted T cells by microbial antigens leads to their clonal expansion and development of CD1d-restricted memory T cells [59].

5.2
Enhanced Autoreactivity of CD1d-Restricted NKT Cells During Infection

TCR-dependent recognition of microbial lipid antigens is one way that CD1d-restricted T cells become activated following infection and is analogous to the way we envision presentation of specific antigens to activate group 1 CD1- and MHC-restricted T cells. However, microbial pathogens or infected cells can activate lymphocytes by signaling pathways that are independent of specific antigen receptors. For example, viral pathogens often interfere with the class I MHC antigen-processing and -presentation pathway, which diminishes class I MHC surface expression by the infected cell and represents a possible mechanism of immune evasion [60]. NK cells express inhibitory receptors that bind to class I MHC, so that class I MHC downregulation releases NK cells from inhibition and activates their killing of virally infected target cells [61, 62]. Thus, NK cells can recognize and kill virally infected cells even though they lack the capacity to recognize virally encoded antigens. Like NK cells, B-1 B cells, and γδ-T cells, NKT cells are lymphocytes that express invariant or semi-invariant immunoglobulin-like receptors and may be important in the innate immune response to infection [5]. NKT cells are postulated to serve a role linking the innate and adaptive responses both temporally and functionally. We will now consider the hypothesis that NKT cells recognize endogenous self-lipid antigens and become activated during infection because microbes induce host-derived factors that co-stimulate weakly autoreactive CD1d-restricted T cells (Fig. 1).

5.2.1
Autoreactivity of CD1d-Restricted T Cells

The self-reactive nature of human and murine CD1d-restricted T cells is an integral part of their original description and autoreactivity is a characteristic of both invariant and diverse CD1d-restricted murine T cells [63–66]. Most studies that detect self-reactivity use sensitive assays that may exaggerate the

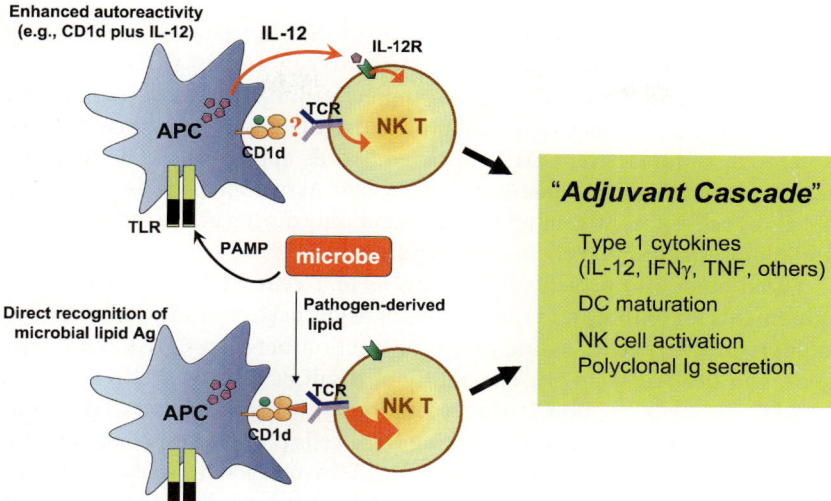

Fig. 1 Alternative mechanisms of CD1d-restricted NKT cell activation by infection. *Top*: activation of NKT cells by enhanced autoreactivity. This occurs when the low-level autoreactivity of most NKT cells synergizes with additional co-stimulatory signals in the environment that are produced by antigen presenting cells (*APCs*) in response to pathogen-associated molecular patterns (*PAMPs*) that are sensed by toll-like receptors (*TLRs*) or other pattern recognition receptors. IL-12 represents one co-stimulatory signal that is induced in the setting of acute infection that has been shown to synergize with TCR-mediated autoreactivity toward CD1d to induce full activation and effector function expression by NKT cells. *Bottom*: activation of NKT cells by direct microbial lipid antigen recognition. This involves direct stimulation of NKT cells by pathogen-derived lipid or glycolipid antigens. The complex formed by the association of the specific microbial lipid antigen is able to engage the TCR of the NKT cell and induce responses that may be less dependent on co-stimulatory signals

degree of autoreactivity. For example, many studies use NKT cell hybridomas that have a low threshold of activation and are relatively co-stimulation-independent [64, 65, 67]. Other studies use tumor cells as APCs that are engineered to express supraphysiological levels of CD1d, which increases the avidity between the NKT cell and the CD1d-expressing APC [66, 68, 69]. Primary NKT cell recognition of CD1d in vitro requires the addition of cytokines such as IL-2 and the use of CD1-transfected tumor cells as APC [68, 70]. Interestingly, the original description that primary NKT cells (from a TCR transgenic mouse) recognize αGalCer used an assay system in which primary dendritic cell and antigen were cultured in the absence of exogenously added cytokines. Under these conditions, no autoreactivity was observed [71]. The molecular basis for the autoreactive nature of CD1d-restricted T cells is now better defined. Some of the self-lipid antigens recognized by CD1d-restricted T cells have been identified, and it is appreciated that accessory signals and CD1d levels affect the activation of autoreactive CD1d-restricted T cells. Thus, potentially autoreactive, CD1d-restricted T cells appear not to be tonically activated but remain in a quiescent state in vivo. Activation of CD1d-restricted T cells by self-lipid antigens appears to occur only during active inflammation and requires additional co-stimulatory signals.

CD1d binds and presents lipid antigens to T cells, and the structural requirements for binding and recognition of α-glycosylceramides lends critical support to the specific nature of the interaction between CD1d, lipid antigens, and the TCR [71–73]. The ability of αGalCer to activate NKT cells in an APC-free plate-bound CD1d presentation assay confirms that CD1d–lipid complexes are key stimuli for activating NK T cells [74, 75]. The characteristic autoreactivity that has been described for CD1d-restricted T cells is antigen-dependent, meaning that recognition of CD1d requires a lipid ligand derived either from the pool of endogenous cellular lipids or from the extracellular milieu [74]. Phosphodiacylglycerols are one physiologically relevant class of endogenous CD1d ligands that are recognized by both human and murine CD1d-restricted T cells [52, 74]. Like αGalCer, phosphatidylethanolamine, phosphatidylcholine, and phosphatidylinositol can activate CD1d-restricted T cell hybridomas in the APC-free plate-bound CD1d assay, and the activation of CD1d-restricted T cells depends on certain structural features such as acyl chain length and the number of carbon double bonds [52, 74]. The lysosomal glycosphingolipid isoglobotrihexosylceramide (iGb3) is another self-lipid molecule that is recognized by CD1d-restricted T cells and is proposed to be the primary self antigen involved in thymic selection of CD1d-autoreactive invariant NKT cells [55, 56]. The lysosomal-glycosphingolipid-degrading enzyme β-hexosaminidase is critical in converting the precursor iGb4 into iGb3, and invariant NKT cells do not recognize APCs from mice genetically deficient in the B subunit of β-hexosaminidase.

Primary NKT cells cultured with APCs that express physiological levels of CD1d do not become activated in the absence of other co-stimulatory or accessory signals. Generally, primary NKT cells require culture with IL-2 or IL-12 for proliferation and the production of IL-4 and interferon-γ [68, 70, 76]. In fact, NKT cell recognition of αGalCer presented by dendritic cells promotes interactions of CD40 with CD40 ligand, which induces dendritic cell maturation and promotes dendritic cell production of IL-12p70 [77]. Dendritic cell production of IL-12 may be critical for optimum activation of CD1d-restricted T cells. Thus, co-stimulatory signals are required for full activation of NKT cells, even by potent antigens such as αGalCer [78].

5.2.2
Co-stimulation of CD1d-Restricted T Cells by Host-Derived Factors Induced by Microbial Pathogens

In contrast to group 1 CD1 expression, CD1d is more widely expressed on different types of leukocytes and other somatic cells. However, CD1d expression varies on different cell types with marginal zone B cells having among the highest CD1d expression [79]. Dendritic cells and macrophages express CD1d; however, its level varies depending on the exposure to cytokines and other signals [68, 80, 81]. APCs expressing higher levels of CD1d more efficiently activate NKT cells both in vitro and in vivo, presumably because increasing CD1d levels raise the avidity of the TCR–CD1d interaction, favoring NKT cell activation [68]. This is true both for CD1d-restricted T cells that are autoreactive, and for those that recognize exogenous antigens such as αGalCer [68]. Regulation of CD1d levels in vivo is one way to regulate the activation of potentially autoreactive T cells. During states of inflammation such as infection, cytokines and TLR signals increase CD1d levels, which promote NKT cell activation.

Transgenic mouse models that allow transient ablation of dendritic cells has facilitated the study of which APCs activate NKT cells in vivo [82, 83]. These models show that in vivo activation of splenic NKT cells by αGalCer is dependent upon CD11c$^+$ cells [84]. However, during infection or other inflammatory states, CD1d expression increases on macrophages and probably other cells, and converts them into APCs capable of presenting antigen and activating CD1d-restricted T cells. Thus, CD1d upregulation may serve as a danger signal to activate NKT cells, which in turn activates the innate and adaptive immune systems. Induction of high CD1d levels on cells other than dendritic cells is especially important if CD1d-restricted T cells are to function as effector cells. Macrophages are particularly vulnerable to infection by intracellular bacteria and protozoan parasites and their CD1d upregulation may flag them as infected cells for recognition by activated CD1d-restricted T cells.

TLR ligands expressed by microbial pathogens can induce cells such as macrophages or dendritic cells to produce soluble mediators that co-stimulate NKT cell activation. Addition of heat-killed bacteria to cultured human CD1d-restricted autoreactive T cell clones and dendritic cells induces T cell proliferation and cytokine production [76]. Although the activation is CD1d-dependent, it does not appear to require presentation of microbial lipid antigens by CD1d. Instead, bacterial products such as LPS induce dendritic cell production of IL-12, which provides a co-stimulatory signal sufficient to activate weakly CD1d-autoreactive T cell clones. Consistent with this hypothesis, activation of NKT cells requires APC with an intact TLR signaling pathway. Heat-killed *Salmonella* cultured with MyD88$^{-/-}$ dendritic cells are unable to activate murine invariant NKT cells [56]. Similarly, dendritic cells lacking the iG3b endogenous antigen are also unable to activate NKT cells, even when cultured in the presence of heat-killed *Salmonella* [56]. These data validate a model in which pathogen-induced TLR-dependent IL-12 production co-stimulates a weak TCR signal generated by the recognition of self antigens such as iG3b presented by CD1d, and leads to invariant NKT cell activation during infection.

5.3
An Integrated Model

Whether self or microbial in origin, lipid antigens promote formation of stable ternary complexes of CD1d, antigen, and TCR. Microbes can lead to the activation of CD1d-restricted T cells either by providing a source of foreign lipid antigens that can be directly presented by CD1d, or by activating APCs, which provide co-stimulation to weakly autoreactive CD1d-restricted NKT cells. For example, microbial TLR ligands activate macrophages and dendritic cells to secrete IL-12 and increase cell-surface expression of CD40. These accessory signals may be required to fully activate weakly autoreactive CD1d-restricted T cells. In contrast, bona fide microbial lipid antigens presented by CD1d can mediate TCR-dependent activation of CD1d-restricted T cells independently of these co-stimulatory signals. CD1d-restricted invariant NKT cells recognize *Sphingomonas* lipid antigens presented by dendritic cells independently of MyD88-dependent TLR signaling [56]. Similarly, the presentation of *Leishmania* antigens is independent of IL-12 [57]. The difference in the co-stimulatory requirements of self and microbial lipid-specific CD1d-restricted T cells could simply reflect a variance in the strength of the TCR signal generated; however, this potential difference and its significance remain to be defined.

Activation of CD1d-restricted NKT cells often results in interferon-γ production, which can further activate APCs. The production interferon-γ by itself, or synergistically with TLR ligand-induced tumor necrosis factor α, can induce high levels of CD1d cell surface expression [68]. For example, *Salmonella* infection, which has been shown to induce interferon-γ secretion by macrophages, NK, and NKT cells [76, 80, 85], is predicted to increase cell surface CD1d expression and lead to a positive feedback loop that would further stimulate autoreactive invariant NKT cells [56]. An increase in CD1d cell surface expression will increase the avidity of NK T cell interaction with APCs, and thereby enhance activation of both autoreactive CD1d-restricted T cells as well as ones that recognize exogenous antigens such as α-glucuronylceramides. Once activated, CD1d-restricted T cells can mediate certain immunological functions that have antimicrobial effects. CD1d-restricted T cells can act as direct effector cells via cytolysis or granulysin [86], and their interferon-γ production can activate macrophages to become more microbicidal.

Activated NKT cells can also have immunoregulatory functions that affect the outcome of infection. For example, NKT cells induce dendritic cell maturation, and this effect may be the basis for the adjuvant-like property of αGalCer when administered during vaccination [87]. The interaction between CD1d-restricted NKT cells and dendritic cells can lead to more rapid or more efficient antigen presentation of protein antigens to conventional CD4+ and CD8+ T cells. Additionally, invariant NKT cells are prodigious cytokine producers and can rapidly generate large amounts of IL-4 and interferon-γ. When made locally, these cytokines can modulate the function of other cells, by activating NK cells [88, 89], inducing MHC on macrophages and dendritic cells, and modulating the Th1/Th2 balance of CD4+ T cell responses.

Although enhanced autoreactivity of CD1d-restricted T cells induced by infection represents an alternative pathway of activation, it is not certain this effect is crucial to the overall outcome of infection. For example, *Salmonella* infection leads to the activation of invariant NKT cells; however, the outcome of infection is not altered in the absence of CD1d or invariant NKT cells [80]. Enhanced autoreactivity of activated CD1d-restricted T cells could even be detrimental since the production of proinflammatory cytokines could lead to excessive tissue injury. One could imagine that the production of IL-4 and IL-10 could lead to a more dominant Th2 response, which may prove less effective against certain pathogens under some conditions. Either of these scenarios could explain why disease caused by certain pathogens is attenuated in the absence of CD1d or NKT cells.

6
Contribution of CD1d-Restricted T Cells to Antimicrobial Immunity in Specific Models of Infectious Diseases

The investigation of how CD1d-restricted T cells contribute to microbial immunity has taken advantage of the mouse model. Numerous studies have addressed the role of CD1d-restricted T cells in a variety of bacterial, viral, mycotic, and parasitic infections (summarized in Table 1). These studies have been summarized by recent reviews [39, 49, 50, 90] and the focus of this section will be limited to studies showing that CD1d-restricted T cells contribute to the natural host response following infection.

Table 1 Contribution of CD1d-restricted T cells to antimicrobial immunity

Pathogen	Outcome[a]	Refs
Mycobacterium tuberculosis[b]	No change	[47, 93–95, 146]
Salmonella	No change	[56, 76, 80, 85, 100]
Listeria moncytogenes	No change	[101–103]
Streptococcus pneumoniae	Shortened survival	[104]
Pseudomonas aeruginosa	Decreased bacterial clearance	[105]
Ehrlichia muris	Decreased bacterial clearance	[56]
Sphingomonas[b]	Decreased bacterial clearance; increased survival	[55, 56, 106]
Borrelia burgdorferi	Decreased myocarditis in CD1d$^{-/-}$ but not Jα18$^{-/-}$ mice	[129, 142]
Chlamydia trachomatis	Increased pathogen clearance, less pathology, less morbidity	[147]
Schistosoma mansoni[c]	Less tissue inflammation	[113, 114]
Leishmania donovani[b]	Increased parasitemia	[13]
Leishmania major[b]	Increased parasitemia	[115, 116]
Trypanosoma cruzi[b, c]	Increased parasitemia; Jα18$^{-/-}$ mice die prematurely from excessive tissue inflammation	[110]
Toxoplasma gondii[d]	Premature death; excessive tissue inflammation [119] Prolonged survival in Jα18$^{-/-}$ [120]	[119,120]
Cryptococcus neoformans	Increased pathogen burden	[145]
HSV-1[d]	Diminished viral clearance [134] No change [135]	[134, 135]
HSV-2	Diminished viral clearance, increased pathology, premature death	[133]
CMV	No change	[139]
Coxsackievirus B3	Similar viral load; less myocarditis	[142]
LCMV[d]	More rapid viral clearance [141] Similar viral clearance [140]	[141]
RSV	Delayed viral clearance	[138]
EMCV	More severe disease in CD1d$^{-/-}$ but not Jα18$^{-/-}$	[137, 148]

[a] "Outcome" refers to the outcome of infection in CD1d$^{-/-}$ or Jα18$^{-/-}$ mice compared to appropriate wild-type control mice [b] Evidence for a microbial lipid antigen presented by CD1d and/or recognized by CD1d-restricted T cells [c] Evidence for enhanced autoreactivity during infection [d] Contradictory studies in literature, or differences in experimental approaches that may include different mouse or pathogen strains, or other variables

6.1
Bacterial Pathogens

The capacity of group 1 CD1 to present mycobacterial lipid antigens to human T cells led to a careful analysis of whether CD1d serves a similar function. Intradermal injection of mycobacterial lipids leads to the local recruitment of invariant NKT cells and to granuloma formation, but interestingly, this phenomenon does not appear to be dependent upon CD1d [91, 92]. Not only are NKT cells found in the lungs of both naïve and *M. tuberculosis*-infected mice, but infection leads to an increase in the cell surface expression of CD1d on macrophages and dendritic cells [68]. Finally, mycobacterial lipid antigens have been described that can be presented by CD1d to NKT cells [58]. However, there is little evidence that CD1d is required for optimum host resistance to *M. tuberculosis* infection in the mouse model [47, 93–96]. This may reflect the critical role that conventional $CD4^+$ T cells play in this model [97]. Clearly, CD1d-restricted T cells are unable to control bacterial replication in the absence of MHC-restricted T cells [98]. Although NKT cells are dispensable for immunity to tuberculosis in the mouse model, it is remarkable that mice treated with the CD1d ligand αGalCer are protected long term [48]. The prolonged duration of the in vivo αGalCer effect in *M. tuberculosis*-infected mice may suggest that an adjuvant-like effect of activated NKT cells modulates the conventional adaptive immune response, although this has not been documented. Activated human NKT cells can act as effector cells and have a direct bactericidal effect when cultured with infected APCs, possibly through the production of the antimicrobial effector protein granulysin [99]. Thus, the possibility that NKT cells contribute to antimycobacterial responses in a significant way needs to be more extensively studied. For example, whether NKT cells could play a role in another phase of infection, such as during latency, has not been fully addressed in the murine model.

Listeria and *Salmonella* are also intracellular pathogens that infect macrophages, but in contrast to *M. tuberculosis*, these pathogens cause an acute gastrointestinal infection. Several studies have examined the role of CD1d-restricted T cells in immunity to these bacteria. Early on in *Salmonella* infection, NKT cells are activated and are an initial source of interferon-γ [76, 80, 85]. However, early control of oral *Salmonella* infection is not impaired in the absence of CD1d [80, 100]. Similarly, NKT cells are activated following *Listeria monocytogenes* infection and although NKT cells can protect immunodeficient mice against this pathogen, there is little evidence that NKT cells are required for protective immunity in mice with an otherwise intact immune system [101–103].

Streptococcus pneumoniae is a common pulmonary pathogen that causes acute pneumonia. Because *S. pneumoniae* is a classic extracellular bacterium, it is somewhat unexpected that host immunity against this pathogen is dependent upon T cells. Nevertheless, invariant NKT cells appear to be required for control of bacterial replication. Following intratracheal infection, mice lacking the Jα18 gene segment necessary for expression of the canonical invariant NK T cell TCR have a greater bacterial burden and a shortened survival compared to normal control mice [104]. Following infection, invariant NKT cells in the lung increase in a monocyte chemotactic protein-1-dependent manner. The invariant NKT cells exert their protective effect by producing cytokines such as tumor necrosis factor and macrophage inflammatory protein-2, which lead to the accumulation of neutrophils in the lung. This proposed mechanism is similar to the events observed following intratracheal infection with *Pseudomonas aeruginosa*, another pulmonary pathogen in which NKT cells play a physiological role in host resistance [105].

The strongest data that CD1d-restricted invariant NKT cells recognize microbial lipid antigens comes from the study of Gram-negative bacteria that do not produce lipopolysaccharide. These include *Ehrlichia muris*, *Sphingomonas capsulata*, and *Sphingomonas yanoikuyae* [55, 56]. The activation of invariant NKT cells by these bacteria is CD1d-dependent, but in contrast to *Salmonella*, is independent of MyD88, IL-12, and iGb3 production [55, 56]. In the presence of β-hexosaminidase B-deficient dendritic cells, which are believed to lack the endogenous antigen iGb3, these bacteria activate invariant NKT cells, which suggests that this is dependent on presentation of microbial lipids and not self lipids by CD1d. Furthermore, *Sphingomonas* species produce α-linked glucuronyl ceramides and other molecules that are structurally related to the synthetic α-glycosylceramides [55, 106, 107]. Many of these analogs bind CD1d and activate NKT cells in vitro. Compared to control mice, Jα18-deficient and CD1d-deficient mice have impaired clearance of *E. muris* and *Sphingomonas* species, respectively. Interestingly, CD1d-deficient mice live longer after challenge with high-dose *Sphingomonas*, which is associated with a lower interferon-γ response. In this case, a robust inflammatory response may be detrimental to the survival of the host.

CD1d-deficient mice develop arthritis, a pathological feature that does not occur in wild type control mice, following infection with the spirochete *Borrelia burgdorferi*, which is the causative agent of Lyme disease [108]. In addition, CD1d-deficient mice have an altered humoral immune response to spirochete antigens with features that are typically observed in susceptible mouse strains. Recent data suggest that marginal zone B cells, which normally express very high CD1d levels, are involved in this pathological response following infection [109]. Thus, CD1d-restricted NKT cells may have an early impact on immunity to *B. burgdorferi*.

6.2
Protozoan and Metazoan Parasites

Trypanosoma cruzi is a protozoan parasite that causes Chagas disease. Murine NKT cells play a protective role in limiting acute parasitemia since CD1d-deficient and Jα18-deficient mice have a greater and more prolonged parasite burden compared to control mice [110]. Interestingly, invariant NKT cells and diverse NKT cells may have distinct roles in immunity to *T. cruzi* infection. Jα18-deficient mice, which lack invariant NKT cells only, succumb rapidly following infection with *T. cruzi*, while the survival of CD1d-deficient mice, which lack both invariant and diverse NKT cells, is similar to control mice [111]. Although parasitemia is similarly increased in CD1d-deficient and Jα18-deficient mice, the latter have greater hepatic and splenic mononuclear cell infiltrates, increased production of tumor necrosis factor, interferon-γ, and nitric oxide, and more muscle inflammation than either CD1d-deficient or control mice, suggesting that the diverse NKT cells may have a distinct function in limiting the inflammatory response [110, 111]. Finally, although GPI-anchored, mucin-like glycoproteins from *T. cruzi* can bind to CD1d, there is no evidence that they or other *T. cruzi* lipids are recognized by CD1d-restricted T cells [54, 112]. Instead, weakly autoreactive CD1d-restricted NKT cells are activated in an IL-12-dependent manner following infection [112].

The eggs of the extracellular metazoan parasite *Schistosoma mansoni* are deposited in the host liver and induce a strong Th2 response, which leads to chronic inflammation and disease. CD1d is essential for the development of a full Th2 response during murine schistosomiasis and contributes to the immunopathology observed following infection [113]. *S. mansoni* infection leads to NKT cell activation and schistosome egg-sensitized dendritic cells induce IL-4 and interferon-γ production by NKT cells [114]. In this case, activation of NKT cells is CD1d-dependent, but appears to be partially dependent on the presence of β-hexosaminidase B, and presumably iGb3 [114]. Thus, NKT cell activation during *S. mansoni* infection may result from the recognition of endogenous lipid ligands, but is independent of co-stimulatory signals mediated by TLR or IL-12.

CD1d-restricted T cells are also required for optimum host defense against both *L. donovani* and *L. major* [13, 115]. As discussed above, CD1d-restricted NKT cells recognize a lipophosphoglycan antigen from Leishmania, and their activation can occur in the absence of IL-12-mediated co-stimulation [57]. Control of cutaneous disease does not require NKT cells; however, NKT cells appear to be critical in limiting visceral involvement [57, 116]. Several mechanisms may account for the protective effect of NKT cells during *Leishmania* infection, including early production of interferon-γ, activation of NK cells, and regulation of chemokine production [116, 117]. Interestingly, *Leishmania* infection of human dendritic cells leads to downregulation of both group 1 CD1 and CD1d, possibly indicating an attempt by the parasite to evade CD1-restricted T cells [13].

CD4$^+$NK1.1$^+$ T cells were proposed to have a possible role in vaccine-induced protection of class II MHC-deficient mice against lethal challenge with the protozoan parasite *Toxoplasma gondii* [118]. When backcrossed to the susceptible C57BL/6 genetic background, CD1d-deficient mice are more susceptible to *T. gondii* than wild type control mice [119]. Despite their increased mortality, the parasite burden in CD1d-deficient mice was modestly increased in the ileum compared to controls, and the number of parasites in the liver and lung was similar to C57BL/6 mice [119]. Infected CD1d-deficient mice exhibit worse ileitis, suggesting that a difference in immunopathology and not in control of parasite numbers leads to the premature mortality of CD1d-deficient mice. Supporting this possibility, more activated CD4$^+$ T cells, NK1.1$^+$ cells, and Gr-1$^+$ (Ly-6C/G, a marker of myeloid lineage cells most often associated with granulocytes) cells are present in the mesenteric lymph nodes of *T. gondii*-infected, CD1d-deficient mice than in C57BL/6 control mice. Depletion of CD4$^+$ T cells increased the survival of infected CD1d-deficient mice. In contrast, Jα18-deficient mice have a milder phenotype, and a protective effect of NKT cells can be demonstrated during the chronic phase of disease. A second study found that Jα18-deficient mice are more resistant to disease and survive longer than control mice, and they have less severe ileitis and produce more interferon-γ, which suggests a possible role for NKT cells in aggravating the inflammatory process [120].

Finally, a possible role for CD1d-restricted T cells in mediating immunity to infections with plasmodia, the protozoan parasites that cause malaria, remains controversial [121–124]. The situation is complicated since the natural killer complex, expressed by NKT cells, is an important genetic locus that modulates host resistance response and disease outcome [125]. Furthermore, as is true with many pathogens, lipid molecules produced by plasmodia are both potential CD1-presented antigens, and also direct activators of immune cells by other means. For example, the glycolipids lipoarabinomannan and LPS activate TLR2 and TLR4, respectively. Thus, detailed studies are required to sort out the pleiotropic effects of microbial lipids on the host immune response following infection.

6.3
Viruses

6.3.1
Modulation of CD1d Levels by Viral Infection

Just as viruses are known to interfere with antigen processing and class I MHC expression, viral infection can also lead to the downregulation of CD1d. CD1d expression by splenic dendritic cells and macrophages following several different viral infections is reduced [126]. Interestingly, viral infection of CD1d-transfected L cells did not alter CD1d surface levels, but antigen presentation was abrogated after infection with vesicular stomatitis and vaccinia virus, an effect that was due to changes in CD1d trafficking [127]. Different viruses may alter CD1d expression by distinct mechanisms. Recognition of the tyrosine-based motif located in the cytoplasmic tail of CD1d allows the Nef protein of HIV-1 to downregulate CD1d expression by increasing its internalization from the cell surface [128]. In contrast, the Kaposi sarcoma-associated herpes virus promotes downregulation of cell surface CD1d due to ubiquitination of its cytoplasmic tail and leads to reduced activation of CD1d-restricted T cells [81]. Not all viruses downregulate CD1d. Following infection with coxsackievirus B3, CD1d levels are increased on cardiac endothelial cells in a TNF-dependent manner [129]. CD1d levels are also strongly upregulated in the liver of patients with chronic hepatitis C virus, both on hepatocytes and infiltrating mononuclear cells [130, 131]. Therefore, similar to the ability of bacterial ligands to synergize with host factors to upregulate CD1d expression [68], viral infection can also increase CD1d levels.

6.3.2
Resolution of Viral Infection

One reason to believe that invariant NKT cells may play a role in immunity to viral infection is the case of an 11-year-old girl who developed disseminated varicella infection after immunization with the varicella-zoster vaccine strain. Upon evaluation, she was found to have a profound deficiency of NKT cells [132]. Whether or not NKT cells play a role in the resolution of viral infections has been addressed for several different viruses using mouse models. Increased susceptibility to viral infection in mice lacking CD1d-restricted NKT cells is predicted because these cells are a source of interferon-γ early after infection, and can promote NK cell activation, as observed in genital herpes simplex virus type 2 infection [133]. Similarly, resolution of herpes simplex virus type 1 depends in part upon NKT cells [134], but it is uncertain whether this is a general phenomenon or whether it depends on the particular viral strain [135]. CD1d-deficient mice are more susceptible to diabetogenic encephalomyocarditis virus (EMCV-D) infection, and interestingly, Jα18-deficient mice are similarly resistant as wild type control mice [136, 137]. This implicates a role for type 2 (diverse TCR) CD1d-restricted T cells in resistance to EMCV-D infection. Finally, CD1d-restricted NKT cells may influence the outcome of respiratory syncytial virus (RSV) infection by enhancing the adaptive immune response following infection [138].

The outcome of several viral infections is unaltered in the absence of CD1d or invariant NKT cells. Using murine cytomegalovirus as a model to evaluate the role of NKT cells in immunity to viral infections, Jα18-deficient mice lacking invariant NKT cells were found to have unaltered clearance of CMV infection [139]. Similarly, the loss of CD1d-restricted NKT cells does not hamper NK cell activation following lymphocytic choriomeningitis virus (LCMV) infection, nor does the absence of CD1d-restricted NKT cells impair the generation of LCMV-specific MHC-restricted cytotoxic T cells [140, 141].

6.3.3
Immunopathology

While CD1d-restricted T cells may have an effector function following certain viral infections, they may also contribute to the immunopathology that sometimes arises during the immune response to viral pathogens. For example, the absence of CD1d-restricted T cells does not have a significant impact on viral titers after coxsackievirus B3 virus. However, the severe myocarditis caused by coxsackievirus B3 in BALB/c mice was not observed in mice lacking CD1d [142]. Type 2 CD1d-resticted T cells are implicated in the development of myocarditis since myocarditis develops in BALB/c and Jα18$^{-/-}$ mice, but not CD1d$^{-/-}$ mice. Similarly, in a transgenic model of hepatitis B virus, CD1d-restricted T cells are activated and lead to hepatic injury [143]. Interestingly, like coxsackievirus-induced myocarditis, the development of hepatitis in this adoptive transfer model appears to be dependent on diverse CD1d-restricted T cells. It will be interesting to determine whether this holds true for human disease since human HCV-infected liver contains large numbers of diverse CD1d-restricted T cells [144].

6.4
Mycotic Infection

Cryptococcus is a fungal pathogen that causes pulmonary disease; Kawakami et al. observed that Jα18-deficient mice are unable to manage the infection as efficiently as control mice and have evidence of impaired immunity to cryptococcal antigen [46,145]. These results suggest that invariant NKT cells play a physiological role in the host response to cryptococcal infection.

7
Conclusions

The discovery that the CD1 proteins are a third distinct lineage of antigen-presenting molecules that evolved to present lipid molecules to T cells fundamentally changed how we view T cell immunity to microbial pathogens. Microbial lipids, which are the products of multistep enzymatic synthesis, and are often significantly different from mammalian lipids, appear to be a perfect target for vaccine development. Furthermore, the minimal polymorphisms present in the CD1 genes suggest that vaccination with microbial lipids has the potential to stimulate protective immunity in ethnically diverse populations. The utopian dream of exploiting the CD1 system for vaccine development has yet to be realized. Understanding the role of CD1 and CD1-restricted T cells in microbial immunity has been impeded by the emergence of two dichotomies. First, group 1 CD1-restricted T cells appear to function primarily in the adaptive immune response, while group 2 CD1-restricted T cells appear to have a greater role in immunoregulation and in innate immunity. The second dichotomy is an experimental issue, namely that rodents only have group 2 CD1, which creates a barrier to the study of group 1 CD1 in the most widely used animal infection models. Some of these issues can be dealt with. There are suitable animal models for the study of group 1 CD1, and mice expressing human group 1 CD1 can be engineered. These alternate approaches are important if the potential role of group 1 CD1 in infectious diseases other than mycobacterial infections is to be determined. For group 2 CD1, the rodent models may be adequate but a more thorough search for microbial lipids that are presented by CD1d and activate NKT cells is needed. Finally, the enhanced autoreactivity model provides an alternative paradigm for the activation of CD1d-restricted T cells by infectious and inflammatory diseases. Whether the activation of self-reactive T cells will be of benefit in eliminating microbial pathogens, or whether such T cells are detrimental and contribute to the tissue injury that often accompanies infectious diseases, remains to be determined.

References

1.   Porcelli SA (1995) The CD1 family: a third lineage of antigen presenting molecules. Adv Immunol 59:1–98

2. Dascher CC, Brenner MB (2003) Evolutionary constraints on CD1 structure: insights from comparative genomic analysis. Trends Immunol 24:412–418
3. Calabi F, Jarvis L, Martin JM, Milstein C (1989) Two classes of CD1 genes. Eur J Immunol 19:285–292
4. Brigl M, Brenner MB (2004) CD1: antigen presentation and T cell function. Ann Rev Immunol 22:817–890
5. Nicolle D, Fremond C, Pichon X, Bouchot A, Maillet I, RyffelB, Quesniaux VJ (2004) Long-term control of *Mycobacterium bovis* BCG infection in the absence of toll-like receptors (TLRs): investigation of TLR2-, TLR6-, or TLR2-TLR4-deficient mice. Infect Immun 72:6994–7004
6. Porcelli SA, Modlin RL (1999) The CD1 system: antigen-presenting molecules for T cell recognition of lipids and glycolipids. Annu Rev Immunol 17:297–329
7. Small TN, Knowles RW, Keever C, Kernan NA, Collins N, O'Reilly RJ, Dupont B, lomenberg NF (1987) M241 (CD1c) expression on B lymphocytes. J Immunol 138:2864–2868
8. Small TN, Keever C, Collins N, Dupont, O'ReillyRJ, Flomenberg N (1989) Characterization of B cells in severe combined immunodeficiency disease. Hum Immunol 25:181–193
9. Hiromatsu K, Dascher CC, Sugita M, Gingrich-Baker C, Behar SM, LeClair KP, Brenner MB, Porcelli SA (2002) Characterization of guinea-pig group 1 CD1 proteins. Immunology 106:159–172
10. Stenger S, Niazi KR, Modlin RL (1998) Down-regulation of CD1 on antigen-presenting cells by infection with *Mycobacterium tuberculosis*. J Immunol 161:3582–3588
11. Giuliani A, Prete SP, Graziani G, Aquino A, Balduzzi A, Sugita M, Brenner MB, Iona E, Fattorini L, Orefici G, Porcelli SA, Bonmassar E (2001) Influence of *Mycobacterium bovis* bacillus Calmette Guerin on in vitro induction of CD1 molecules in human adherent mononuclear cells. Infect Immun 69:7461–7470
12. Prete SP, Giuliani A, Iona E, Fattorini L, Orefici G, Franzese O, Bonmassar E, Graziani G (2001) Bacillus Calmette-Guerin down-regulates CD1b induction by granulocyte-macrophage colony stimulating factor in human peripheral blood monocytes. J Chemother 13:52–58
13. Amprey JL, Spath GF, Porcelli SA (2004) Inhibition of CD1 expression in human dendritic cells during intracellular infection with *Leishmania donovani*. Infect Immun 72:589–592
14. Roura-Mir C, Wang L, Cheng TY, Matsunaga I, Dascher CC, Peng SL, Fenton MJ, Kirschning C, Moody DB (2005) *Mycobacterium tuberculosis* regulates CD1 antigen presentation pathways through TLR-2. J Immunol 175:1758–1766
15. Sieling PA, Jullien D, Dahlem M, Tedder TF, Rea TH, Modlin RL, Porcelli SA (1999) CD1 expression by dendritic cells in human leprosy lesions: correlation with effective host immunity. J Immunol 162:1851–1858
16. Krutzik SR, Tan B, Li H, Ochoa MT, Liu PT, Sharfstein SE, Graeber TG, Sieling PA, Liu YJ, Rea TH, Bloom BR, Modlin RL (2005) TLR activation triggers the rapid differentiation of monocytes into macrophages and dendritic cells. Nat Med 11:653–660

17. Dascher CC, Hiromatsu K, Naylor JW, Brauer PP, Brown KA, Storey JR, Behar SM, Kawasaki ES, Porcelli SA, Brenner MB, LeClair KP (1999) Conservation of a CD1. Multigene family in the guinea pig. J Immunol 163:5478–5488

18. Hiromatsu K, Dascher CC, LeClair KP, Sugita M, Furlong ST, Brenner MB, Porcelli SA (2002) Induction of CD1-restricted immune responses in guinea pigs by immunization with mycobacterial lipid antigens. J Immunol 169:330–339

19. Hayes SM, Knight KL (2001) Group 1 CD1 genes in rabbit. J Immunol 166:403–410

20. Van Rhijn I, Koets AP, Im JS, Piebes D, Reddington F, Besra GS, Porcelli SA, van Eden W, MGRutten VP (2006) The bovine CD1 Family contains group 1 CD1 proteins, but no functional CD1d. J Immunol 176:4888–4893

21. Castillo F, Guerrero C, Trujillo E, Delgado G, Martinez P, Salazar LM, Barato P, Patarroyo ME, Parra-Lopez C (2004) Identifying and structurally characterizing CD1b in *Aotus nancymaae* owl monkeys. Immunogenetics 56:480–489

22. Porcelli S, Morita CT, Brenner MB (1992) CD1b restricts the response of human CD4(-)8(-) T lymphocytes to a microbial antigen. Nature 360:593–597

23. Moody DB, Besra GS (2001) Glycolipid targets of CD1-mediated T-cell responses. Immunology 104:243–251

24. Sieling PA, Chatterjee D, Porcelli SA, Prigozy TI, Mazzaccaro RJ, Soriano T, Bloom BR, Brenner MB, Kronenberg M, Brennan PJ (1995) CD1-restricted T cell recognition of microbial lipoglycan antigens. Science 269:227–230

25. Beckman EM, Melian A, Behar SM, Sieling PA, Chatterjee D, Furlong ST, Matsumoto R, Rosat JP, Modlin RL, Porcelli SA (1996) CD1c restricts responses of mycobacteria-specific T cells. Evidence for antigen presentation by a second member of the human CD1 family. J Immunol 157:2795–2803

26. Beckman EM, Porcelli SA, Morita CT, Behar SM, Furlong ST, Brenner MB (1994) Recognition of a lipid antigen by CD1-restricted alpha beta+ T cells. Nature 372:691–694

27. Thomssen H, Ivanyi J, Espitia C, Arya A, Londei M (1995) Human CD4-CD8-alpha beta + T-cell receptor T cells recognize different mycobacteria strains in the context of CD1b. Immunology 85:33–40

28. Rosat JP, Grant EP, Beckman EM, Dascher CC, Sieling PA, Frederique D, Modlin RL, Porcelli SA, Furlong ST, Brenner MB (1999) CD1-restricted microbial lipid antigen-specific recognition found in the CD8+ alpha beta T cell pool. J Immunol 162:366–371

29. Sieling PA, Ochoa MT, Jullien D, Leslie DS, Sabet S, Rosat JP, Burdick AE, Rea TH, Brenner MB, Porcelli SA, Modlin RL (2000) Evidence for human CD4+ T cells in the CD1-restricted repertoire: derivation of mycobacteria-reactive T cells from leprosy lesions. J Immunol 164:4790–4796

30. Stenger S, Mazzaccaro RJ, Uyemura K, Cho S, Barnes PF, Rosat JP, Sette A, Brenner MB, Porcelli SA, Bloom BR, Modlin RL (1997) Differential effects of cytolytic T cell subsets on intracellular infection. Science 276:1684–1687

31. Grant EP, Beckman EM, Behar SM, Degano M, Frederique D, Besra GS, Wilson IA, Porcelli SA, Furlong ST, Brenner MB (2002) Fine specificity of TCR complementarity: determining region residues and lipid antigen hydrophilic moieties in the recognition of a CD1-lipid complex. J Immunol 168:3933–3940

32. Ulrichs T, Moody DB, Grant E, Kaufmann SH, and Porcelli SA (2003) T-cell responses to CD1-presented lipid antigens in humans with *Mycobacterium tuberculosis* infection. Infect Immun 71:3076–3087

33. Gilleron M, Stenger S, Mazorra Z, Wittke F, Mariotti S, Bohmer G, Prandi J, Mori L, Puzo G, De Libero G (2004) Diacylated sulfoglycolipids are novel mycobacterial antigens stimulating CD1-restricted T cells during infection with *Mycobacterium tuberculosis*. J Exp Med 199:649–659

34. Moody DB, Ulrichs T, Muhlecker W, Young DC, Gurcha SS, Grant E, Rosat JP, Brenner MB, Costello CE, Besra GS, Porcelli SA (2000) CD1c-mediated T-cell recognition of isoprenoid glycolipids in *Mycobacterium tuberculosis* infection. Nature 404:884–888

35. Kawashima T, Norose Y, Watanabe Y, Enomoto Y, Narazaki H, Watari E, Tanaka S, Takahashi H, Yano I, Brenner MB, Sugita M (2003) Cutting edge: major CD8 T cell response to live bacillus Calmette-Guerin is mediated by CD1 molecules. J Immunol 170:5345–5348

36. Sieling PA, Torrelles JB, Stenger S, Chung W, Burdick AE, Rea TH, Brennan PJ, Belisle JT, Porcelli SA, Modlin RL (2005) The human CD1-restricted T cell repertoire is limited to cross-reactive antigens: implications for host responses against immunologically related pathogens. J Immunol 174:2637–2644

37. Dascher CC, Hiromatsu K, Xiong X, Morehouse C, Watts G, Liu G, McMurray DN, LeClair KP, Porcelli SA, Brenner MB (2003) Immunization with a mycobacterial lipid vaccine improves pulmonary pathology in the guinea pig model of tuberculosis. Int Immunol 15:915–925

38. Fairhurst RM, Wang CX, Sieling PA, Modlin RL, Braun J (1998) CD1 presents antigens from a Gram-negative bacterium *Haemophilus influenzae* type b. Infect Immun 66:3523–3526

39. Brigl M, Brenner MB (2004) CD1: antigen presentation and T cell function. Annu Rev Immunol 22:817–890

40. Kaufmann SH (2001) How can immunology contribute to the control of tuberculosis? Nat Rev Immunol 1:20–30

41. Gumperz JE, Miyake S, Yamamura T, Brenner MB (2002) Functionally distinct subsets of CD1d-restricted natural killer T cells revealed by CD1d tetramer staining. J Exp Med 195:625–636

42. Behar SM, Cardell S (2000) Diverse CD1d-restricted T cells: diverse phenotypes, and diverse functions. Semin Immunol 12:551–560

43. Godfrey DI, MacDonald HR, Kronenberg M, Smyth MJ, Kaer LV (2004) NKT cells: what's in a name? Nat Rev Immunol 4:231–237

44. Gonzalez-Aseguinolaza G, de Oliveira C, Tomaska M, Hong S, Bruna-Romero O, Nakayama T, Taniguchi M, Bendelac A, Van Kaer L, Koezuka Y, Tsuji M (2000) Alpha-galactosylceramide-activated Valpha 14 natural killer T cells mediate protection against murine malaria. Proc Natl Acad Sci U S A 97:8461–8466

45. Kakimi K, Guidotti LG, Koezuka Y, Chisari FV (2000) Natural killer T cell activation inhibits hepatitis B virus replication in vivo. J Exp Med 192:921–930

46. Kawakami K, Kinjo Y, Yara S, Koguchi Y, Uezu K, Nakayama T, Taniguchi M, Saito A (2001) Activation of Valpha14(+) natural killer T cells by alpha-galactosylceramide results in development of Th1 response and local host resistance in mice infected with *Cryptococcus neoformans*. Infect Immun 69:213–220

47. Behar SM, Dascher CC, Grusby MJ, Wang CR, Brenner MB (1999) Susceptibility of mice deficient in CD1D or TAP1 to infection with *Mycobacterium tuberculosis*. J Exp Med 189:1973–1980

48. Chackerian A, Alt J, Perera V, Behar SM (2002) Activation of NKT cells protects mice from tuberculosis. Infect Immun 70:6302–6309

49. Skold M, Behar SM (2003) Role of CD1d-restricted NKT cells in microbial immunity. Infect Immun 71:5447–5455

50. Yu KO, Porcelli SA (2005) The diverse functions of CD1d-restricted NKT cells and their potential for immunotherapy. Immunol Lett 100:42–55

51. Gumperz JE (2006) The Ins and outs of CD1 molecules: bringing lipids under immunological surveillance. Traffic 7:2–13

52. Rauch J, Gumperz J, Robinson C, Skold M, Roy C, Young DC, Lafleur M, Moody DB, Brenner MB, Costello CE, Behar SM (2003) Structural features of the acyl chain determine self-phospholipid antigen recognition by a CD1d-restricted invariant NKT (iNKT) cell. J Biol Chem 278:47508–47515

53. Benlagha K, Weiss A, Beavis A, Teyton L, Bendelac A (1999) In vivo identification of glycolipid antigen-specific T cells using fluorescent CD1d tetramers. J Exp Med 191:1895–1903

54. Procopio DO, Almeida IC, Torrecilhas AC, Cardoso JE, Teyton L, Travassos LR, Bendelac A, Gazzinelli RT (2002) Glycosylphosphatidylinositol-anchored mucin-like glycoproteins from *Trypanosoma cruzi* bind to CD1d but do not elicit dominant innate or adaptive immune responses via the CD1d/NKT cell pathway. J Immunol 169:3926–3933

55. Kinjo Y, Wu D, Kim G, Xing GW, Poles MA, Ho DD, Tsuji M, Kawahara K, Wong CH, Kronenberg M (2005) Recognition of bacterial glycosphingolipids by natural killer T cells. Nature 434:520–525

56. Mattner J, Debord KL, Ismail N, DGoff R, Cantu C III, Zhou D, Saint-Mezard P, Wang V, Gao Y, Yin N, Hoebe K, Schneewind O, Walker D, Beutler B, Teyton L, Savage PB, Bendelac A (2005) Exogenous and endogenous glycolipid antigens activate NKT cells during microbial infections. Nature 434:525–529

57. Amprey JL, Im JS, Turco SJ, Murray HW, Illarionov PA, Besra GS, Porcelli SA, Spath GF (2004) A subset of liver NKT cells is activated during *Leishmania donovani* infection by CD1d-bound lipophosphoglycan. J Exp Med 200:895–904

58. Fischer K, Scotet E, Niemeyer M, Koebernick H, Zerrahn J, Maillet S, Hurwitz R, Kursar M, Bonneville M, Kaufmann SH, Schaible UE (2004) Mycobacterial phosphatidylinositol mannoside is a natural antigen for CD1d-restricted T cells. Proc Natl Acad Sci U S A 101:10685–10690

59. Dascher CC, Hiromatsu K, Xiong X, Morehouse C, Watts G, Liu G, McMurray DN, LeClair KP, Porcelli SA, Brenner MB (2003) Immunization with a mycobacterial lipid vaccine improves pulmonary pathology in the guinea pig model of tuberculosis. Int Immunol 15:915–925

60. Basta S, Bennink JR (2003) A survival game of hide and seek: cytomegaloviruses and MHC class I antigen presentation pathways. Viral Immunol 16:231–242

61. Hamerman JA, Ogasawara K, Lanier LL (2005) NK cells in innate immunity. Curr Opin Immunol 17:29–35

62. Cerwenka A, Lanier LL (2003) NKG2D ligands: unconventional MHC class I-like molecules exploited by viruses and cancer. Tissue Antigens 61:335–343

63. Balk SP, Ebert EC, Blumenthal RL, McDermott FV, Wucherpfennig KW, Landau SB, Blumberg RS (1991) Oligoclonal expansion and CD1 recognition by human intestinal intraepithelial lymphocytes. Science 253:1411–1415

64. Bendelac A, Lantz O, Quimby ME, Yewdell JW, Bennink JR, Brutkiewicz RR (1995) CD1 recognition by mouse NK1+ T lymphocytes. Science 268:863–865

65. Cardell S, Tangri S, Chan S, Kronenberg M, Benoist C, Mathis D (1995) CD1-restricted CD4+ T cells in major histocompatibility complex class II-deficient mice. J Exp Med 182:993–1004

66. Behar SM, Podrebarac TA, Roy CJ, Wang CR, Brenner MB (1999) Diverse TCRs recognize murine CD1. J Immunol 162:161–167

67. Park SH, Roark JH, Bendelac A (1998) Tissue-specific recognition of mouse CD1 molecules. J Immunol 160:3128–3134

68. Skold M, Xiong X, Illarionov PA, Besra GS, Behar SM (2005) Interplay of cytokines and microbial signals in regulation of CD1d expression and NKT cell activation. J Immunol 175:3584–3593

69. Chiu YH, Jayawardena J, Weiss A, Lee D, Park SH, Dautry-Varsat A, Bendelac A (1999) Distinct subsets of CD1d-restricted T cells recognize self-antigens loaded in different cellular compartments. J Exp Med 189:103–110

70. Chen H, Paul WE (1997) Cultured NK1.1+ CD4+ T cells produce large amounts of IL-4 and IFN-gamma upon activation by anti-CD3 or CD1. J Immunol 159:2240–2249

71. Kawano T, Cui J, Koezuka Y, Toura I, Kaneko Y, Motoki K, Ueno H, Nakagawa R, Sato H, Kondo E, Koseki H, Taniguchi M (1997) CD1d-restricted and TCR-mediated activation of valpha14 NKT cells by glycosylceramides. Science 278:1626–1629

72. Kamada N, Iijima H, Kimura K, Harada M, Shimizu E, Motohashi S, Kawano T, Shinkai H, Nakayama T, Sakai T, Brossay L, Kronenberg M, Taniguchi M (2001) Crucial amino acid residues of mouse CD1d for glycolipid ligand presentation to V(alpha)14 NKT cells. Int Immunol 13:853–861

73. Cantu C III, Benlagha K, Savage PB, Bendelac A, Teyton L (2003) The paradox of immune molecular recognition of alpha-galactosylceramide: low affinity low specificity for CD1d high affinity for alpha beta TCRs. J Immunol 170:4673–4382

74. Gumperz JE, Roy C, Makowska A, Lum D, Sugita M, Podrebarac T, YKoezuka T, Porcelli SA, Cardell S, Brenner MB, Behar SM (2000) Murine CD1d-restricted T cell recognition of cellular lipids. Immunity 12:211–221

75. Naidenko OV, Maher JK, Ernst WA, Sakai T, Modlin RL, Kronenberg M (1999) Binding and antigen presentation of ceramide-containing glycolipids by soluble mouse and human CD1d molecules. J Exp Med 190:1069–1080

76. Brigl M, Bry L, Kent SC, Gumperz JE, Brenner MB (2003) Mechanism of CD1d-restricted natural killer T cell activation during microbial infection. Nat Immunol 4:1230–1237

77. Fujii S, Liu K, Smith C, Bonito AJ, Steinman RM (2004) The linkage of innate to adaptive immunity via maturing dendritic cells in vivo requires CD40 ligation in addition to antigen presentation and CD80/86 costimulation. J Exp Med 199:1607–1618

78. Kitamura H, IwakabeK, Yahata T, Nishimura S, Ohta A, Ohmi Y, Sato M, Takeda K, Okumura K Van Kaer L, Kawano T, Taniguchi M, Nishimura T (1999) The natural killer T (NKT) cell ligand alpha-galactosylceramide demonstrates its immunopotentiating effect by inducing interleukin (IL)-12 production by dendritic cells and IL-12 receptor expression on NKT cells. J Exp Med 189:1121–1128

79. Roark JH, Park SH, Jayawardena J, Kavita U, Shannon M, Bendelac A (1998) CD1.1 expression by mouse antigen-presenting cells and marginal zone B cells. J Immunol 160:3121–3127

80. Berntman E, Rolf J, Johansson C, Anderson P, Cardell SL (2005) The role of CD1d-restricted NKT lymphocytes in the immune response to oral infection with *Salmonella typhimurium*. Eur J Immunol 35:2100–2109

81. Sanchez DJ, Gumperz JE, Ganem D (2005) Regulation of CD1d expression and function by a herpesvirus infection. J Clin Invest 115:1369–1378

82. Probst HC, van den Broek MF (2005) Priming of CTLs by lymphocytic choriomeningitis virus depends on dendritic cells. J Immunol 174:3920–3924

83. Van Rijt LS, Jung S, Kleinjan A, Vos N, Willart M, Duez C, Hoogsteden HC, Lambrecht BN (2005) In vivo depletion of lung CD11c+ dendritic cells during allergen challenge abrogates the characteristic features of asthma. J Exp Med 201:981–991

84. Bezbradica JS, Stanic AK, Matsuki N, Bour-Jordan H, Bluestone JA, Thomas JW, Unutmaz D, Van Kaer L, Joyce S (2005) Distinct roles of dendritic cells and B cells in Va14Ja18 natural T cell activation in vivo. J Immunol 174:4696–4705

85. Kirby AC, Yrlid U, Wick MJ (2002) The innate immune response differs in primary and secondary *Salmonella* infection. J Immunol 169:4450–4459

86. Gansert JL, Kiebler V, Engele M, Wittke F, Rollinghoff M, Krensky AM, Porcelli SA, Modlin RL, Stenger S (2003) Human NKTCells express granulysin and exhibit antimycobacterial activity. J Immunol 170:3154–3161

87. Kamath AB, Alt J, Debbabi H, Taylor C, Behar SM (2004) The major histocompatibility complex haplotype affects T-cell recognition of mycobacterial antigens but not resistance to *Mycobacterium tuberculosis* in C3H mice. Infect Immun 72:6790–6798

88. Carnaud C, Lee D, Donnars O, Park SH, Beavis A, Koezuka Y, Bendelac A (1999) Cutting edge: cross-talk between cells of the innate immune system: NKT cells rapidly activate NK cells. J Immunol 163:4647–4650

89. Kamath AB, Woodworth J, Xiong X, Taylor C, Weng Y, Behar SM (2004) Cytolytic CD8+ T cells recognizing CFP10 are recruited to the lung after *Mycobacterium tuberculosis* infection. J Exp.Med 200:1479–1489

90. Skold M, Behar SM (2005) The role of group 1 and group 2 CD1-restricted T cells in microbial immunity. Microbes Infect 7:544–551

91. Apostolou I, Takahama Y, Belmant C, Kawano T, Huerre M, Marchal G, Cui J, Taniguchi M, Nakauchi H, Fournie JJ, Kourilsky P, Gachelin G (1999) Murine natural killer T(NKT) cells [correction of natural killer cells] contribute to the granulomatous reaction caused by mycobacterial cell walls. Proc Natl Acad Sci U S A 96:5141–5146

92. Mempel M, Ronet C, Suarez F, Gilleron M, Puzo G, Van Kaer L, Lehuen A, Kourilsky P, Gachelin G (2002) Natural killer T cells restricted by the monomorphic MHC class 1b CD1d1 molecules behave like inflammatory cells. J Immunol 168:365–371

93. Sugawara I, Yamada G, Mizuno S, Li CY, Nakayama T, Taniguchi M (2002) Mycobacterial infection in natural killer T cell knockout mice. Tuberculosis 82:97–104

94. Sousa AO, Mazzaccaro RJ, Russell RG, Lee FK, Turner OC, Hong S, Van Kaer L, Bloom BR (2000) Relative contributions of distinct MHC class I-dependent cell populations in protection to tuberculosis infection in mice. Proc Natl Acad Sci U S A 97:4204–4208

95. D'Souza CD, Cooper AM, Frank AA, Ehlers S, Turner J, Bendelac A, Orme IM (2000) A novel nonclassic beta2-microglobulin-restricted mechanism influencing early lymphocyte accumulation and subsequent resistance to tuberculosis in the lung. Am J Respir Cell Mol Biol 23:188–193

96. Kawakami K, Kinjo Y, Uezu K, Yara S, Miyagi K, Koguchi Y, Nakayama T, Taniguchi M, Saito A (2002) Minimal contribution of Valpha14 natural killer T cells to Th1 response and host resistance against mycobacterial infection in mice. Microbiol Immunol 46:207–210

97. Mogues T, Goodrich M, Ryan L, LaCourse R, North R (2001) The relative importance of T cell subsets in immunity and immunopathology of airborne *Mycobacterium tuberculosis* infection in mice. J Exp Med 193:271–280

98. Flynn JL, Chan J (2001) Immunology of tuberculosis. Annu Rev Immunol 19:93–129

99. Gansert JL, Kiessler V, Engele M, Wittke F, Rollinghoff M, Krensky AM, Porcelli SA, Modlin RL, Stenger S (2003) Human NKT cells express granulysin and exhibit antimycobacterial activity. J Immunol 170:3154–3161

100. Ishigami M, Nishimura H, Naiki Y, Yoshioka K, Kawano T, Tanaka Y, Taniguchi SKakumu M, Yoshikai Y (1999) The roles of intrahepatic Valpha14(+) NK1.1(+) T cells for liver injury induced by *Salmonella* infection in mice. Hepatology 29:1799–1808

101. Arrunategui-Correa V, Lenz L, Kim HS (2004) CD1d-independent regulation of NKT cell migration and cytokine production upon Listeria monocytogenes infection. Cell Immunol 232:38–48

102. Ranson T, Bregenholt S, Lehuen A, Gaillot O, Leite-de-Moraes MC, Herbelin A, Berche P, Di Santo JP (2005) Invariant V alpha 14+ NKT cells participate in the early response to enteric *Listeria* monocytogenes infection. J Immunol 175:1137–1144

103. Szalay G, Ladel CH, Blum C, Brossay L, Kronenberg M, Kaufmann SH (1999) Cutting edge: anti-CD1 monoclonal antibody treatment reverses the production patterns of TGF-beta 2 and Th1 cytokines and ameliorates listeriosis in mice. J Immunol 162:6955–6958

104. Kawakami K, Yamamoto N, Kinjo Y, Miyagi K, Nakasone C, Uezu K, Kinjo T, Nakayama T, Taniguchi M, Saito A (2003) Critical role of Valpha14+ natural killer T cells in the innate phase of host protection against *Streptococcus pneumoniae* infection. Eur J Immunol 33:3322–3330

105. Nieuwenhuis EE, Matsumoto T, Exley M, Schleipman RA, Glickman J, Bailey DT, Corazza N, Colgan SP, Onderdonk AB, Blumberg RS (2002) CD1d-dependent macrophage-mediated clearance of *Pseudomonas aeruginosa* from lung. Nat Med 8:588–593

106. Sriram V, Du W, Gervay-Hague J, Brutkiewicz RR (2005) Cell wall glycosphingolipids of *Sphingomonas paucimobilis* are CD1d-specific ligands for NKT cells. Eur J Immunol 35:1692–1701

107. Wu D, Xing GW, Poles MA, Horowitz A, Kinjo Y, Sullivan B, Bodmer-Narkevitch V, Plettenburg O, Kronenberg M, Tsuji M, Ho DD, Wong CH (2005) Bacterial glycolipids and analogs as antigens for CD1d-restricted NKT cells. PNAS 102:1351–1356

108. Kumar H, Belperron A, Barthold SW, Bockenstedt LK (2000) Cutting edge: CD1d deficiency impairs murine host defense against the spirochete Borrelia burgdorferi. J Immunol 165:4797–4801

109. Belperron AA, Dailey CM, Bockenstedt LK (2005) Infection-induced marginal zone B cell production of *Borrelia hermsii*-specific antibody is impaired in the absence of CD1d. J Immunol 174:5681–5686

110. Duthie MS, Wleklinski-Lee M, Smith S, Nakayama T, Taniguchi M, Kahn SJ (2002) During *Trypanosoma cruzi* infection CD1d-restricted NKT cells limit parasitemia and augment the antibody response to a glycophosphoinositol-modified surface protein. Infect Immun 70:36–48

111. Duthie MS, Kahn M, White M, Kapur RP, Kahn SJ (2005) Critical proinflammatory and anti-inflammatory functions of different subsets of CD1d-restricted natural killer T cells during *Trypanosoma cruzi* infection. Infect Immun 73:181–192

112. Duthie MS, Kahn M, White M, Kapur RP, Kahn SJ (2005) Both CD1d antigen presentation and interleukin-12 are required to activate natural killer T cells during *Trypanosoma cruzi* infection. Infect Immun 73:1890–1894

113. Faveeuw C, Angeli V, Fontaine J, Maliszewski C, Capron A, Van Kaer L, Moser M, Capron M, Trottein F (2002) Antigen presentation by CD1d contributes to the amplification of Th2 responses to *Schistosoma mansoni* glycoconjugates in mice. J Immunol 169:906–912

114. Mallevaey T, Zanetta JP, Faveeuw C, Fontaine J, Maes E, Platt F, Capron M, de Moraes ML, Trottein F (2006) Activation of Invariant NKT cells by the helminth parasite *Schistosoma mansoni*. J Immunol 176:2476–2485

115. Ishikawa H, Hisaeda H, Taniguchi M, Nakayama T, Sakai T, Maekawa Y, Nakano Y, Zhang M, Zhang T, Nishitani M, Takashima M, Himeno K (2000) CD4(+) v(alpha)14 NKT cells play a crucial role in an early stage of protective immunity against infection with *Leishmania major*. Int Immunol 12:1267–1274

116. Mattner J, Donhauser N, Werner-Felmayer G, Bogdan C (2006) NKT cells mediate organ-specific resistance against *Leishmania major* infection. Microbes Infect 8:354–362

117. Svensson M, Zubairi S, Maroof A, Kazi F, Taniguchi M, Kaye PM (2005) Invariant NKT cells are essential for the regulation of hepatic CXCL10 gene expression during *Leishmania donovani* infection. Infect Immun 73:7541–7547

118. Denkers EY, Scharton-Kersten T, Barbieri S, Caspar P, Sher A (1996) A role for CD4+ NK1.1+ T lymphocytes as major histocompatibility complex class II independent helper cells in the generation of CD8+ effector function against intracellular infection. J Exp Med 184:131–139

119. Smiley ST, Lanthier PA, Couper KN, Szaba FM, Boyson JE, Chen W, Johnson LL (2005) Exacerbated susceptibility to infection-stimulated immunopathology in CD1d-deficient mice. J Immunol 174:7904–7911

120. Ronet C, Darche S, de Moraes ML, Miyake S, Yamamura T, Louis JA, Kasper LH, Buzoni-Gatel D (2005) NKT cells are critical for the initiation of an inflammatory bowel response against *Toxoplasma gondii*. J Immunol 175:899–908

121. Romero JF, Eberl G, MacDonald HR, Corradin G (2001) CD1d-restricted NKT cells are dispensable for specific antibody responses and protective immunity against liver stage malaria infection in mice. Parasite Immunol 23:267–269

122. Schofield L, McConville MJ, Hansen D, Campbell AS, Fraser-Reid B, Grusby MJ, Tachado SD (1999) CD1d-restricted immunoglobulin G formation to GPI-anchored antigens mediated by NKT cells. Science 283:225–229

123. Mannoor MK, Weerasinghe A, Halder RC, Reza S, Morshed M, Ariyasinghe A, Watanabe H, Sekikawa H, Abo T (2001) Resistance to malarial infection is achieved by the cooperation of NK1.1(+) and NK1.1(−) subsets of intermediate TCR cells which are constituents of innate immunity. Cell Immunol 211:96–104

124. Adachi K, Tsutsui H, Kashiwamura SI, Seki E, Nakano H, Takeuchi O, Takeda K, Okumura K, Van Kaer L, Okamura H, Akira S, Nakanishi K (2001) *Plasmodium berghei* infection in mice induces liver injury by an IL-12- and toll-like receptor/myeloid differentiation factor 88-dependent mechanism. J Immunol 167:5928–5934

125. Hansen DS, Siomos MA, Buckingham L, Scalzo AA, Schofield L (2003) Regulation of murine cerebral malaria pathogenesis by CD1d-restricted NKT cells and the natural killer complex. Immunity 18:391–402

126. Lin Y, Roberts TJ, Wang CR, Cho S, Brutkiewicz RR (2005) Long-term loss of canonical NKT cells following an acute virus infection. Eur J Immunol 35:879–889

127. Renukaradhya GJ, Webb TJ, Khan MA, Lin YL, Du W, Gervay-Hague J, Brutkiewicz RR (2005) Virus-induced inhibition of CD1d1-mediated antigen presentation: reciprocal regulation by p38 and ERK. J Immunol 175:4301–4308

128. Chen N, McCarthy C, Drakesmith H, Li D, Cerundolo V, McMichael AJ, Screaton GR, Xu XN (2006) HIV-1 down-regulates the expression of CD1d via Nef. Eur J Immunol 36:278–286

129. Huber SA, Sartini D (2005) Roles of tumor necrosis factor alpha (TNF-alpha) and the p55 TNF receptor in CD1d induction and coxsackievirus B3-induced myocarditis. J Virol 79:2659–2665

130. Durante-Mangoni E, Wang R, Shaulov A, He Q, Nasser I, Afdhal N, Koziel MJ, Exley MA (2004) Hepatic CD1d expression in hepatitis C virus infection and recognition by resident proinflammatory CD1d-reactive T cells. J Immunol 173:2159–2166

131. De Lalla C, Galli G, Aldrighetti L, Romeo R, Mariani M, Monno A, Nuti S, Colombo M, Callea F, Porcelli SA, Panina-Bordignon P, Abrignani S, Casorati G, Dellabona P (2004) Production of profibrotic cytokines by invariant NKT cells characterizes cirrhosis progression in chronic viral hepatitis. J Immunol 173:1417–1425

132. Levy O, Orange JS, Hibberd P, Steinberg S, LaRussa P, Weinberg A, Wilson SB, Shaulov A, Fleisher G, Geha RS, Bonilla FA, Exley M (2003) Disseminated varicella infection due to the vaccine strain of varicella-zoster virus, in a patient with a novel deficiency in natural killer T cells. J Infect Dis 188:948–953

133. Ashkar AA, Rosenthal KL (2003) Interleukin-15 and natural killer and NKT cells play a critical role in innate protection against genital herpes simplex virus type 2 infection. J Virol 77:10168–10171

134. Grubor-Bauk B, Simmons A, Mayrhofer G, Speck PG (2003) Impaired clearance of herpes simplex virus type 1 from mice lacking CD1d or NKT cells expressing the semivariant Valpha14-Jalpha281 TCR. J Immunol 170:1430–1434

135. Cornish AL, Keating R, Kyparissoudis K, Smyth MJ, Carbone FR, Godfrey DI (2006) NKT cells are not critical for HSV-1 disease resolution. Immunol Cell Biol 84:13–19

136. Exley MA, Bigley NJ, Cheng O, Tahir SM, Smiley ST, Carter QL, Stills HF, Grusby MJ, Koezuka Y, Taniguchi M, Balk SP (2001) CD1d-reactive T-cell activation leads to amelioration of disease caused by diabetogenic encephalomyocarditis virus. J Leukoc Biol 69:713–718

137. Exley MA, Bigley NJ, Cheng O, Shaulov A, Tahir SM, Carter QL, Garcia J, Wang C, Patten K, Stills HF, Alt FW, Snapper SB, Balk SP (2003) Innate immune response to encephalomyocarditis virus infection mediated by CD1d. Immunology 110:519–526

138. Johnson TR, Hong S, Van Kaer L, Koezuka Y, Graham BS (2002) NKT cells contribute to expansion of CD8(+) T cells and amplification of antiviral immune responses to respiratory syncytial virus. J Virol 76:4294–4303

139. Van Dommelen SLH, Tabarias HA, Smyth MJ, Degli-Esposti MA (2003) Activation of natural killer (NK) T cells during murine cytomegalovirus infection enhances the antiviral response mediated by NK cells. J Virol 77:1877–1884

140. Spence PM, Sriram V, Van Kaer L, Hobbs JA, Brutkiewicz RR (2001) Generation of cellular immunity to lymphocytic choriomeningitis virus is independent of CD1d1 expression. Immunology 104:168–174

141. Roberts TJ, Lin Y, Spence PM, Van Kaer L, Brutkiewicz RR (2004) CD1d1-dependent control of the magnitude of an acute antiviral immune response. J Immunol 172:3454–3461

142. Huber S, Sartini D, Exley M (2003) Role of CD1d in coxsackievirus B3-induced myocarditis. J Immunol 170:3147–3153

143. Baron JL, Gardiner L, Nishimura S, Shinkai K, Locksley R, Ganem D (2002) Activation of a nonclassical NKT cell subset in a transgenic mouse model of hepatitis B virus infection. Immunity 16:583–594

144. Exley MA, He Q, Cheng O, Wang RJ, Cheney CP, Balk SP, Koziel MJ (2002) Cutting edge: compartmentalization of Th1-like noninvariant CD1d-reactive T cells in hepatitis C virus-infected liver. J Immunol 168:1519–1523

145. Kawakami K, Kinjo Y, Uezu K, Yara S, Miyagi K, Koguchi Y, Nakayama T, Taniguchi M, Saito A (2001) Monocyte chemoattractant protein-1-dependent increase of Valpha14 NKT cells in lungs and their roles in Th1 response and host defense in cryptococcal infection. J Immunol 167:6525–6532
146. Szalay G, Zugel U, Ladel CH, Kaufmann SH (1999) Participation of group 2 CD1 molecules in the control of murine tuberculosis. Microbes Infect 1:1153–1157
147. Bilenki L, Wang S, Yang J, Fan Y, Joyee AG, Yang X (2005) NKT cell activation promotes *Chlamydia trachomatis* infection in vivo. J Immunol 175:3197–3206
148. Exley MA, Bigley NJ, Cheng O, Tahir SM, Smiley ST, Carter QL, Stills HF, Grusby MJ, Koezuka Y, Taniguchi M, Balk SP (2001) CD1d-reactive T-cell activation leads to amelioration of disease caused by diabetogenic encephalomyocarditis virus. J Leukoc Biol 69:713–718

CTMI (2007) 314:251–265

NKT Cells and Autoimmune Diseases: Unraveling the Complexity

S. Miyake (✉) · T. Yamamura

Department of Immunology, National Institute of Neuroscience, NCNP, 4-1-1, Ogawahigashi, Kodaira, 187-8502 Tokyo, Japan
miyake@ncnp.go.jp

Abstract CD1d-restricted invariant natural killer T (NKT) cells emerge as unique lymphocyte subsets implicated in the regulation of autoimmunity. Abnormalities in the numbers and functions of NKT cells have been observed in patients with diverse autoimmune diseases as well as in animal models of autoimmune diseases. NKT cells recognize glycolipid antigens presented by the nonpolymorphic MHC class I-like protein CD1d and participate in various kinds of immunoregulation due to a potent ability to produce a variety of cytokines. In this review, we examine the potential roles of NKT cells in the regulation and pathogenesis of autoimmune disease and the recent advances in glycolipid therapy for autoimmune disease models.

1
Introduction

Autoimmunity is not forbidden in the healthy immune system and may target peptide or lipid antigens. However, in most healthy individuals, autoimmunity does not manifest its dangerous nature, but rather it plays an essential role in maintaining the immunological homeostasis as a physiological regulator. As evidenced by a number of studies of autoimmune disease models, "dangerous" autoimmunity appears to be controlled by "protective" autoimmunity in the physiological immune network [1, 2].

Although the functional dichotomy of autoimmunity has been documented mostly in peptide and MHC-reactive T cells, it may also hold true for lipid-specific T cells. In fact, opposing functions mediated by lipid-reactive, CD1-restricted T cells have been documented in recently published studies on autoimmune disease models [3–8] (Table 1). Namely, CD1d-restricted invariant $V\alpha14^+$ NKT cells (*NKT*) play a protective role in experimental autoimmune encephalomyelitis (EAE) or type I diabetes in NOD mice, whereas they appear to be involved in mediating the inflammatory pathology of arthritis models. Whatever mechanism may be operative in polarizing *NKT* cells toward being protective or pathogenic, it is obvious that autoimmunity to lipid antigens is not always beneficial for our health. Here we review the recent publications on lipid-reactive T cells, particularly CD1d-restricted *NKT* cells and autoimmune diseases.

2
The Role of NKT Cells in Animal Models of Autoimmune Diseases

2.1
NKT Cells in Experimental Autoimmune Encephalomyelitis

After transgenic mice overexpressing or lacking $V\alpha14$–$J\alpha18$ T cell receptors (TCRs), which define invariant NKT cells, were established, the role of CD1d-restricted *NKT* cells was studied in depth in various autoimmune conditions. Amongst these, EAE is a prototypical model for multiple sclerosis (MS) mediated by Th1 autoimmune cells, which can be induced by immunization with central nervous system (CNS) antigens such as myelin oligodendrocyte glycoprotein (MOG) or myelin basic protein (MBP) in mycobacterium-containing adjuvant. Approximately 2–3 weeks after sensitization, susceptible mice would manifest MS-like ascending limb paralysis due to inflammatory lesions within the brain and spinal cord. However, as seen with human MS, EAE mice usually recover from paralysis, which is thought to involve elaborate immune regulatory processes. Several research groups have investigated the possible involvement of *NKT* cells in the regulation of EAE using transgenic or gene knockout mice. In TCR $V\alpha14$–$J\alpha18$ transgenic NOD mice, bearing an increased number of *NKT* cells, MOG-induced EAE was significantly suppressed in association with inhibition of antigen-specific IFN-γ production in the spleen [9]. Consistent with this, another study showed that $CD1d^{-/-}$ mice developed a more severe EAE compared to C57BL/6 mice [10], suggesting the

Table 1 iNKT cells in autoimmune disease models

The role of iNKT cells in autoimmune disease models		Effect of glycolipid ligand on disease	
Type I diabetes			
NOD mice		NOD mice	
Protection by transfer of NKT enriched thymocytes	[27]	Protection by α-GalCer	[24, 25, 29, 30]
Protection in Vα14 Jα18Tg	[28]	Protection by OCH	[31]
Protection in CD1Tg	[26]		
Exacerbation in CD1 KO	[23–25]		
Transfer of BDC2.5 T cells		Transfer of AI4 T cells	
Protection by increase of iNKT cells	[33]	Protection by α-GalCer	[34]
Transfer of AI4 T cells			
Exacerbation by increase of iNKT cells	[35]		
Experimental autoimmune encephalomyelitis (EAE)		MOG-induced EAE in C57BL/6	
Protection in Vα14 Jα18Tg/NOD	[9]	Protection by OCH	[15]
Exacerbation in CD1 KO	[10]	Protection by α-GalCer co-immunization	[11–13]
No difference in CD1 KO	[11, 12]	MBP-induced EAE in B.10PL	
No difference in Jα18 KO	[12]	Protection by α-GalCer pretreatment	[13]
Protection in CD1 KO(C57BL/6,B10.PL.)	[11]	MBP-induced EAE in PL/J	
		Protection by α-GalCer co-immunization	[11]
		MBP-induced EAE in SLJ/J	
		Exacerbation by α-GalCer co-immunization	[11, 13]

Table 1 (continued)

The role of iNKT cells in autoimmune disease models		Effect of glycolipid ligand on disease	
Arthritis models			
Collagen-induced arthritis		CIA in C57BL/6	
Protection in Jα18 KO	[37, 39, 40]	Protection by OCH	[39]
Protection by anti-CD1d mAb	[37]	CIA in SJL	
Antibody-induced arthritis		Protection by OCH	[39]
Protection in Jα18 KO	[37, 41]		
Protection in CD1 KO	[37]		
Lupus models			
MRLlpr/lpr		Dermatitis in MRLlpr/lpr	
Exacerbation of dermatitis in CD1 KO	[50]	Protection by α-GalCer	[52]
No difference in dermatitis in CD1 KO	[51]	Nephritis in MRLlpr/lpr	
No difference in nephritis in CD1 KO	[50, 51]	No effect by α-GalCer	[52]
Pristane-induced nephritis		Pristane-induced nephritis in Balb/c	
Exacerbation in CD1 KO	[49]	Protection by α-GalCer	[53]
		Pristane-induced nephritis in SJL/J	
		Exacerbation by α-GalCer	[53]
Nephritis in (NZBxW)F1		Nephritis in (NZBxW)F1	
Protection by anti-CD1d mAb	[56]	Exacerbation by α-GalCer	[56]
Inflammatory bowel disease model			
Oxazalone-induced protection in Jα18 KO		Dextran sodium sulfate-induced colitis	
Protection in CD1 KO or Jα18 KO	[59]	Protection by α-GalCer	[57]
		Protection by OCH	[58]

KO, knockout mice; *Tg*, transgenic mice

immunoregulatory role of NKT cells. We could not rule out the possibility that NKT cells take the space of pathogenic MHC-restricted T cells. Other groups, however, reported that there was no difference in disease course between wild type and mice lacking all CD1d-restricted T cells (CD1d$^{-/-}$) or selectively lacking invariant NKT cells (Jα18$^{-/-}$) [11, 12] in ameliorating disease in C57BL/6. CD1d$^{-/-}$ and B10.PL.CD1d$^{-/-}$ mice [13]. Although the basis for these inconsistencies is not clear, it is possible that the role of NKT cells in each EAE system is critically determined by various ill-defined factors such as non-MHC genes that result from different levels of back-crossing to the C57BL/6 background, the breeding environment (cleanliness, serenity), or dose and quality of adjuvant used for EAE induction.

After α-galactosylceramide (α-GalCer) was identified as the efficacious glycolipid ligand for NKT cells, this glycolipid was widely used as a pharmacological reagent to explore the potential for NKT cells to regulate autoimmunity. The results obtained from α-GalCer treatment of EAE also generated conflicting results. Intraperitoneal injection of α-GalCer before immunization led to suppression of EAE in B.10 PL mice induced with a peptide from MBP [13]. Co-immunization of α-GalCer with an encephalitogenic MOG peptide ameliorated EAE induced in C57BL/6 mice, as compared to MOG immunization without α-GalCer [13]. This co-immunization protocol was adopted by others and proved effective in suppressing EAE in MBP-immunized PL/J mice [11, 12]. However, exacerbation of EAE was observed by a similar co-immunization with α-GalCer in MBP-immunized B10.PL and SJL/L mice [11, 12].

Accompanying ex vivo analysis showed that the protective effect of α-GalCer seemed to correlate with the differential abilities of the mouse strains to produce IL-4 upon stimulation with α-GalCer. For, example, protection was seen in strains secreting higher levels of IL-4 in response to α-GalCer. Moreover, the protective effect of α-GalCer in EAE was not observed in IL-4- or IL-10-deficient mice [11], whereas disease was ameliorated in IFN-γ-deficient mice [13, 14]. Taken together, this suggests that EAE protection by α-GalCer is mediated by Th2 cytokines produced by NKT cells, although one study demonstrated that IFN-γ but not IL-4 is critical for the disease protection by α-GalCer in C57BL/6 mice [13]. Another line of evidence to support Th2-mediated protection is that in vivo injection of α-GalCer-pulsed antigen-presenting cells (APCs) with CD86 blockade (treated with anti-B7.2 antibodies does not only polarize NKT cells toward a Th2-like phenotype but mediates concomitant suppression of EAE, whereas α-GalCer presented by anti-CD40 activated APC induces a bias of NKT cells toward a Th1-like phenotype and exacerbated EAE [14].

Further support for Th2-mediated suppressive effect on EAE by NKT cells has been shown using OCH, a sphingosine truncated analog of α-GalCer, which preferentially induces IL-4 from NKT cells [15–18]. OCH has been shown to be more effective than α-GalCer in preventing EAE in C57BL/6 mice, and it possesses some efficacy even when treatment was initiated several days after EAE induction. OCH was also effective when administrated orally, which is the favored treatment route for humans. The protective effect by OCH was abrogated by neutralization of IL-4 [15].

Taken together, NKT cells appear to work as a regulatory cells in EAE and a proper activation of NKT cells could lead to amelioration of EAE.

2.2
NKT Cells in Diabetes Models

Nonobese diabetic (NOD) mice develop spontaneous autoimmune diabetes that is similar to the human disease, insulin-dependent type 1 diabetes mellitus. In parallel with effector cells such as Th1 type CD4+ cells and CD8+ T cells, regulatory cells including *NKT* cells have been suggested to inhibit the development of diabetes. While a deficit in the number and function of *NKT* cells has been indicated in NOD mice [19–22], further deletion of *NKT* cells by genetic ablation expression accelerated onset and increased incidence of diabetes [23–25]. Protection against diabetes in transgenic NOD mice overexpressing CD1d molecules within the pancreatic islets further supports a CD1d-dependent regulatory function of *NKT* cells [26].

Consistent with the hypothesis that NKT cells are protective in experimental models of diabetes, NOD mice were also protected against diabetes by increasing the number of *NKT* cells either by infusion of *NKT* cell-enriched thymocyte preparations [27] or by the introduction of the Vα14 Jα18 gene into NOD mice [28]. Moreover, activation of *NKT* cells with synthetic glycolipid ligands such as α-GalCer or OCH has been shown to prevent the development of diabetes in NOD mice [24, 25, 29–31].

In many studies, protection from diabetes by *NKT* cells is associated with the induction of Th2 response to islet autoantigens. Neutralization of IL-4 and IL-10 abolished the protection from diabetes by transferred CD4−CD8− TCRαβ+ (NKT) thymocytes [27]. In Vα14 Jα18 transgenic mice, the response to the pancreatic autoantigen, glutamic acid decarboxylase (name autoantigen) response was shifted toward Th2 phenotype and neutralization of IL-4 abrogated protection from cyclophosphamide-induced diabetes [32]. Th2 polarization was also observed in mice treated with glycolipid ligands for NKT cells [24, 25, 29–31]. Treatment with α-GalCer ameliorated cyclophosphamide-induced diabetes in an IL-4-dependent manner [32], though the role of IL-10 is controversial [30, 32]. Th2-independent mechanisms underlying *NKT* cell-mediated suppression have been reported in a different system using TCR transgenic mice. The BDC2.5 TCR was cloned from an MHC class II-restricted T cell clone specific to an islet-derived antigen. Diabetogenic CD4 T cells from BDC2.5 NOD mice were unable to induce diabetes when transferred into mice with increased *NKT* cell numbers [33]. The presence of *NKT* cells inhibited the differentiation of BDC2.5 T cells into IFN-γ producing cells without a Th2 shift. BDC2.5 T cells were initially activated in pancreatic lymph nodes and then became anergic. The regulation of BDC2.5 T cells by *NKT* cells was not dependent on IL-4, IL-10, IL-13, or TGF-β [34]. A similar mechanism was implied in the transfer of diabetogenic transgenic $CD8^+$ AI4 T cells expressing the β cell-autoreactive TCR to sublethally irradiated NOD mice when *NKT* cells had been activated with α-GalCer [35]. Activation of *NKT* cells enhanced the apoptosis and induced anergy of AI4 T cells. Even though several different mechanisms might be involved, NKT cell seems to work as regulatory cells in diabetes models. Recently however, the opposing effect of *NKT* cells on $CD8^+$ MHC-restricted T cells was reported. In diabetes induced by the transfer of $CD8^+$ T cells specific for the influenza virus hemagglutinin into mice expressing the hemagglutinin antigen in pancreatic cells, a high frequency of *NKT* cells exacerbated diabetes by enhancing CD8 T cell activation, expansion, and differentiation into effector cells producing IFN-γ [36]. Acceleration of disease by the presence of *NKT* cells was also observed in other autoimmune models such as arthritis.

2.3
NKT Cells in Arthritis Models

Collagen-induced arthritis (CIA) is an animal model for human rheumatoid arthritis induced by immunizing susceptible mouse strains with type II collagen (CII) with adjuvant. When mice develop arthritis, the proportions of *NKT* cells in liver and peripheral blood have been reported to be increased, even though it is not clear what stimulates *NKT* cells to proliferate or if *NKT* cells are generated in situ or recruited from other organs [37]. Since it has been shown that activation of *NKT* cells can be enhanced by non-TCR stimulation such as IL-12 and possibly other cytokines [38], it might be possible that *NKT* cells proliferate in CIA by stimulation of inflammatory cytokines elevated in this model. The protective effect of blocking anti-CD1 monoclonal antibody on CIA has revealed that *NKT* cells contributed to the development of arthritis [37]. Furthermore, amelioration of arthritis is seen in mice lacking all *NKT* cells ($CD1d^{-/-}$) or invariant NK T cells ($Jα18^{-/-}$), further supported the important role of *NKT* cells in the development of arthritis [37, 39, 40]. The reduction of disease severity in $Jα18^{-/-}$ mice was associated with a decrease in IL-10 or IL-1β production in response to antigen stimulation, suggesting that NK T cells directly or indirectly control the levels of these cytokines [37, 40].

Recent advances in the use of anti-inflammatory drugs such as anti-TNF reagents reminded us of the importance of the later occurring inflammatory phase in the pathogenesis of arthritis in which cytokines amplify local tissue destruction. The K/BxN serum transfer model of arthritis allows arthritis to be induced in a manner that bypasses the initial T cell and B cell interactions necessary to promote autoantibodies and instead measures the downstream events involved in antibody-induced, cytokine-mediated joint destruction. To more specifically investigate the more distal inflammatory phase of arthritis, K/BxN serum transfer arthritis or anti-CII antibody-induced arthritis preferable to CIA [42, 43]. The proportion of *NKT* cells was increased in the lymph nodes and peripheral blood of mice receiving K/BxN serum similar to CIA [39]. Arthritis induced either by injection of K/BxN serum or CII antibody in *NKT*-deficient mice was ameliorated [39, 41]. Regarding the mechanisms that *NKT* cells contribute to the development of arthritis in K/BxN serum transfer model, production of IFN- γ and IL-4 from *NKT* cells has been implicated in the suppression of TGF-β1 [41]. TGF-β is known to inhibit arthritis, especially when administrated systemically [44–46]. TGF-β inhibits T cell proliferation and downregulates the expression of IL-1 receptor, which may result in the suppression of arthritis. Even though *NKT* cells appear to contribute to the pathogenesis of arthritis, activation of *NKT* cells by synthetic glycolipid ligands protected mice against CIA [37]. Repeated injections of OCH, the Th2 polarizing form of an αGalCer, inhibited the clinical course of CIA, whereas α-GalCer administration exhibited a mild suppression of disease. Interestingly, OCH treatment suppressed CIA in SJL mice that have defects in numbers and functions of *NKT* cells. Moreover, OCH treatment ameliorated disease even after arthritis had developed. Suppression of arthritis was associated with the elevation of the IgG1:IgG2a ratio, suggesting a Th2 bias of CII-reactive T cells in OCH-treated mice. Furthermore, neutralization of IL-10 or IL-4 by monoclonal antibody reversed the beneficial effect of OCH treatment. In contrast to CIA, the treatment of α-GalCer has been shown to exacerbate disease in K/BxN serum transfer arthritis [41]. In our study, however, administration of α-GalCer efficiently inhibited K/BxN serum transfer arthritis by a Th2-independent mechanism [75]. The protective effect of arthritis by synthetic glycolipid ligands in arthritis models seems inconsistent with the reduction of disease severity in *NKT*-deficient mice. It is possible that activation of *NKT* cells by synthetic glycolipid is different from the physiological activation of *NKT* cells with endogenous ligands under pathogenic conditions such as arthritis.

2.4
NKT Cells in Lupus Models

Early studies in mice strains which spontaneously develop lupus-like disease such as MRL lpr/lpr mice, C3H gld/gld mice, and (NZBxNZW)F1 mice demonstrated a decrease in *NKT* cell number before the onset of disease, suggesting a preventive effect of *NKT* cells, although NKT cells were not well defined in these studies [47, 48]. The studies using *NKT*-deficient mice revealed a functional role for *NKT* cells in lupus animal models. CD1d deficiency led to exacerbation of pristine-induced nephritis in Balb/c mice [49] and skin disease in MRL lpr/lpr mice without inducing significant differences in nephritis and production of autoantibodies to nuclear antigens [50]. Another group, however, demonstrated that CD1d deficiency neither accelerated skin disease nor ameliorated kidney disease in MRL/lpr mice [51]. Stimulation of *NKT* cells with α-GalCer ameliorated dermatitis in MRL lpr/lpr mice in association with expansion of *NKT* cells and increased Th2 responses, while treatment with α-GalCer had no effect on kidney disease and serum anti-DNA antibody level [52]. In pristine-induced nephritis models, the effect of α-GalCer differs, depending on the strains of mice used. In Balb/c mice, treatment with α-GalCer promoted Th2 responses and protected mice against nephritis. Conversely, treatment with α-GalCer promoted Th1 responses and exacerbated disease in SJL/J mice [53]. The difference in the effect of α-GalCer seems to correlate with the ability to produce Th2 cytokines by activated *NKT* cells, similar to the phenomenon observed in EAE models.

Enhancement of disease rather than protection was observed in (NZB x NZW)F1 mice. In wild-type mice, *NKT* cells increased in number after the onset of disease [54, 55], and the transfer of NK1.1[+] T cells from diseased mice to young F1 mice (before the onset of renal failure) induced proteinuria and swelling of the glomeruli [56]. Moreover, treatment with anti-CD1d monoclonal antibody augmented Th2-type responses, increased serum levels of IgE, decreased levels of IgG2a and IgG2a anti-double-stranded DNA (dsDNA) antibodies, and ameliorated lupus [56]. Consistent with these results, activation of *NKT* cells with α-GalCer accelerated nephritis in correlation with enhancement of Th1 responses [56]. Despite the differences in the outcome of disease treatment following *NKT* cell activation, one consistent finding in the above studies is that *NKT* cell-driven Th1 responses lead to disease exacerbation, whereas *NKT* cell-driven Th2 responses lead to disease amelioration. One future direction may be to concentrate on which strain-dependent factors promote *NKT* cell-induced Th1 or Th2 responses.

2.5
NKT Cells in Colitis

Dextran sodium sulfate (DSS) -induced colitis is an experimental model for Crohn's disease mediated by Th1 cells. Activation of *NKT* cells with α-GalCer or OCH has been shown to protect mice against DSS-induced colitis [57, 58]. While treatment with both glycolipids induced higher amounts of IFN-γ and IL-4 than controls, the IFN-γ:IL-4 ratio was decreased compared to the control group [58]. The level of IL-10 in the supernatants of colon organ cultures after the injection of OCH was increased [58]. Treatment with OCH induced higher IL-10 production than did α-GalCer, which is consistent with the stronger inhibitory effect of OCH in this model of colitis [58]. Conversely, *NKT* cells have been proposed to act as effector cells in oxazalone-induced colitis [59]. Oxazalone-induced colitis is an experimental colitis model of human ulcerative colitis and is dependent on IL-13. This model of colitis was effectively blocked by neutralizing the IL-13 or depleting *NKT* cells. Moreover, the colitis did not develop in mice deficient in *NKT* cells, indicating the crucial pathological role of *NKT* cells in this model, similar to asthma models which *NKT* cells play an important role in the pathogenesis through IL-13 production.

3
NKT Cells in Human Autoimmune Diseases

Previous studies have documented a reduced number of *NKT* cells in the peripheral blood of patients suffering from systemic sclerosis [60], type 1 diabetes [61,62], multiple sclerosis (MS) [63–65], and other autoimmune disease conditions [66–68]. However, in type 1 diabetes, inconsistent results (decreased [61, 62], normal [69] or increased [70] number of *NKT* cells) were obtained by three independent groups, which led to considerable argument on the role of *NKT* cells in autoimmunity. To identify *NKT* cells, recent studies used α-GalCer-loaded CD1d tetramers, the most reliable tool for staining *NKT* cells, and confirmed a reduced number of *NKT* cells in the peripheral blood from untreated MS patients in remission [64] compared to healthy subjects. Unexpectedly, the number of *NKT* cells tended to increase in the relapse phase of MS and that the deficiency of *NKT* cells may become normalized in the patients treated with low doses of oral corticosteroids (unpublished results). These results imply that disease activity as well as prescribed medications would greatly influence on the number of *NKT* cells, which may provide some clue to designing future studies.

Production of Th2 cytokines was previously described as a cardinal feature of *NKT* cells. Now it is widely accepted that anti-inflammatory Th2 cytokines are secreted from CD4$^+$ *NKT* cells, but not from CD4$^-$ *NKT* cells [71, 72]. Namely, CD4$^+$ *NKT* cells are able to produce both Th1 and Th2 cytokines, whereas CD4$^-$ *NKT* cells selectively produce proinflammatory Th1 cytokines TNF-α and IFN-γ. Given this important dichotomy of *NKT* cells, we have re-analyzed the number and functions of *NKT* cells from untreated MS patients after sorting the cells into CD4$^+$ and CD4$^-$ populations [64]. CD4$^-$ *NKT* cells were greatly reduced in the peripheral blood of the untreated patients in remission, whereas a reduction of CD4$^+$ *NKT* cells was only marginal. Moreover, CD4$^+$ *NKT* cells from the patients were Th2-biased, as evidenced by enhancement of IL-4, whereas CD4$^-$ *NKT* cells were not. As both of the observed changes, Th2 bias of CD4$^+$ and a great reduction of CD4$^-$ *NKT* cells, could be regarded as disease stabilizing changes, we interpreted that this finding to suggest that the role of *NKT* cells in remission of MS is protective against disease development. In contrast, Th1 bias, as evidenced by loss of IL-4 secretion, was confirmed in *NKT* cell clones derived from peripheral blood [61] as well as draining lymph nodes [73] of type 1 diabetes. Although it remains unclear why *NKT* cells from MS and type 1 diabetes are biased toward opposing directions, it is possible that it may reflect the differential disease activity at the time of examination or due to differences in disease pathogenesis.

4
Concluding Remarks and Future Research

The research of the last decade has firmly established that *NKT* cells have the potential to either drive or suppress autoimmune conditions, although we know very little about the precise rules of how the regulation of *NKT* cells in vivo. Despite previous controversies, it now seems that numerical or functional changes of NKT cells may be associated with certain stages of autoimmune diseases, as has been revealed in MS [64] Therapeutic effects of glycolipid ligands for *NKT* cells have indicated that these lymphocytes bridging innate and adaptive immunity may be an excellent target for immune intervention. In particular, the design of "altered" CD1 glycolipid ligands has been shown in many models to alter the outcomes of disease. Meanwhile, it is much less clear how *NKT* cells regulate unwanted autoimmunity taking place in the context of the physiological immune network. It is likely that *NKT* cells produce Th2 cytokines to achieve this, and that the trigger of cytokine production may be an encounter of *NKT* cells with an endogenous ligand bound to CD1d. However, one known endogenous ligand, iGb3, seems to provoke

Th1 cytokines from *NKT* cells [74]. In this regard, there is room for a seeking Th2-inducing natural ligand. Not mutually exclusive to this is the theory that cytokines produced in the inflammatory site together with endogenous antigen and TCR-mediated signals may play a key role in conducting *NKT* cells [38] to secrete Th2 cytokines (Sakuishi et al., unpublished data). To gain deeper insights into the role of *NKT* cells in autoimmunity, the details of natural regulation needs to be clarified in the future.

References

1. Cohen IR, Young DB (1991) Autoimmunity, microbial immunity and the immunological homunculus. Immunol Today 12:105–110
2. Kuchroo VK, Anderson AC, Waldner H, Munder M, Bettelli E, Nicholson LB (2002) T cell response in experimental autoimmune encephalomyelitis (EAE): role of self and cross-reactive antigens in shaping, tuning, and regulating the autopathogenic T cell repertoire. Annu Rev Immunol 20:101–123
3. Wilson SB, Delovitch TL (2003) Janus-like role of regulatory NKT cells in autoimmune disease and tumour immunity. Nat Rev Immunol 3:211–222
4. Mars LT, Novak J, Liblau RS, Lehuen A (2004) Therapeutic manipulation of NKT cells in autoimmunity: modes of action and potential risks. Trends Immunol 25:471–476
5. Kronenberg M (2005) Toward an understanding of NKT cell biology: progress and paradoxes. Annu Rev Immunol 26:877–900
6. Kaer LV (2005) α-Galactosylceramide therapy for autoimmune diseases: prospects and obstacles. Nat Rev Immunol 5:31–42
7. Yu KOA, Porcelli SA (2005) The diverse functions of CD1d-restricted NKT cells and their potential for immunotherapy. Immmunol Lett 100:42–55
8. Cardell SL (2005) The natural killer T lymphocyte: a player in the complex regulation of autoimmune diabetes in non-obese diabetic mice. Clin Exp Immmunol 143:197–202
9. Mars LT, Laloux V, Goude K, Desbois S, Saoudi A, Van Kaer L, Lassmann H, Herbelin A, Lehuen A, Liblau RS (2002) Vα14-Jα281. NKT cells naturally regulate experimental autoimmune encephalomyelitis in nonobese diabetic mice. J Immunol 168:6007–6011
10. Teige A, Teiga I, Savasani S, Bockermann R, Mondoc E, Holmdahl R, Issazadel-Navikas S (2004) CD1-dependent regulation of chronic central nervous system inflammation in experimental autoimmune encephalomyelitis. J Immunol 172:186–194
11. Singh AK, Wilson MT, Hong S, Oliveres-Villagomez D, Du C, Stanic AK, Joyce S, Siriam S, Koezka Y, Van Kaer L (2001) Natural killer T cell activation protects mice against experimental autoimmune encephalomyelitis. J Exp Med 194:1801–1811
12. Furlan R, Bergami A, Cantarella D, Brambilla E, Taniguchi M, Dellabona P, Casorati G, Martino G (2003) Activation of invariant NKT cells by αGalCer administration protects mice from MOG_{35-55}-induced EAE: critical roles for administration route and IFN-γ. Eur J Immunol 33:1830–1838

13. Jahng AW, Maricic I, Pedersen B, Burdin N, Naidenko O (2001) Activatin of natural killer T cells potentiates or prevents experimental autoimmune encephalomyelitis. J Exp Med 194:1789–1799
14. Pal E, Tabira T, Kawano T, Taniguchi M, Miyake S, Yamamura T (2001) Costimulation-dependent modulation of experimental autoimmune encephalomyelitis by ligand stimulation of Vα 14 NKT cells. J Immunol 166:662–668
15. Miyamoto K, Miyake S, Yamamura T (2001) A synthetic glycolipid prevents autoimmune encephalomyelitis by inducing Th2 bias of natural killer T cells. Nature 413:531–534
16. Oki S, Chiba A, Yamamura T, Miyake S (2004) The clinical implication and molecular mechanism of preferential IL-4 production by modified glycolipid-stimulated NKT cells. J Clin Inv 113:1631–1640
17. Goff RD, Gao Y, Mattner J, Zhou D, Yin N, Cantu C, Teyton L, Bendelac A, Savage PB (2004) Effects of lipid chain lengths in α-galactosylceramides on cytokine release by natural killer T ells. J Am Chem Soc 126:13602–13603
18. Oki S, Tomi C, Yamamura T, Miyake S (2005) Preferential Th2 polarization by OCH is supported by incompetent NKT cell induction of CD40L and following production of inflammatory cytokines by bystander cells in vivo. Int Immunol 17:1619–1629
19. Gombert JM, Herbelin A, Tancrede-Bohin E, Dy M, Carnaud C, Bach JF (1996) Early quantitative and functional deficiency of NK1+-like thymocytes in the NOD mouse. Eur J Immunol 126:2989–2998
20. Falcone M, Yeung B, Tucker L, Rodriguez E, Sarvetnick N (1999) A defect in interleukin 12-induced activation and interferon gamma secretion of peripheral natural killer T cells in nonobese diabetic mice suggests new pathogenic mechanisms for insulin-dependent diabetes mellitus. J Exp Med 190:963–972
21. Godfrey DI, Kinder SJ, Silvera P, Baxter AG (1997) Flow cytometric study of T cell development in NOD mice reveals a deficiency in alpha-beta TCR+CDR-CD8-tymocytes. J Autoimmun 10:279–285
22. Poulton LD, Smyth MJ, Hawke CG, Silveira P, Shepherd D, Naidenko OV, Godfrey DI, Baxter AG (2001) Cytometric and functional analyses of NK and NKT cell deficiencies in NOD mice. Int Immunol 13:887–896
23. Shi FD, Flodstrom M, Balasa B, Kim SH, van Gunst K, Strominger JL, Wilson SB, Sarvetnick N (2001) Germ line deletion of the CD1 locus exacerbates diabetes in the NOD mouse. Proc Natl Acad Sci U S A 98:6777–6782
24. Naumov YN, Bahjat KS, Gausling R, Abraham R, Exley MA, Koezuka Y, Balk SB, Stominger JL, Clare-Salzer M, Wilson SB (2001) Activation of CD1d-restricted T cells protects NOD mice from developing diabetes by regulating dendritic cell subsets. Proc Natl.Acad Sci U S A 98:13838–13843
25. Wang B, Geng Y-B, Wang C-R (2001) CD1-restricted NKT cells protect nonobese diabetic mice from developing diabetes. J Exp Med 194:313–320
26. Falcone M, Facciotti F, Ghidoli N, Monti P, Olivieri S, Zaccagnino L, Bonifacio E, Casorati G, Sanvito F, Sarventrick N (2004) Up-regulation of CD1d expression restores the immunoregulatory function of NKT cells and prevents autoimmune diabetes in nonobese diabetic mice. J Immunol 172:5908–5916

27. Hammond KJL, Poulton LD, Almisano LJ, Silveira PA, Godrey DI, Bazter AG (1998) α/β-T cell receptor (TCR)$^+$ CD4$^-$CD8$^-$ (NKT) thymocytes prevent insulin-dependent diabetes mellitus in nonobese diabetic (NOD)/Lt mice by the influence of interleukin (IL)-4 and/or IL-10. J Exp Med 187:1047–1056

28. Lehuen A, Lantz O, Beaudoin L, Laloux V, Carnaud C, Bendelac A, Bach J-F, Monteriro RC (1998) Overexpression of natural killer T cells protects Vα14-Jα18 transgenic nonobese diabetic mice against diabetes. J Exp Med 188:1831–1839

29. Hong S, Wilson MT, Serizawa I, Wu L, Singh N, Naidenko OV, Miura T, Haba T, Scherer DC, Wei J, Kronenberg M, Koezuka Y, Van Kaer L (2001) The natural killer T-cell ligand α-galactosylceramide prevents autoimmune diabetes in non-obese diabetic mice. Nat Med 7:1052–1056

30. Sharif S, Arreaza GA, Zucker P, Mi Q-S, Sondhi J, Naidenko OV, Kronenberg M, Koezuka Y, Delovitch TL, Gombert J-M, Leite-de-Moraes M, Gouarin C, Zhu R, Hameg A, Nakayama T, Taniguchi M, Lepault F, Lehuen A, Bach J-F, Herbelin A (2001) Activation of natural killer T cells by α-galactosylceramide treatment prevents the onset and recurrence of autoimmune tye1 diabetes. Nat Med 7:1057–1062

31. Mizuno M, Masumura M, Tomi C, Chiba A, Oki S, Yamamura T, Miyake S (1997) Synthetic glycolipid OCH prevents insulitis and diabetes in NOD mice. J Autoimmun 10:279–285

32. Laloux V, Beaudoin L, Jeske D, Carnaud C, Lehuen A (2001) NKT cell-induced protection against diabetes in Vα14-Jα281 transgenic nonobese diabetic mice is associated with a Th2 shift circumscribed regionally to the islets and functionally to islet autoantigen. J Immunol 166:3749–3756

33. Beaudoin L, Laloux V, Novak J, Lucas B, Lehuen A (2002) NKT cells inhibit the onset of diabetes by impairing the development of pathogenic T cells specific for pancreatic beta cells. Immunity 17:725–736

34. Novak J, Beaudoin L, Griseri T, Lehuen A (2005) Inhibition of T cells differentiation into effectors by NKT cells requires cell contacts. J Immunol 174:1954–1961

35. Chen YG, Choisy-Rossi CM, Holl TM, Champan HD, Besra GS, Porcelli SA, Shaffer DJ, Roopenian D, Wilson SB, Serreze DV (2005) Activated NKT cells inhibit autoimmune diabetes through tolerogenic recruitment of dendritic cells to pancreatic lymph nodes. J Immunol 174:1196–1204

36. Griseri T, Beaudoin L, Novak J, Mars LT, Lepault F, Liblau R, Lehuen A (2005) Invariant NKT cells exacerbate type 1 diabetes induced by CD8 T cells. J Immunol 175:2091–2101

37. Chiba A, Kaieda S, Oki S, Yamamura T, Miyake S (2005) The involvement of Vα14 natural killer T cells in the pathogenesis of murine models of arthritis. Arthritis Rheum 52:1941–1948

38. Brigl M, Bry L, Kent SC, Gumperz JE, Brenner MB (2003) Mechanism of CD1d-restricted natural killer T cell activation during microbial infection. Nat Immunol 4:1230–1237

39. Chiba A, Oki S, Miyamoto K, Hashimoto H, Yamamura T, Miyake S (2004) Suppression of collagen-induced arthritis by natural killer activation with OCH, a sphingosine-truncated analog of α-galactosylceramide. Arthritis Rheum 50:305–313

40. Ohnishi Y, Tsutsumi A, Goto D, Itoh S, Matsumoto I, Taniguchi M, Sumida T (2005) TCRVα14+ natural killer T cell function and effector T cells in mice with collagen-induced arthritis. Clin Exp Immunol 141:47–53

41. Kim HY, Kim HJ, Min HS, Park ES, Park SH, Chung DH (2005) NKT cells promote antibody-induced arthritis by suppressing transforming growth β1 production. J Exp Med 201:41–47

42. Korganow AS, Ji H, Mangialaio S, Dchatelle V, Pelanda R, Martin T, Degott C, Kikutani H, Rajewsky K, Pasquali JL, Benoist C, Mathis D (1999) From systemic T cell self-reactivity to organ-specific autoimmune disease via immunoglobulins. Immunity 10:451–461

43. Terato K, Hasty KA, Reife RA, Cremer MA, Kang H, Stuart JM (1992) Induction of arthritis with monoclonal antibodies to collagen. J Immunol 148:2103–2108

44. Brandes ME, Allen JB, Ogawa Y, Wahl SM (1991) Transforming growth factor β1 suppresses acute and chronic arthritis in experimental animals. J Clin Invest 87:1108–1113

45. Kuruvilla AP, Shah R, Hochwald GM, Liggitt HD, Palladino MA et al (1991) Protective effect of transforming growth factor β1 on experimental autoimmune diseases in mice. Proc Natl Acad Sci U S A 88:2918–2921

46. Thorbecke GJ, Shah R, Leu CH, Kuruvilla AP, Hardison AM et al (1992) Involvement of endogenous tumor necrosis factor alpha and transforming growth factor β during induction of collagen type II arthritis in mice. Proc Natl Acad Sci U S A 189:7375–7379

47. Takeda K, Dennert G (1993) The development of autoimmunity in C57BL/6 lpr mice correlates with the disappearance of natural killer type 1-positive cells: evidence for their suppressive action on bone marrow stem cell proliferation B cell immunoglobulin secretion, and autoimmune symptoms. J Exp Med 177:155–164

48. Mieza MA, Itoh T, Cui JQ, Makino Y, Kawano T, Tsuchida K, Koike AT, Shirai T, Yagita H, Matsuzawa A, Koseki H, Taniguchi M (1996) Selective reduction of Vα14+ NKT cells associated with disease development in autoimmune-prone mice. J Immunol 156:4035–4040

49. Yang J-Q, Saxena V, Xu H, Van Kaer L, Wang C-R, Singh RR (2003) Immunoregulatory role of CD1d in the hydrocarbon oil-induced model of lupus nephritis. J Immunol 171:4439–4446

50. Yang JQ, Singh AK, Wilson MT, Satoh M, Stanic AK, Par J-J, Hong S, Gadola SD, Mizutani A, Kakumanu SR, Reeves W, Cerundolo V, Joyce S, Van Kaer L, Singh RR (2003) Repeated α-galactosylceramide administration results in expansion of NKT cells and alleviates inflammatory dermatitis in MRL-lpr/lpr mice. J Immunol 171:2142–2153

51. Chan OTM, Paliwal V, Mcniff JM, Park SH, Bendelac A, Schlomchik MJ (2001) Deficiency in β2-microglobulin, but not CD1, accelerates spontaneous lupus skin disease while inhibiting nephritis in MRL-Fas[lpr] mice: an example of disease regulation at the organ level. J Immunol 167:2985–2990

52. Yang JQ, Saxena V, Xu H, van Kaer L, Wang C-R, Singh RR (2003) Repeated α-galactosylceramide administration results in expansion of NKT cells and alleviates inflammatory dermatitis in MRL-lpr/lpr mice. J Immunol 171:4439–4446

53. Singh AK, Yang JQ, Parekh VV, Wei J, Wang CR, Joyce S, Singh RR, van Kaer L (2005) The natural killer T cell ligand α-galactosylceramide prevents or promotes pristine-induced lupus in mice. Eur J Immunol 35:1143–1154

54. Morshe SRM, Mannoor K, Halder RC, Kawamura H, Bannai M, Sekikawa H, Watanabe H, Abo T (2002) Tissue-specific expansion of NTK and CD5+B cells at the onset of autoimmune disease in (NZB x NZW)F1 mice. Eur J Immunol 32:2551–2561

55. Firestier C, Molano A, Im JS, Dutronc Y, Diamond B, Davidson A, Illarionov PA, Besra GS, Porcelli SA (2005) Expansion and hyperactivity of CD1d-restricted NKT cells during the progression of systemic lupus erythematosus in (New Zealand Black x New Zealand White) F_1 mice. J Immunol 175:763–770

56. Zeng D, Liu Y, Sidobre S, Kronenberh M, Strober S (2003) Activation of natural killer T cells in NZB/W mice induces Th1-type immune responses exacerbating lupus. J Clin Invest 112:1211–1222

57. Saubermann LJ, Beck P, Jong YPD, Pitman RS, Ryan MS, Kim HS, Exley M, Snapper S, Balk SP, Hagen SJ, Kanauchi O, Motoki K, Sakai T, Terhorst C, Koezuka Y, Podolsky DK, Blumerg RS (2000) Activation o f natural killer T cells by α-galactosylceramide in the presence of CD1d provides protection against colitis in mice. Gastroenterology 119:119–128

58. Ueno Y, Tanaka S, Sumi M, Miyake S, Tazuma S, Taniguchi M, Yamamura T, Chyayama K (2005) Single dose of OCH improves mucosal T helper type 1/T helper type 2 cytokine balance and prevents experimental colitis in the presence of Vα14 natural killer T cells in mice. Inflamm Bowel Dis 11:35–41

59. Heller F, Fuss IJ, Nieuwenhuis EE, Blumberg RS, Strober W (2002) Oxazolone colitis, a Th2 colitis model resembling ulcerative colitis, is mediated by IL-13-producing NK-T cells. Immunity 17:629–638

60. Sumida T, Sakamoto A, Murata H, Makino Y, Takahashi H, Yoshida S, Nishioka K, Iwamoto I, Taniguchi M (1995) Selective reduction of T cells bearing invariant Vαa24 JαQ antigen receptor in patients with systemic sclerosis. J Exp Med 182:1163–1168

61. Wilson SB, Kent SC, Patton KT, Orban T, Jackson RA, Exley M, Porcelli S, Schatz DA, Atkinson MA, Balk SP, Strominger JL, Hafler DA (1998) Extreme Th1 bias of invariant Vα24 JαQT cells in type 1 diabetes. Nature 391:177–181

62. Kukreja A, Cost G, Marker J, Zhang C, Sun Z, Lin-Su K, Ten S, Sanz M, Exley M, Wilson B, Porcelli S, Maclaren N (2002) Multiple immuno-regulatory defects in type-1 diabetes. J Clin Invest 109:131–140

63. Illes Z, Kondo T, Newcombe J, Oka N, Tabira T, Yamamura T (2000) Differential expression of NKT cell Vα24JαQ invariant TCR chain in the lesions of multiple sclerosis and chronic inflammatory demyelinating polyneuropathy. J Immunol 164:4375–4381

64. Araki M, Kondo T, Gumperz JE, Brenner MB, Miyake S, Yamamura T (2003) Th2 bias of CD4+ NKT cells derived from multiple sclerosis in remission. Int Immunol 15:279–288

65. Demoulins T, Gachelin G, Bequet D, Dormont D (2003) A biased Vα24+ T-cell repertoire leads to circulating NKT-cell defects in a multiple sclerosis patient at the onset of his disease. Immunol Lett 90:223–228

66. Oishi Y, Sumida T, Sakamoto A, Kita Y, Kurasawa K, Nawata Y, Takabayashi K, Takahashi H, Yoshida S, Taniguchi M, Saito Y, Iwamoto I (2001) Selective reduction and recovery of invariant Vα24JαQT cell receptor T cells in correlation with disease activity in patients with systemic lupus erythematosus. J Rheumatol 28:275–283

67. Kojo S, Adachi Y, Keino H, Taniguchi M, Sumida T (2001) Dysfunction of T cell receptor AV24AJ18+, BV11+ double-negative regulatory natural killer T cells in autoimmune diseases. Arthritis Rheum 44:1127–1138

68. Van der Vliet HJ, von Blomberg BM, Nishi N, Reijm M, Voskuyl AE, van Bodegraven AA, Polman CH, Rustemeyer T, Lips P, van den Eertwegh AJ, Giaccone G, Scheper RJ, Pinedo HM (2001) Circulating Vα24$^+$ Vβ11$^+$ NKT cell numbers are decreased in a wide variety of diseases that are characterized by autoreactive tissue damage. Clin Immunol 100:144–148

69. Lee PT, Putnam A, Benlagha K, Teyton L, Gottlieb PA, Bendelac A (2002) Testing the NKT cell hypothesis of human IDDM pathogenesis. J Clin Invest 110:793–800

70. Oikawa Y, Shimada A, Yamada S, Motohashi Y, Nakagawa Y, Irie J, Maruyama T, Saruta T (2002) High frequency of Vα24$^+$ Vβ11$^+$ T-cells observed in type 1 diabetes. Diabetes Care 25:1818–1823

71. Gumperz JE, Miyake S, Yamamura T, Brenner MB (2002) Functionally distinct subsets of CD1d-restricted natural killer T cells revealed by CD1d tetramer staining. J Exp Med 195:625–636

72. Lee PT, Benlagha K, Teyton L, Bendelac A (2002) Distinct functional lineages of human Vα24 natural killer T cells. J Exp Med 195:637–641

73. Kent SC, Chen Y, Clemmings SM, Viglietta V, Kenyon NS, Ricordi C, Hering B, Hafler DA (2005) Loss of IL-4 secretion from human type 1a diabetic pancreatic draining lymph node NKT cells. J Immunol 175:4458–4464

74. Zhou D, Mattner J, Cantu C 3rd, Schrantz N, Yin N, Gao Y, Sagiv Y, Hudspeth K, Wu YP, Yamashita T, Teneberg S, Wang D, Proia RL, Levery SB, Savage PB, Teyton L, Bendelac A (2004) Lysosomal glycosphingolipid recognition by NKT cells. Science 306:1786–1789

75. Kaleda S, Tom C, Oki S, Yamamura T, Miyake S (2007) Activation of iNKT cells by synthetic glycolipid ligands supresses autoantibody-induced arthritis. Arthritis Rheum (in press)

CTMI (2007) 314:269–289

*i*NKT Cells in Allergic Disease

E. H. Meyer[1,2] · R. H. DeKruyff[1] · D. T. Umetsu[1] (✉)

[1] Division of Immunology, Children's Hospital Boston, Harvard Medical School, One Blackfan Circle, Boston, MA 02115, USA
dale.umetsu@childrens.harvard.edu

[2] Immunology Program and the Department of Pediatrics, Stanford University, Stanford, CA 94305, USA

Abstract Recent studies indicate that invariant TCR$^+$ CD1d-restricted natural killer T (*i*NKT) cells play an important role in regulating the development of asthma and allergy. *i*NKT cells can function to skew adaptive immunity toward Th2 responses, or can act directly as effector cells at mucosal surfaces in diseases such as ulcerative colitis and bronchial asthma. In mouse models of asthma, NKT cell-deficient strains fail to develop allergen-induced airway hyperreactivity (AHR), a cardinal feature of asthma, and NKT cells are found in the lungs of patients with chronic asthma, suggesting a critical role for NKT cells in the development of AHR. However, much work remains in characterizing iNKT cells and their function in asthma, and in understanding the relationship between the iNKT cells and conventional CD4$^+$ T cells.

1
Introduction

Atopic diseases such as allergic rhinitis, acute contact sensitivity, chronic atopic dermatitis, and asthma have increased dramatically in worldwide prevalence over the past two decades, particularly in industrialized countries such as the United States, Europe, and Japan [1–3]. Atopic diseases are complex traits caused by immune responses to environmental factors such as allergens among genetically susceptible individuals [1]. Roughly one in six individuals in the United States has some form of allergic disease [4]. As a result, allergic diseases have reached epidemic proportions, and current health care expenditure for allergic disease, particularly asthma, is enormous [5].

At least a dozen polymorphic genes regulate allergic diseases like asthma, controlling the inflammatory response, IgE, and cytokine and chemokine production [4, 6–8]. In addition, the environment in industrialized cultures has changed dramatically over recent years, in ways that appear to directly exaggerate the environmental effects on the pathogenesis of allergic disorders [9]. These environmental and genetic factors lead to the development of a Th2-biased immune responses and the overproduction of cytokines such as IL-4, IL-5, IL-9, and IL-13. This inappropriate Th2 inflammatory response causes many of the symptoms seen in allergy, including vascular and pulmonary inflammation, eosinophilia, mucous production, rashes, swelling, itching, wheezing, and progressive tissue remodeling [11–15]. NKT cells, which comprise a newly described, unique subset of lymphocytes that express features of both classical T cells and natural killer (NK) cells are capable of rapidly producing large amounts of Th2 cytokines and appear to play a critical role in this allergic inflammatory response, particularly in the development of asthma and airway hyperreactivity (AHR) [16–18], a cardinal feature of asthma.

Asthma is a chronic inflammatory disease of the respiratory tract that affects one in eight to ten individuals in the United States [2, 19]. Examination of the lungs of patients with asthma has shown that the inflammation in asthma is characterized by large numbers of eosinophils and CD4$^+$ T lymphocytes [20]. The pulmonary CD4$^+$ cells in asthmatic subjects produce predominantly Th2 cytokines, which play essential roles in asthma by enhancing the growth, differentiation, and recruitment of eosinophils, basophils, mast cells, and IgE producing B cells, and by directly inducing AHR [20]. Thus, MHC class II restricted CD4$^+$ Th2 cells, which have been observed in the airways of virtually all patients with asthma, are thought to play an obligatory role in the pathogenesis of bronchial asthma [21]. However, the CD4 cell surface marker is expressed not only by conventional protein antigen-specific class II-restricted CD4$^+$ T cells, but also by NKT cells, which play an important role in the pathogenesis of asthma [16–18, 22].

In this review, we focus specifically on the role of invariant NKT cells (*i*NKT or type 1 NK T cells) in inducing Th2 inflammation and allergic pathology, with particular attention to asthma where the contribution of *i*NKT cells to allergic pathology is best characterized. We also review the general idea that *i*NKT cells can serve as critical Th2-like effector cells and explore the factors that contribute to the production of IL-4 by *i*NKT cells as well as the possibility that a Th2-like subset of *i*NKT cells may be particularly important in the pathogenesis of asthma. We believe that a greater understanding of the mechanisms governing the function of *i*NKT cells will likely contribute to a greater comprehension of allergic diseases and to the development of new therapeutic approaches.

2
The Major Subsets of NKT Cells

The term "NKT cell" was first coined in 1995 and classification of NKT cells is complicated by the fact that NKT cells consist of a heterogenous group of cell types that sometimes share surface makers. Nonetheless, NKT cells fall generally into three major categories [23].

2.1
Type I NKT Cells

Type I (or classical) NKT cells were first recognized in the late 1980s as a distinct subset of T cells expressing a highly restricted T cell receptor (TCR) repertoire consisting of Vα14-Jα18 (in mice) or Vα24-Jα18 (in humans). It was not until later that these invariant TCR$^+$ cells were recognized to be NKT cells and are now often referred to as *i*NKT cells [24]. *i*NKT cells are CD4$^+$ or CD4$^-$/CD8$^-$ (double negative), and in humans a small subset of *i*NKT cells express CD8. Through their invariant TCRs, *i*NKT cells recognize bacterial and endogenous glycolipid antigens presented by the nonpolymorphic MHC class I-like protein, CD1d [25–27]. CD1d is widely expressed, for example by gut and airway epithelial cells, T cells, hepatocytes, B cells, macrophages, and dendritic cells [25, 28]. Recognition of CD1d presented glycolipids, such as α-galactosylceramide (α-GalCer), by *i*NKT cells is highly conserved across phylogeny, suggesting that these cells play a pivotal role in immunity [28]. The type 1 *i*NKT cells have been shown to be involved in asthma and AHR (see below).

2.2
Type II NKT Cells

Type II (or nonclassical or noninvarient) NKT cells have a diverse TCR repertoire but still recognize the CD1d molecule. These cells are exceedingly rare in the spleens and livers of mice (<0.1% of lymphocyte gate) but are more common in the bone marrow [24]. Type II NKT cells are found in humans and may be more prevalent in the liver and bone marrow than type I NKT. Type II NKT cells have been associated in human and mice with some diseases such as ulcerative colitis or with suppression of tumor growth [29, 30]. Since many type II NKT cells do not recognize α-GalCer, when presented by CD1d, it is thought that they may be particularly important for the recognition of exogenous glycolipid antigens. Since the year 2000, fluorochrome-conjugated CD1d-tetramers loaded with various glycolipid antigens have been used to identify type I and type II NKT cells, revolutionizing how we understand these cell populations [28].

2.3
Type III NKT Cells

Type III (or CD1d-independent) NKT cells express a diverse TCR repertoire restricted to classical MHC class I and II molecules but not CD1d molecule, and might be more common than type I and II NKT cells. They are often classified by surface expression of Ly49 or NK1.1 (CD161 in humans) and CD3 but not the CD1d-restricted TCRs. The study of type III cells is complicated by the fact that some mice strains, such as BALB/c, do not express NK1.1, and therefore NK1.1+ NKT cells cannot be easily identified. While type III NKT cells are thought to be important for many immune functions such as antitumor responses or hepatic inflammation [23, 31], in this review, we will primarily focus upon type I *i*NKT cells, which appear to be critical for the development of asthma.

Because *i*NKT cells rapidly produce large quantities of cytokines such as IL-4 and IFN-γ within minutes of stimulation as a manifestation of innate-like immunity, they can critically amplify and regulate adaptive immune responses by enhancing the function of DCs, NK cells, B cells, as well as conventional CD4$^+$ and CD8$^+$ T cells, and thus link innate and adaptive immunity [27, 28, 31, 32]. Moreover, the rapid production of cytokines by *i*NKT cells has been shown to regulate the development of autoimmune, antimicrobial, anti-tumor and anti-transplant immune responses [25, 33, 34], providing either disease-causing or disease-protective effects. For example, depending upon their activation state, *i*NKT cells can either promote or prevent tumor growth, colitis, experimental autoimmune encephalomyelitis (EAE) and airway hyper-reactivity (AHR) in mouse models of asthma [16, 22, 31].

3
*i*NKT Cells and Th2 Immune Deviation

3.1
Asthma and AHR

Bronchial asthma is characterized by the presence in the airways of large numbers of CD4$^+$ T cells producing IL-4 and IL-13. The pulmonary CD4$^+$ T cells have been thought to be conventional allergen-specific CD4$^+$ MHC class II-restricted T cells, which orchestrate the inflammation in the airways in response to environmental allergens. However, because the CD4 antigen is also expressed by NKT cells, and because NKT cells produce large amounts of IL-4 and IL-13, their role in the development of allergen-induced AHR is under investigated. In mice, several groups investigators have shown that *i*NKT cells were absolutely required for the development of AHR [17, 18]. In these models, CD1d$^{-/-}$ mice, which are deficient in type 1 and type 2 NKT cells, showed reduced eosinophilic inflammation and failed to develop allergen-induced AHR, as measured by whole body plethysmograph or by direct measurement of airway resistance and dynamic compliance in intubated and mechanically ventilated mice [17, 18]. Wild type mice treated with anti-CD1d blocking mAbs prior to allergen sensitization and challenge also failed to develop AHR [18].

The requirement for *i*NKT cells in the development of AHR was confirmed by experiments evaluating allergen-induced AHR in another *i*NKT cell-deficient mouse strain, Jα18$^{-/-}$ mice. These mice lack the α-chain of the invariant TCR, and therefore specifically lack type I or *i*NKT cells [35]. Similar to CD1d$^{-/-}$ mice, these mice showed reduced eosinophilic inflammation in the lungs and failed to develop AHR as measured by whole body plethysmography and by direct examination of airway resistance and dynamic compliance [17]. Moreover, the adoptive transfer of purified WT *i*NKT cells into the Jα18$^{-/-}$ mice prior to allergen challenge fully reconstituted lung inflammation and AHR [17], indicating that *i*NKT cells were specifically required for the development of AHR. Production by the iNKT cells of IL-4 and IL-13 but not IFN-γ was required for the development of AHR since adoptive transfer of iNKT cells from IL-4$^{-/-}$IL-13$^{-/-}$ into Jα18$^{-/-}$ mice failed to restore AHR [17]. Taken together, these studies demonstrated that iNKT cells producing IL-4 and IL-13 are required for the development of AHR.

While studies carried out in different laboratories with any of several mouse strains and experimental protocols have confirmed the requirement for iNKT cells in the development of AHR, a few other studies have concluded that iNKT cells may not be necessary for the development of asthma in murine models. For example, one study showed that allergen-induced airway inflammation was normal in CD1d$^{-/-}$ mice, although data from this study showed a reduction in airway eosinophilia in CD1d$^{-/-}$ mice that did not reach statistical significance [36]. Importantly, AHR, which is the critical feature that is absent in CD1d$^{-/-}$ mice, was not assessed in these studies [36]. Other studies that have questioned the role of iNKT cells in AHR examined allergen-induced AHR in β2-microglobulin-deficient mice. Such mice lack all class I molecules, including CD1d, which associates with β2-microglobulin to form the complete CD1d heterodimer molecule, and thus the mice have been assumed to lack both CD8$^+$ cells as well as NKT cells. Sensitization and challenge of these mice with allergen resulted in normal airway eosinophilia and AHR [37, 38]. However, it is difficult to interpret these studies because it has become apparent that CD1d molecules can be expressed in the absence of the β2-microglobulin chain [39] and that CD1d-independent NKT are present in the β2-microglobulin$^{-/-}$ mice [40, 41]. The functionality of such possible CD1d-independent NKT cells in β2-microglobulin$^{-/-}$ mice in asthma is not yet clear. Thus, it is possible that while iNKT cells are required for the development of allergen-induced AHR in most circumstances that have been studied experimentally, there may be some situations in which some form of airway inflammation or AHR develops without iNKT cells.

The requirement of iNKT cells for the development of AHR is independent of Th2 responses, since antigen-induced Th2 responses and antigen-specific Th2 polarized MHC II-restricted CD4$^+$ T cells develop normally but perhaps with less intensity in CD1d$^{-/-}$ and Jα18$^{-/-}$ mice [17]. However, while iNKT cells are not absolutely required for certain types of Th2 responses [42], iNKT cells have been shown to play a critical role in regulating innate and adaptive Th2 immune responses, particularly as iNKT cells are a critically important source of Th2 cytokines [24, 31]. For example, investigators have found that co-administration α-GalCer, which specifically activates iNKT cells, along with exogenous antigen results in enhanced sensitization of mice to these antigens and the subsequent development of AHR [43]. These studies demonstrate that the pharmacological activation of iNKT cells can function in the immune response as an adjuvant and lead to the development of immunological memory and maturation of antigen-specific conventional CD4$^+$ T cells that can later participate in allergen-induced AHR.

3.2
iNKT Cells and IgE

Although initial reports indicated that iNKT cells were important for IgE production in response to treatment with anti-IgD or anti-CD3 activating mAbs [44–46], subsequent reports showed that isotype switching and antigen-specific IgE production in the context of adaptive immunity does not require iNKT cells [42]. Thus iNKT cell deficient CD1d$^{-/-}$ and Jα18$^{-/-}$ mice develop normal antigen-specific IgE responses [17, 36, 42]. However, Vα14-Jα18 transgenic mice, which contain increased numbers of iNKT cells, exhibit significantly higher serum levels of Th2-associated immunoglobulins, IgG1 and IgE [47], suggesting that iNKT cells may modulate total serum levels of Th2-related immunoglobulins. Similarly, activation of iNKT cells with α-GalCer or other glycolipid antigens results in a rapid rise in total serum IgE that remains elevated with chronic activation of iNKT cells with glycolipids [22]. However, the effects of iNKT cells on IgE production are likely independent of the NKT cell effect on AHR, since AHR can develop in the absence of IgE. Nevertheless, it is likely that understanding the mechanism whereby iNKT cells might regulate the production of IgE will improve our understanding of hyper-IgE states and atopy, and therefore further experimental studies examining the interaction of iNKT cells with B cell populations are needed in this regard.

3.3
Endogenous Glycolipids and Asthma

In murine models of allergen-induced AHR, administration of protein antigens such as ovalbumin, bovine serum albumin, or ragweed antigen led to the activation of iNKT cells and the development of AHR. Because no exogenous glycolipids were administered to these mice, it is likely that endogenous glycolipids are released or exposed in the inflammatory environment elicited by protein allergens and these glycolipid antigens are recognized by iNKT cells, which then become activated [17, 22]. Recognition of glycolipid antigens distinguishes iNKT cells from conventional MHC class II restricted CD4$^+$ T cells, which recognize protein antigens. Because of their restricted TCR repertoire, iNKT cells are also relatively restricted in their antigen-recognition and are considered a part of the innate-adaptive or early adaptive system, in which repertoire-limited B and T cell populations respond to evolutionarily conserved self and non-self antigens as a means to rapidly respond to immunological danger [49]. Thus, it is believed that a few special endogenous glycolipids are produced by cells in the body and serve as early indicators of "threatened, damaged or altered self." In vitro experiments have shown that these iNKT activating glycolipids are processed and presented by both professional bone marrow-derived APCs as well as nonprofessional tissue cells such as hepatic or epithelial cells during inflammation [25, 27, 32]. The full range of endogenous glycolipid antigens is not yet known, but one endogenous glycolipid has been identified, called isoglobotrihexosylceramide, or iGb3 [27, 32].

iGb3 is important for the development of iNKT cells, because mice with a deficient β-hexoseaminidase b subunit cannot make iGb3, and show a 95% reduction in iNKT cell numbers [27, 32]. The identification of iGb3 as an endogenous glycolipid is an important advance, but there is some thought that iGb3 may perhaps be more important for the thymic maturation of iNKT cells, and that other endogenous ligands may function to activate iNKT cells in the periphery. This may explain why intranasal administration of iGb3 does not induce AHR in mice in contrast to other glycolipid antigens that more strongly activate iNKT cells (E.H. Meyer, unpublished observations) [22]. Nonetheless, iGb3 may be produced in an inflammatory setting and has recently been shown to be upregulated endogenously and loaded in CD1d by DCs pretreated with *Salmonella typhimurium* extract, which then activate iNKT cells [27, 32, 48]. The precise role of iGb3 in asthma has not been determined, and other endogenous glycolipids, perhaps expressed primarily in the tissues in response to environmental insults, may also be important in asthma. Understanding the mechanisms that regulate the expression of these endogenous glycolipids will likely be critical in understanding the regulation of asthma.

Glycolipids presented by the CD1d molecule can also originate exogenously, and these exogenous glycolipids may be recognized as dangerous non-self antigens [28, 49]. These exogenous glycolipids include the bacterial membrane constituents from the *Sphingomonadaceae* and *Rickettsiaceae* families [26, 32, 50]. Many of these species are Gram-negative LPS-negative bacteria and include human bacteria such as *Sphingomonas paucimobilis* and *Ehrlichia chaffeensis*. Recently, it has been speculated that α-GalCer itself may in fact be derived from the *Sphingomonas* bacterial family, which commonly infects marine sponges. If we assume that these exogenous membrane glycolipids possess pathogen-associated molecular patterns (PAMPs), then it is possible that iNKT cells may be important for the immune recognition of potential pathogens that are not recognized by the currently catalogued innate pathogen pattern recognition receptors [26]. The range of pathogens expressing glycolipids recognized by NKT cells is not known, but may include *Borrelia burgdorferi*, *Cryptococcus neoformans*, *Plasmodium falciparum*, *Trypanosoma cruzi*,

Leishmania major, and *Schistosoma mansoni* [25, 26, 28, 32, 51, 52]. Whether pathogens encountered in the respiratory tract may also express glycolipids recognized by NKT cells, or whether antigen-presenting cells recognize these pathogens through TLRs or other unknown receptors and then produce endogenous glycolipids that activate iNKT cells is not yet clear. In either case, this line of reasoning opens up the exciting possibility that some microbes and/or abnormalities in function of glycolipid danger signaling pathways may be acting upon iNKT cells in the pathogenesis of allergic disorders.

Exogenous glycolipids that directly activate iNKT cells may also be expressed by plants. For example, cypress tree pollen contains lipids that have been shown to directly activate human iNKT cells in vitro [53]. The cypress tree pollen-derived lipids were recognized in the context of CD1a as well as CD1d, and induced the proliferation of CD4$^+$ αβTCR$^+$, γδTCR$^+$ and some Vα24$^+$ iNKT cells [53]. These cypress responsive T cells could provide help for IgE production, and were more evident in the peripheral blood of allergic subjects during the pollinating season. Finally, injection of the glycolipids induced cutaneous wheal and flare reactions, indicating that anti-cypress lipid IgE antibodies were present in cypress allergic patients [53]. These results suggest that plant pollens may be an important and previously unrecognized source of lipid antigens that can directly activate iNKT cells and that pollen-associated lipids or other environmental lipids may play an important role in the development of some forms of asthma and allergy.

3.4
iNKT Cells as Effector Cells of AHR

As discussed above, iNKT cells are absolutely necessary for the development of AHR in many mice models and, as a source of large amounts of IL-4 and IL-13, can function to enhance antigen sensitization. However, since iNKT cells can directly respond to exogenous antigens from pathogens and pollens, it was of interest to determine whether the activation of iNKT cells alone might be sufficient for the induction of AHR. In fact, when pulmonary iNKT cells were directly activated by glycolipid antigens, these antigens could indeed induce the rapid development of AHR in mice [22]. Thus, intranasal administration of glycolipids that activate iNKT cells (such as α-GalCer or a *Sphingomonas* glycolipid membrane constituent) resulted in the rapid induction of AHR, eosinophilic airway inflammation, and IgE production, which typify the Th2-driven response normally associated with protein allergen administration. In addition, the induction of AHR occurred in the absence of eosinophils in mice treated with anti-IL-5 blocking mAb or of B cells in B cell-deficient mice. Moreover, these glycolipids induced AHR in MHC class II$^{-/-}$ mice, which do not contain conventional CD4$^+$ T cells, but which have increased numbers of iNKT cells [22], demonstrating that iNKT cell-driven AHR can occur in the complete absence of conventional CD4$^+$ T cells and adaptive immunity.

These results together indicate that iNKT cells are potent effector cells in the lungs and are entirely sufficient for inducing AHR under the experimental conditions studied. In addition, the direct activation of AHR by *Sphingomonas* suggests that glycolipids from respiratory pathogens might directly activate iNKT cells and cause wheezing and AHR. Moreover, as mentioned above, lipids from cypress pollen can directly activate iNKT cells [53], which suggests that lipids from many pollens or plants that enter the lungs may directly activate pulmonary iNKT cells and drive the development of wheezing, airway inflammation, and asthma. Given evidence that iNKT cells are both necessary and sufficient for AHR, future studies examining the capacity of glycolipids from respiratory pathogens and plant pollens in activating iNKT cells and in inducing AHR could greatly alter our understanding of respiratory pathobiology.

3.5
iNKT Cells in Human Asthma

In follow-up to studies of allergen-induced AHR in mice, the possibility that iNKT cells might be important in human asthma has now been assessed in human clinical studies. Using CD1d-tetramers loaded with α-GalCer, mAb specific for the invariant TCR of NKT cells, and RT-PCR analysis for the invariant TCR of iNKT cells, the frequency and distribution of iNKT cells in the lungs and in the circulating blood of patients with moderate to severe persistent asthma was assessed [16]. Surprisingly, approximately 60% of the pulmonary CD4$^+$CD3$^+$ cells in the lungs of these patients with asthma were not class II MHC-restricted CD4$^+$ T cells, but rather iNKT cells. The NKT cells expressed the invariant Vα24$^+$ TCR and produced IL-4 and IL-13, but not IFN-γ. In contrast, the CD4$^+$ T cells found in the lungs of patients with sarcoidosis, an inflammatory disease in which large numbers of CD4$^+$ Th1 cells are found in the lungs, were conventional CD4$^+$ CD3$^+$ T cells, and not iNKT cells. While other studies have found lower numbers of iNKT cells in patients with mild and moderate asthma, the presence of iNKT cells the lungs of patients with moderate to severeasthma strongly suggests that iNKT cells play a prominent pathogenic role in human asthma, although further research is needed to clarify under what conditions and in which asthmatic populations (if not all) iNKT cells may be most involved.

The presence of large numbers of iNKT cells in the lungs of patients with asthma is surprising, and suggests that these cells may have been mistakenly identified in the past as conventional CD4$^+$ Th2 cells. Most of the iNKT cells in the lungs of patients with asthma expressed CD4, and produced IL-4, IL-13, but not IFN-γ, suggesting that a Th2-like subset of iNKT cells was recruited or expanded in the lungs of patients with asthma. In this and another study, iNKT cells were not increased in the peripheral blood of patients with asthma nor did circulating iNKT show any change in functionality [16, 54], indicating that the immunology of asthma must be studied not by the examination of peripheral blood alone but rather by the evaluation of cells from within the lung. The specific mechanisms by which the Th2-like subset of iNKT cells enters or expands in the lungs, and whether the number of iNKT cells in the lungs correlate with disease severity, are not yet clear, although recent experiments in mouse models of AHR indicate that chemokine pathways, particularly the chemokine receptor CCR4 may play a major role (Meyer et al., unpublished data).

Although iNKT cells appear to outnumber conventional CD4$^+$ T cells in the airways of patients with moderate to severe asthma, conventional CD4$^+$ Th2 cells remain an important regulatory population in asthma. For example, Th2 cells recognize environmental protein allergens that drive the development of allergic asthma, suggesting that Th2 cells might enhance the production or expression of endogenous glycolipids, which then activate iNKT cells to induce AHR. Alternatively, iNKT cells may amplify the function of Th2 cells, perhaps by "licensing" conventional CD4$^+$ Th2 effectors cells to induce AHR [17]. This possibility is supported by the observation that pulmonary iNKT cells and conventional CD4$^+$ T cells appear to directly interact with each other [55]. Alternatively, it is possible that iNKT cells and conventional CD4$^+$ Th2 cells may have overlapping functions, such that both are able to induce AHR, since Th2 CD4$^+$ T cells have been shown to act as effector cells in the induction of AHR, particularly in adoptive transfer models. Clearly, additional studies are required to clarify the precise relationship between conventional CD4$^+$ T cells and iNKT cells in the development of AHR and asthma.

It is possible that iNKT cells could drive particular forms of asthma. For example, in the limited number of patients with asthma studied, the frequency of iNKT cells in the lungs did not appear to be affected by treatment with inhaled corticosteroids [16], perhaps because iNKT cells are relatively resistant to corticosteroid treatment [56, 57]. The relative resistance of iNKT cells to corticosteroids and the importance of iNKT cells in the pathogenesis of asthma may reflect the fact that 10%–25% of patients with asthma have corticosteroid-resistant disease, which may account for half or more of the healthcare costs related to asthma [58, 59]. Therefore, treatment of asthma with medications that may diminish the function or reduce the number of iNKT cells in the lungs of these patients may provide more effective therapy for asthma, particularly in those patients with the especially difficult and costly corticosteroid-resistant form.

3.6
Therapies for Asthma

Since *i*NKT cells appear to play such an important role in the development of asthma, several studies have begun to demonstrate how inactivation of *i*NKT cells might form the basis for the treatment of asthma. One approach is to block the activation of *i*NKT cells by blockade of CD1d with neutralizing mAb. When given early during the development of allergen-induced AHR, anti-CD1d mAb has been shown to prevent the development of AHR [18]. The effectiveness of this approach, however, is limited, because it appears that *i*NKT effector cells, after initial activation, are less dependent on CD1d-TCR signaling and may function normally when anti-CD1d blocking mAb is given later during the development of AHR (E.H. Meyer, unpublished observations).

Another approach involves the administration of α-GalCer, intravenously or intraperitoneally 24 h prior to respiratory challenge of sensitized mice with OVA. This treatment reduces airway inflammation and inhibits allergen-induced AHR [60–62]. The mechanism by which AHR is suppressed by the administration of α-GalCer is not clear, but appears to involve the production of IFN-γ, and/or the development of inhibitory/suppressor cells [60–62]. In addition, because the administration of α-GalCer renders *i*NKT cells unresponsive to further stimulation for a period of days to weeks [63], α-GalCer treatment may involve *i*NKT cell anergy, thereby preventing *i*NKT cells from inducing AHR [22, 43]. This therapeutic approach with α-GalCer, however, is problematic in that α-GalCer can function as an adjuvant to enhance allergen sensitization, and can by itself induce AHR. Therefore, other therapeutic approaches focused on selectively eliminating *i*NKT cells in the lungs or selectively reducing their function must be developed for optimal treatment of asthma.

4
Toward Understanding Th2-Like *i*NKT Cells

Until recently, some investigators have proposed that subsets of *i*NKT cells producing restricted cytokine profiles did not exist. In general, activation of *i*NKT cells with α-GalCer results in the production of both Th1 and Th2 cytokines. This cytokine profile is relatively fixed in mice, even in IL-4$^{-/-}$ and IL-12$^{-/-}$ mice, which lack Th2 and Th1 cells respectively [64]. Moreover, resting Vα14i T cells from different organs of wild type mice such as the liver and spleen contain mRNA for both IFN-γ and IL-4, and both types of cells produce both cytokines at the same ratios following in vivo activation with α-GalCer or other glycolipids [64]. The persistence of an often fixed cytokine profile in iNKT cells in contrast to polarized conventional T cells may result from the fact that control of cytokine production in iNKT cells is quite distinct from that of conventional T cells. Notably IL-4 production in iNKT cells does not require STAT6 signaling or the transcription factor GATA3 [65], and post-transcriptional regulation of IL-4 may be important, similar to situations in other cell types of the innate immune system such as mast cells [66].

More recently, subsets of iNKT cells have been described, some of which have restricted cytokine profiles. For example, human iNKT cells have been shown to segregate into a CD4$^+$ population, which produce both Th1 and Th2 cytokines (unrestricted profile) and a double-negative population (CD4$^-$ CD8$^-$) or CD8$^+$ population, which produces only Th1 cytokines and exhibiting greater cytotoxic activity [67, 68]. Additional human CD4$^+$ iNKT cell subsets may exist: for example, the CD4$^+$ iNKT cells in the lungs of patients with asthma have the phenotype of Th2 cells, and produce only Th2 cytokines when evaluated by intracellular cytokine staining [16]. These Th2-like iNKT cells in the lungs may represent a tissue-specific iNKT subpopulation, especially since it was shown in mice that iNKT cell populations in different tissue locations appear to be discrete subpopulations based upon their TCRβ chain usage [69].

Recent and important evidence that functional iNKT cell subsets exist by anatomical location in mice come from studies in which liver-derived iNKT cells were shown to be distinct from those in the thymus or spleen in being better able to inhibit tumor growth [34]. Inhibition of tumor growth was associated with iNKT cells that did not produce IL-4, for example those that resided in the liver. In contrast, iNKT cells taken from the thymus produce IL-4 and fail to inhibit tumor growth. In addition, thymic iNKT cells from IL-4$^{-/-}$ mice were more effective than thymic-derived WT iNKT cells in mediating anti-tumor responses. While the production of IL-4 by tissue subsets appears to differ, the anatomic location of the iNKT cells did not appear to alter the expression of CD4, which does not appear to segregate with cytokine profiles in mice, as it does in humans, although murine CD4$^+$ iNKT cells may produce higher levels of IL-4 than CD4$^-$ iNKT cells.

The recent findings that iNKT cells from different tissue locations have different functionality suggests that a Th2 inducing or Th2-like iNKT cells may express distinct chemokine receptor profiles. Some evidence suggests that iNKT cells likely express distinct chemokine receptor profiles by tissue location [70]. Likewise, in one study of human blood-derived NKT cells, only CD4$^+$CCR4$^+$ produced IL-4 [67]. Recent studies of mouse models of AHR suggest a potentially important role for CCR4 in the recruitment of *i*NKT cells to the airways in the induction of AHR (Meyer et al., unpublished data).

The mechanisms by which Th2-like *i*NKT cells might develop are not understood. However, the identification and study of Th2-like *i*NKT cells represents an important research topic in allergy and immunology. There are a number of observed associative factors that have been linked to the appearance of Th2-like *i*NKT cells that may be relevant. First, greater IL-4 with reduced IFN-γ production by *i*NKT cells occurs with chronic stimulation of *i*NKT cells. In many situations, repeated dosing with α-GalCer causes *i*NKT cells to favor the production of IL-4 but not IFN-γ [71, 72]. This may be related to the fact that immature murine *i*NKT cells produce more IL-4 than IFN-γ [73, 74], and the replacement of older, anergic *i*NKT cells with fresh cells from the thymus could explain, to some extent, why chronic *i*NKT cell activation is associated with increased IL-4 production by these cells.

Second, analysis of glycolipid molecules structurally related to α-GalCer indicates that the manner in which *i*NKT cells are activated can affect how they produce cytokines and affect immune responses. Analogs with shorter fatty-acyl chains and sphingosine chains (e.g., OCH) induce greater amounts of IL-4 in *i*NKT cells [75]. The increased capacity of OCH to induce production of IL-4 is thought to be due to a reduced affinity of OCH for CD1d, resulting in reduced stability of the OCH-CD1d complex, and reduced interaction with the invariant TCR, akin to altered peptide ligands [75]. In contrast to OCH, another α-GalCer related molecule, α-C-GalCer (which has a single atomic substitution of C for O at the bond attaching the glycosyl head to the lipid tail) and other analogs more hydrophobic then α-GalCer may induce more IFN-γ then α-GalCer [75, 76]. The capacity of α-C-GalCer to induce more IFN-γ, however, may be related to the capacity of α-C-GalCer to engage NK cells to produce IFN-γ. When NK cells are eliminated, the IFN-γ response to α-C-GalCer (and to α-GalCer) is greatly reduced [75, 76], because NK cells are stimulated to rapidly produce IFN-γ by CD8α$^+$ DCs, which have interacted with *i*NKT cells [76]. In contrast to this interaction with DCs, studies have shown that when *i*NKT cells interact with B cells, *i*NKT cells produce IL-4 (weakly) rather than IFN-γ [77–79]. Thus, the type of and/or way in which APCs activate *i*NKT cells could elicit Th2-like *i*NKT cells.

Third, Th2 cytokine producing *i*NKT cells are found in contexts where there is an increased homeostatic expansion of T cells, for example in transgenic mice expressing the invariant TCR of *i*NKT cells [47], or following transplantation conditioning regimes [47, 80, 81]. Finally, Th2 cytokine producing *i*NKT cells appear especially linked to mucosal immune responses in mouse models of colitic inflammation and airway inflammation [16, 22, 82, 83]. These general observations suggest that many factors that foster IL-4$^+$

production in iNKT cells may be relevant in the development of asthma and other allergic diseases.

5
iNKT Cells in Allergic Diseases Other than Asthma

5.1
iNKT Cells and Contact Sensitivity

The discovery that iNKT cells as play an active role in asthma and AHR suggests that iNKT cells may be important in the context other allergic diseases. For example, contact sensitivity (allergic contact dermatitis, contact hypersensitivity), which has increased in prevalence over the past few decades [84], is a delayed-type hypersensitivity (DTH) reaction in the skin rapidly mediated by conventional CD4$^+$ T cells in response to re-exposure to environmental haptens which conjugate to self-protein antigens. Contact sensitivity cannot occur without the initial exposure to environmental haptens and sensitization of conventional CD4$^+$ T cells. This initial sensitization has been recently shown in mouse models of contact sensitivity to depend upon the presence of IL-4$^+$ iNKT cells [85] and CD1d glycolipid presentation [86].

In a series of experiments, it was shown that CD1d$^{-/-}$ and Jα18$^{-/-}$ failed to develop significant contact sensitivity, but that contact sensitivity was restored by adoptive transfer of iNKT cells into Jα18$^{-/-}$ mice [85]. Furthermore, iNKT cells from wild type but not IL-4$^{-/-}$ reconstituted contact sensitivity following adoptive transfer into Jα18$^{-/-}$ mice, indicating that the production of IL-4 by iNKT cells is essential for contact sensitivity [85]. The production of IL-4 by iNKT cells presumed reside the liver occurred within 10 min after the initial hapten exposure. This early burst of IL-4 alone is probably the major mechanism whereby iNKT cells contribute to contact sensitivity, because the contact sensitivity was restored in CD1d$^{-/-}$ and Jα18$^{-/-}$ following administration of rIL-4 alone at early time points during the initial hapten sensitization phase. The IL-4 produced by iNKT acted upon B1 B cells and was eventually critical for the sensitization of conventional T cells, which are thought to be the primary effector cells at the skin in the development of contact sensitivity. The early IL-4 produced by iNKT cells following hapten exposure was required for B1 B cells to rapidly produce large quantities of nonspecific IgM [85]. This IgM, in turn, was shown to be a critical inflammatory signal that contributed to the homing and sensitization of conventional T cells in the skin. Without IL-4 from iNKT cells acting on B1 B cells, production of IgM and T cell sensitization did not occur in CD1d$^{-/-}$ or Jα18$^{-/-}$ mice. However, adoptive transfer of activated IgM-secreting B1 B cells alone into Jα18$^{-/-}$ mice restored contact sensitivity, indicating that B1 B cells are critical cells that act downstream of IL-4 produced by iNKT cells. Without the production of IgM by B cells, the sensitization of conventional T cells to hapten antigens in the skin fails to occur.

The importance of iNKT cells in the priming phase of contact sensitivity is reinforced by experiments in which contact sensitivity was disrupted by the administration of lipid antagonists (polyethylene glycol (PEG)2000 dipalmitoyl-l-α-phosphatidylethanolamine (DPPE-PEG) and (PEG)2000 ceramide), which presumably disrupt glycolipid presentation by CD1d [86]. An outstanding question in this field now concerns the relative importance of iNKT cells in mediated contact sensitivity during secondary hapten challenge in which conventional CD4$^+$ T cells play an important regulatory role. It has been suggested that iNKT cells play an important role in intensifying DTH, potentially by interacting with CD1d$^+$ cells such as DCs and even epithelial cells, but the actual experimental evidence is scant in this regard.

5.2
*i*NKT Cells and Atopic Dermatitis

Atopic dermatitis (AD) is a chronic atopic inflammatory disease closely associated with allergic rhinitis and asthma that presents in infancy and afflicts between 10%–20% of children and 2%–5% of adults in developed countries. Little is known about what role, if any, iNKT cells play in AD. A number of studies have examined iNKT cells in the peripheral blood of human individuals with AD, two of which found that AD patients have fewer circulating CD4$^-$CD8$^-$ Vα24$^+$ iNKT cells but roughly equivalent CD4+ Vα24$^+$ iNKT when compared to normal controls [87, 88], and one of which found that AD patients had more CD4$^+$ Vα24$^+$ iNKT cells that produced IL-4 [89]. While these studies may indicate an imbalance in CD4$^+$ iNKT cells in AD patients, trends in peripheral blood iNKT cells often do not relate to increases in iNKT cell numbers or CD4 expression at the actual anatomical site of allergic inflammation. Further work in humans will need to be performed to understand the role of iNKT cells in atopic dermatitis.

5.3
Allergic Colitis

Mouse models of colitis reveal a dichotomy in the contribution of iNKT cells in disease based upon the production of IL-4 and IFN-γ. This is because there are both Th1-driven and Th2-driven colitic diseases. In dextran sodium sulfate models of colitis, which were associated with Th1-type colitis in C57BL/6J mice, treatment with α-GalCer induced IL-4 and IL-10, which, in this case, was protective against colitis [90]. The type of colitis induced in another model system, oxazalone-induced colitis (a model for human ulcerative colitis), depends upon genetic background and immune predisposition of the mouse strain being treated, with BALB/c or C57BL/6J mice showing mixed Th1 and Th2 type colitis, whereas SJL/J mice showed primarily Th2 type colitis. In SJL/J mice with oxazalone-induced colitis, *i*NKT cells are needed for the pathology to occur, and it is the production of IL-4 and IL-13, induced by in vivo treatment with α-GalCer exacerbates the disease [82]. In fact, IL-13 has been demonstrated to be cytotoxic to epithelial cells in some circumstances of ulcerative human colitis [83]. Interestingly, there is evidence in human patients with allergic ulcerative colitis that noninvariant or type 2 CD1d-restricted cells that produce IL-13 may drive pathology [91].

These results clearly indicate that *i*NKT cells situated in the gut mucosa can influence the type of colitis observed and can contribute to allergic colitis. Furthermore, there is some experimental evidence for the contention that *i*NKT cells within the gut mucosa consistently appear to be biased toward the production of Th2 cytokines such as IL-4 and IL-13 [83]. Further work is needed to document the presence and functionality of *i*NKT cells or type 2 CD1d-restricted *i*NKT cells, which may be infiltrating the gut mucosa in patients with colitic diseases.

6
Are *i*NKT Cells Involved in Other Allergic Diseases?

The relatively recent discoveries that *i*NKT cells play an active role in atopic disease progression, such as contact sensitivity and asthma and AHR, suggest the *i*NKT cell population needs to be evaluated in the context of other allergic diseases. Given the importance of *i*NKT cells in rapidly initiating allergic inflammation, *i*NKT cells could contribute to other clinical pathologies such as drug allergic hypersensitivity reactions, allergic interstitial nephritis, Stevens-Johnson syndrome, and a host of other pathologies that are often triggered rapidly, that affect a large number of patients and are not well understood. While speculative, we think it is clear that the contribution of *i*NKT cells to allergic responses can and should be studied more broadly and doing so could provide new understanding and improved therapeutic options for clinical allergic diseases and their complications.

7
Summary and Conclusion

From studies conducted over the past 5 years, it has become clear that invariant TCR$^+$ CD1d-restricted *i*NKT cells (*i*NKT or type I NKT cells) play a very important role in Th2 inflammation and asthma. *i*NKT cells can function to skew adaptive immunity toward Th2 or can act directly as effector cells, particularly in mediating skin and mucosal allergic responses, in diseases such as contact sensitivity, contact dermatitis, ulcerative colitis, in addition to bronchial asthma. However, much more work remains to be done in identifying and further characterizing the role of *i*NKT cells in allergic diseases, particularly the role and characteristics of Th2-like subsets of *i*NKT cells and their relationship to conventional CD4$^+$ T cells. We believe that a greater understanding of the mechanisms governing the function of *i*NKT cells will contribute to a greater comprehension of allergic diseases and to the development of new therapeutic approaches for asthma and possibly for other allergic diseases.

References

1. Umetsu DT, McIntire JJ, Akbari O, Macaubus C, DeKruyff RH (2002) Asthma: an epidemic of dysregulated immunity. Nat Immunol 3:715–720
2. Mannino DM, Homa DM, Pertowski CA et al (1998) Surveillance for asthma – United States, 1960–1995. MMWR CDC Surveill Summ 47:1–27
3. McNally N, Philips D, Williams H (1998) The problem of atopic eczema: aetiological clues from the environment and lifestyles. Soc Sci Med 46:729–741
4. Blumenthal J, Blumenthal MN (1996) Immunogenetics of allergy and asthma. Immunol Allergy Clin North Am 16:517–534
5. Weiss KB, Sullivan SD (2001) The health economics of asthma and rhinitis. I. Asssessing the economic impact. J Allergy Clin Immunol 107:3–8
6. Zaas D, Schwartz DA (2003) Genetics of environmental asthma. Semin Respir Crit Care Med 24:185–195
7. McIntire JJ, Umetsu DT, DeKruyff RH (2004) TIM-1, a novel allergy and asthma susceptibility gene. Springer Semin Immunopathol 25:335–348
8. Blumenthal MN (2005) The role of genetics in the development of asthma and atopy. Curr Opin Allergy Clin Immunol 5:141–145
9. McIntire JJ et al (2005) Hepatitis A virus link to atopic disease. Nature 425:576
10. Umetsu SE, Lee WL, McIntire JJ et al (2005) TIM-1 induces T cell activation and inhibits the development of peripheral tolerance. Nat Immunol 6:447–454
11. Maizels RM (2005) Infections and allergy—helminths, hygiene and host immune regulation. Curr Opin Immunol 17:656–661
12. Blaser K (2004) Allergy and hypersensitivity—From genes to phenotype—Editorial overview. Curr Opin Immunol 16:685–688
13. Upham JW, Holt PG (2005) Environment and development of atopy. Curr Opin Allergy Clin Immunol 5:167–172

14. Kay AB (2001) Advances in immunology: allergy and allergic diseases: first of two parts. N Engl J Med 344:30–37

15. Kay AB (2001) Advances in immunology—allergy and allergic diseases—second of two parts. N Engl J Med 344:109–113

16. Akbari O et al (2006) CD4+ invariant T-cell-receptor plus natural killer T cells in bronchial asthma. N Engl J Med 354:1117–1129

17. Akbari O et al (2003) Essential role of NKT cells producing IL-4 and IL-13 in the development of allergen-induced airway hyperreactivity. Nat Med 9:582–588

18. Lisbonne M et al (2003) Cutting edge: invariant V alpha 14. NKT cells dare required for allergen-induced airway inflammation and hyperreactivity in an experimental asthma model. J Immunol 171:1637–1641

19. Mannino DM et al (2002) Surveillance for asthma – United States 1980–1999. MMWR CDC Surveill Summ 51:1

20. Herrick CA, Bottomly K (2003) To respond or not to respond: T cells in allergic asthma. Nat Rev Immunol 3:405–412

21. Robinson DS et al (1992) Predominant Th2-like bronchoalveolar lymphocyte-t population in atopic asthma. N Engl J Med 326:298–304

22. Meyer EH et al (2006) Glycolipid activation of invariant T cell receptor(+) NKT cells is sufficient to induce airway hyperreactivity independent of conventional CD4(+) T cells. Proc Natl Acad Sci U S A 103:2782–2787

23. Godfrey DI, MacDonald HR, Kronenberg M, Smyth MJ, Van Kaer L (2004) Opinion—NKT cells: what's in a name? Nat Rev Immunol 4:231–237

24. Taniguchi M, Harada M, Kojo S, Nakayama T, Wakao H (2003) The regulatory role of Valpha14 NKT cells in innate and acquired immune response. Ann Rev Immunol 21:483

25. Brigl M, Brenner MB (2004)CD1: antigen presentation and T cell function. Ann Rev Immunol 2:557

26. Kinjo Y et al (2005) Recognition of bacterial glycosphingolipids by natural killer T cells. Nature 434:520–525

27. Zhou DP et al (2004) Lysosomal glycosphingolipid recognition by NKT cells. Science 306:1786–1789

28. Kronenberg M (2005) Toward an understanding of NKT cell biology: progress and paradoxes. Ann Rev Immunol 23:877–900

29. Exley MA, Koziel MJ (2004) To be or not to be NKT: natural killer T cells in the liver. Hepatology 40:1033–1040

30. Seino K, Taniguchi M (2005) Functionally distinct NKT cell subsets and subtypes. J Exp Med 202:1623–1626

31. Godfrey DI, Kronenberg M (2004)Going both ways: immune regulation via CD1d-dependent NKT cells. J Clin Invest 114:1379–1388

32. Mattner J et al (2005) Exogenous and endogenous glycolipid antigens activate NKT cells during microbial infections. Nature 434:525–529

33. Zeng DF et al (1999) Bone marrow NK1.1- and NK1.1+ T cells reciprocally regulate acute graft versus host disease. J Exp Med 189:1073–1081

34. Crowe NY et al (2005) Differential antitumor immunity mediated by NKT cell subsets in vivo. J Exp Med 202:1279–1288

35. Cui JQ et al (1999) Inhibition of T helper cell type 2 cell differentiation and immunoglobulin E response by ligand-activated Valpha14 natural killer T cells. J Exp Med 190:783–792

36. Korsgren M et al (1999) Natural killer cell determine development of allergen-induced eosinophilic airway inflammation in mice. J Exp Med 189:553–562

37. Brown DR et al (1996) Beta-2-microglobulin-dependent NK1.1+ T cells are not essential for T helper cell 2 immune responses. J Exp Med 184:1295–1304

38. Zhang Y, Rogers KH, Lewis DB (1996) Beta-2-microglobulin-dependent T cells are dispensable for allergen-induced T helper 2 responses. J Exp Med 184:1507–1512

39. Kim HS et al (1999) Biochemical characterization of CD1d expression in the absence of beta(2)-microglobulin. J Biol Chem 274:9289–9295

40. Amano M et al (1998) CD1 expression defines subsets of follicular and marginal zone B cells in the spleen: beta(2)-microglobulin-dependent and independent forms. J Immunol 161:1710–1717

41. Maeda M, Shadeo A, MacFadyen AM, Takei F (2004) CD1d-independent NKT cells in beta(2)-microglobulin-deficient mice have hybrid phenotype and function of NK and T cells. J Immunol 172:6115–6122

42. Smiley ST, Kaplan MH, Grusby MJ (1997) Immunoglobulin E production in the absence of interleukin-4-secreting CD1-dependent cells. Sci (Washington DC) 275:977–979

43. Kim JO et al (2004) Asthma is induced by intranasal coadministration of allergen and natural killer T-cell ligand in a mouse model. J Allergy Clin Immunol 114:1332–1338

44. Yoshimoto T, Bendelac A, Watson C, Hu-Li K, Paul W (1995) Role of NK1.1+ T cells in Th2 responses and in immunoglobulin E production. Science 270:1845–1847

45. Vonderweid T, Beebe AM, Roopenian DC, Coffman RL (1996) Early production of IL-4 and induction of Th2 responses in the lymph node originate from an MHC class I-independent CD4(+)NK1.1(–)T cell population. J Immunol 157:4421–4427

46. Yoshimoto T, Bendelac A, Huli J, Paul WE (1995) Defective IgE production by SJL mice is linked to the absence of CD4+, NK1.1+ T cells that promptly produce interleukin 4. Proc Natl Acad Sci U S A 92:11931–11934

47. Bendelac A, Hunziker RD, Lantz O (1996) Increased interleukin 4 and immunoglobulin E production in transgenic mice overexpressing NK1 T cells. J Exp Med 184:1285–1293

48. Mattner J et al (2005) Exogenous and endogenous glycolipid antigens activate NKT cells during microbial infections. Nature 434:525–529

49. Stein-Streilein J (2003) Invariant NKT cells as initiators, licensors, and facilitators of the adaptive immune response. J Exp Med 198:1779–1783

50. Lin M, Rikihisa Y (2003) *Erlichia chaffeensis* and *Anaplasma phaocytophilum* lack genes for lipid A biosynthesis and incorporate cholesterol for their survival. Infect Immun 71:5325

51. Trottein F, Mallevaey T, Faveeuw C, Capron M, Leite-de-Moraes M (2006) Role of the natural killer T lymphocyte in Th2 responses during allergic asthma and helminth parasitic diseases. Chem Immunol Allergy 90:113–127

52. Mallevaey T et al (2006) Activation of invariant NKT cells by the helminth parasite *gl Schistosoma mansoni*. J Immunol 176:2476–2485

53. Agea E et al (2005) Human CD1-restricted T cell recognition of lipids from pollens. J Exp Med 202:295–308
54. Ikegami Y, Yokoyama A, Haruta Y, Hiyama K, Kohno N (2004) Circulating natural killer T cells in patients with asthma. J Asthma 41:877–882
55. Sen Y et al (2005) V alpha 24-invariant NKT cells from patients with allergic asthma express CCR9 at high frequency and induce Th2 bias of CD3(+) T cells upon CD226 engagement. J Immunol 175:4914–4926
56. Milner JD et al (1999) Differential responses of invariant V alpha 24J alpha QT cells and MHC class II-restricted CD4(+) T cells to dexamethasone. J Immunol 163:2522–2529
57. Tamada K, Harada M, Abe K, Li TL, Nomoto K (1998) IL-4-producing NK1.1(+) T cells are resistant to glucocorticoid-induced apoptosis: implications for the Th1/Th2 balance. J Immunol 161:1239–1247
58. Adcock IM, Ito K (2004) Steroid resistance in asthma: a major problem requiring novel solutions or a non-issue? Curr Opin Pharmacol 4:257–262
59. Ito K, Chung KF, Adcock IM (2006) Update on glucocorticoid action and resistance. J Allergy Clin Immunol 117:522–543
60. Hachem P et al (2005) Alpha-galactosylceramide-induced iNKT cells suppress experimental allergic asthma in sensitized mice: role of IFN-gamma. Eur J Immunol 35:2793–2802
61. Matsuda H et al (2005) Alpha-galactosylceramide, a ligand of natural killer T cells, inhibits allergic airway inflammation. Am J Respir Cell Mol Biol 33:22–31
62. Morishima Y et al (2005) Suppression of eosinophilic airway inflammation by treatment with alpha-galactosylceramide. Eur J Immunol 35:2803–2814
63. Parekh VV, Wilson MT, Van Kaer L (2005) iNKT-cell responses to glycolipids. Crit Rev Immunol 25:183–213
64. Matsuda JL et al (2003) Mouse V alpha 14i natural killer T cells are resistant to cytokine polarization in vivo. Proc Natl Acad Sci U S A 100:8395–8400
65. Wang ZY et al (2006) Regulation of Th2 cytokine expression in NKT cells: unconventional use of Stat6, GATA-3, and NFAT2. J Immunol 176:880–888
66. Sherman MA, Secor VH, Lee SK, Lopez RD, Brown MA (1999) STAT6-independent production of IL-4 by mast cells. Eur J Immunol 29:1235–1242
67. Kim CH, Johnston B, Butcher EC (2002) Trafficking machinery of NKT cells: shared and differential chemokine receptor expression among V alpha 24(+)V beta 11(+) NKT cell subsets with distinct cytokine-producing capacity. Blood 100:11–16
68. Gumperz JE, Miyake S, Yamamura T, Brenner MB (2002) Functionally distinct subsets of CD1d-restricted natural killer T cells revealed by CD1d tetramer staining. J Exp Med 195:625–636
69. Matsuda JL et al (2001) Natural killer T cells reactive to a single glycolipid exhibit a highly diverse T cell receptor beta repertoire and small clone size. Proc Natl Acad Sci U S A 98:12636–12641
70. Johnston B et al (2003) Differential chemokine responses and homing patterns of murine TCR alpha beta NKT cell subsets. J Immunol 171:2960–2969
71. Mi QS, Ly D, Zucker P, McGarry M, Delovitch TL (2004) Interleukin-4 but not interleukin-10 protects against spontaneous and recurrent type 1 diabetes by activated CD1d-restricted invariant natural killer T-cells. Diabetes 53:1303–1310

72. Sharif S et al (2001) Activation of natural killer T cells by alpha-galactosylceramide treatment prevents the onset and recurrence of autoimmune type 1 diabetes. Nat Med 7:1057–1062

73. Benlagha K, Kyin T, Beavis A, Teyton L, Bendelac A (2002) A thymic precursor to the NKT cell lineage. Science 296:481–482

74. MacDonald HR (2002) Development and selection of NKT cells. Curr Opin Immunol 14:250–254

75. Schmieg J, Yang GL, Franck RW, Tsuji M (2003) Superior protection against malaria and melanoma metastases by a C-glycoside analogue of the natural killer T cell ligand alpha-galactosylceramide. J Exp Med 198:1631–1641

76. Schmieg J, Yang GG, Franck RW, Van Rooijen NV, Tsuji M (2005) Glycolipid presentation to natural killer T cells differs in an organ-dependent fashion. Proc Natl Acad Sci U S A 102:1127–1132

77. Bezbradica JS et al (2005) Distinct roles of dendritic cells and B cells in Va14Ja18 natural T cell activation in vivo. J Immunol 174:4696–4705

78. Fujii SI, Liu K, Smith C, Bonito AJ, Steinman RM (2004) The linkage of innate to adaptive immunity via maturing dendritic cells in vivo requires CD40 ligation in addition to antigen presentation and CD80/86 costimulation. J Exp Med 199:1607–1618

79. Fujii S, Shimizu K, Kronenberg M, Steinman RM (2002) Prolonged IFN-gamma-producing NKT response induced with alpha-galactosylceramide-loaded DCs. Nat Immunol 3:867–874

80. Lan FS, Zeng DF, Higuchi M, Higgins JP, Strober S (2003) Host conditioning with total lymphoid irradiation and antithymocyte globulin prevents graft-versus-host disease: the role of CD1-reactive natural killer T cells. Biol Blood Marrow Transplant 9:355–363

81. Lowsky R et al (2005) Protective conditioning for acute graft-versus-host disease. N Engl J Med 353:1321–1331

82. Heller F, Fuss IJ, Nieuwenhuis EE, Blumberg RS, Strober W (2002) Oxazolone colitis, a Th2 colitis model resembling ulcerative colitis, is mediated by IL-13-producing NK-T cells. Immunity 17:629–638

83. Kaser A et al (2004) Natural killer T cells in mucosal homeostasis. In: Weiner H, Mayer L, Strober W (eds) Oral tolerance: new insights and prospects for clinical application. Ann N Y Acad Sci 1029:154–168

84. Hopkin JM (1997) Mechanisms of enhanced prevalence of asthma and atopy in developed countries. Curr Opin Immunol 9:788–792

85. Campos RA et al (2003) Cutaneous immunization rapidly activates liver invariant V alpha-14. NKT cells stimulating B-1B cells to initiate T cell recruitment for elicitation of contact sensitivity. J Exp Med 198:1785–1796

86. Nieuwenhuis EES et al (2005) CD1d and CD1d-restricted iNKT-cells play a pivotal role in contact hypersensitivity. Exp Dermatol 14:250–258

87. Oishi Y et al (2000) CD4(-)CD8(-) T cells bearing invariant V alpha 24J alpha QTCR alpha-chain are decreased in patients with atopic diseases. Clin Exp Immunol 119:404–411

88. Takahashi T et al (2003) V alpha 24(+) natural killer T cells are markedly decreased in atopic dermatitis patients. Hum Immunol 64:586–592

89. Magnan A et al (2000) Relationships between natural T cells, atopy IgE levels, and IL-4 production. Allergy (Copenhagen) 55:286–290
90. Saubermann LJ et al (2000) Activation of natural killer T cells by alpha-galactosylceramide in the presence of CD1d provides protection against colitis in mice. Gastroenterology 119:119–128
91. Fuss IJ et al (2004) Nonclassical CD1d-restricted NKT cells that produce IL-13 characterize an atypical Th2 response in ulcerative colitis. J Clin Invest 113:1490–1497

CTMI (2007) 314:293–321
© Springer-Verlag Berlin Heidelberg 2007

CD1-Restricted T Cells and Tumor Immunity

J. B. Swann[2] · J. M. C. Coquet[1] · M. J. Smyth[2] · D. I. Godfrey[1] (✉)

[1]Department of Microbiology and Immunology, University of Melbourne,
3010 Parkville, Victoria, Australia
godfrey@unimelb.edu.au

[2]Cancer Immunology Program, Trescowthick Laboratories, Peter MacCallum Cancer Centre, St. Andrews Place, East Melbourne, Victoria, Australia

Abstract CD1d-restricted T cells (NKT cells) are potent regulators of a broad range of immune responses. In particular, an abundance of research has focussed on the role of NKT cells in tumor immunity. This field of research has been greatly facilitated by the finding of agonist ligands capable of potently stimulating NKT cells and also animal models where NKT cells have been shown to play a natural role in the surveillance of tumors. Herein, we review the capability of NKT cells to promote the rejection of tumors and the mechanisms by which this occurs. We also highlight a growing field of research that has found that NKT cells are capable of suppressing anti-tumor immunity and discuss the progress to date for the immunotherapeutic use of NKT cells.

1
Introduction

The CD1 gene family – comprising CD1a, CD1b, CD1c, CD1d, and CD1e – encodes a group of antigen-presenting molecules, which, unlike the conventional class I and class II MHC molecules, are specialized to present lipid, rather than peptide antigens to T cells. Although T cells restricted to various CD1 family members have been described, only CD1d-restricted T cells have been implicated in the control of tumor immunity to date. This may be due to the fact that the study of CD1d-restricted T cells is more easily addressed experimentally than that of the other CD1 family members, as CD1d is the only member present in the mouse genome. The availability of mouse models, including CD1d$^{-/-}$ mice which lack all CD1d-restricted T cells, and TCR.Jα18$^{-/-}$ mice, which lack only invariant Vα14-Jα18$^+$ NKT cells, has allowed detailed experimental investigation of CD1d-restricted T cells and the CD1d molecule in vivo. In addition, the identification of several antigens presented by CD1d to T cells, together with tetramer technology to specifically identify such T cells, has greatly facilitated the study of NKT cells in tumor immunity.

2
CD1d-Restricted T Cells

In both mice and humans, the CD1d-restricted T cell receptor (TCR) repertoire consists of a number of different TCR rearrangements capable of recognizing CD1d-antigen complexes. CD1d-restricted T cells can be divided into at least two distinct populations: invariant NKT cells, which express the canonical Vα14-Jα18 (mice) or Vα24-Jα18 (humans) TCR rearrangement, and noninvariant NKT cells, which appear to have slightly more diverse TCRs. For a detailed review on the subject of NKT cell nomenclature, refer to [1]. Here, for the sake of clarity, we will refer to invariant NKT cells as simply NKT cells, and when referring to noninvariant NKT cells we will specify noninvariant NKT cells.

Early studies of the TCR repertoire demonstrated that Vα14+ T cells almost exclusively used the Jα18 junctional region [2], and it was also suggested that the Vα14+ T cell population developed independently of the known major histocompatibility complex antigens. It was subsequently discovered that Vα14+-NK1.1+ cells were CD1d-specific [3] and that CD1d was required for the development of this distinct subset [4–6]. Investigation of the potent immunostimulatory and anti-tumor activity of the glycolipid compound α-galactosylceramide (α-GalCer), also known as KRN7000, led to the finding that α-GalCer is presented by CD1d and exclusively recognized by Vα14-Jα18+ NKT cells [7]. α-GalCer has proven to be an invaluable reagent in dissecting the biology of this unique T cell subset, facilitating both specific identification (by tetramer technology [8, 9]) and activation of NKT cells. Both CD1d and the NKT cell receptor are highly conserved between mice and humans, such that mouse CD1d can present α-GalCer to human NKT cells and vice versa [10]. More recently, glycolipid antigens that are presented by CD1d to NKT cells have been described [11–17], and other ligands are likely to be discovered.

Noninvariant NKT cells have been less well characterized, largely due to the lack of a method for specifically identifying cells of this subset. Unlike the invariant NKT cell subset, the antigen specificity of noninvariant NKT cells is currently unknown, although experimental evidence demonstrates that noninvariant NKT cells are capable of recognizing self-derived glycolipid antigens that differ from those recognized by invariant NKT cells [18, 21, 124].

To date, both invariant and noninvariant NKT cells have been identified as potent modifiers of anti-tumor immune responses, although the two subsets may have opposite, if not opposing functions. Invariant NKT cells have been implicated in the natural promotion of anti-tumor immunity, as well as being potent drivers of anti-tumor immune responses when artificially activated by stimulation with a synthetic antigen, while noninvariant NKT cells have been shown to suppress anti-tumor immunity in some settings.

3
A Natural Role for NKT Cells in Tumor Immunity

3.1
Immunosurveillance

NKT cells are important modulators of immunosurveillance, and mice deficient for both NKT cell subsets (CD1d−/−) or only the invariant NKT subset

(TCR.Jα18$^{-/-}$ mice) display an increased susceptibility to tumor induction. When challenged with the chemical carcinogen methylcholanthrene (MCA), mice lacking NKT cells are more susceptible to tumor growth, with both an earlier onset of tumor development, as well as a higher tumor incidence [19]. These tumors exhibit an unedited phenotype, since while they grow progressively in NKT cell-deficient hosts, they are rejected by an IFN-γ and CTL-dependent mechanism when transplanted into WT mice [20]. Tumor protection is dependent on NKT cells, as adoptive transfer of these cells into TCR.Jα18$^{-/-}$ mice is sufficient for protection from tumor growth [20]. It seems that direct recognition of tumor cells by NKT cells is not required for rejection, as sarcomas that lack expression of CD1d can be rejected in WT mice [20]. It is also clear that downstream effector cells, including NK cells, are required for tumor rejection [20]. These studies have raised several questions, namely how do NKT cells trigger downstream activation of the anti-tumor immune response, and which antigen or antigens drive this response?

The identity and source of the antigen that drives the NKT cell response, which is presumably some form of lipid molecule, is currently under investigation. There are two potential sources of antigen. Firstly, tumor-derived glycolipids may be taken up by an antigen-presenting cell (APC) and presented to NKT cells via CD1d. To test this hypothesis, glycolipid extracts from MCA-induced sarcoma lines are currently being used to stimulate NKT cells in vitro, an approach which has been used previously to investigate the antigenic properties of cellular lipids from the RMA-S lymphoma [21]. Alternatively, the inflammatory response associated with tumor cells may provide additional signals that complement APC-mediated presentation of an endogenous glycolipid such as isoglobotrihexosylceramide (iGb3), as appears to occur in the setting of *Salmonella typhimurium* infection [16, 22]. Regardless of the identity of the possible antigens that drive NKT cell responses, it seems that only particular subsets of NKT cells are capable of mediating the anti-tumor response [23].

A role for NKT cells in protection from sarcoma growth following the depletion of regulatory T cells (Treg) has also been elucidated. In this model, it was demonstrated that rather than having a protective effect, vaccination with the SEREX-defined tumor-derived antigen DNA J-like 2, significantly enhances metastasis of the CMS5m fibrosarcoma to the lung. The enhanced tumor growth following vaccination was associated with a decrease in NKT cell proportions in the lung, and the induction of Treg activity. Depletion of Treg before tumor challenge abrogated the ability of vaccination to enhance tumor metastasis, but this effect required the presence of NKT cells [24]. Additionally, suppression of NKT cells by vaccination-induced Treg was also observed in mice challenged with MCA [25], and this study also independently verified the role of NKT cells in controlling induction of MCA-induced sarcomas. In addition, it is interesting to note that human Treg are also capable of suppressing NKT cell activity in vitro [26]; however, others have hypothesized that the reverse may be true and that NKT cells may in fact promote Treg function through the production of IL-2 [27].

3.2
NKT Cells in Experimental Tumor Models

One tumor-derived glycolipid that is recognized by NKT cells is the ganglioside (GD3). Immunization of mice with either a GD3$^+$ human melanoma line, or with GD3-loaded syngeneic dendritic cells (DCs) effectively induced CD1d-dependent activation of a subset of NKT cells [11]. This study provides evidence that tumors can produce glycolipids capable of being recognized by NKT cells, and similar antigens may play a role in immunosurveillance models. Both this study and studies in the MCA model suggest that tumor-derived lipid-based antigens are cross-presented to NKT cells by APCs, rather than directly by tumor cells themselves. In contrast to the ability of GD3 to induce IFN-γ secretion by NKT cells, recent in vitro studies have suggested that other ganglioside family members may bias cytokine secretion toward a Th2 profile in a CD1d-dependent manner [28].

GM-CSF-secreting irradiated whole cell tumor vaccines have shown good efficacy in mouse models [29], and have some potential in clinical settings [30]. Studies in the B16F10 melanoma model have demonstrated that successful protection from tumor challenge after vaccination with GM-CSF-secreting B16F10 cells requires NKT cells, as the vaccine failed to induce anti-tumor immunity in CD1d$^{-/-}$ and TCR.Jα18$^{-/-}$ mice [31]. The defect in NKT cell-deficient mice was linked to impaired DC maturation and decreased production of Th2-associated cytokines.

Overall, a number of studies now support a role for NKT cells in immunosurveillance; however, it remains unclear as to what triggers these cells to become activated and initiate downstream effector functions in these settings.

4
Induction of Anti-tumor Immunity by Exogenous Activation of NKT Cells

4.1
Soluble α-GalCer Therapy

α-GalCer is a synthetic glycolipid isolated during a screen for anti-cancer agents derived from the marine sponge *Agelas mauritianus* [32, 33]. Many studies have now investigated the potent anti-tumor activity of α-GalCer in experimental and spontaneous mouse tumor models, including thymoma, melanoma, carcinoma, and sarcoma [34–37]. In these settings, treatment of mice with α-GalCer leads to the potent suppression of tumor growth. Importantly, treatment of NKT cell-deficient mice with α-GalCer fails to induce any anti-tumor response [36, 38], implicating NKT cells as crucial effectors of α-GalCer-mediated anti-tumor immunity.

The mechanism of α-GalCer-mediated tumor rejection involves the complex interplay of a number of effector cells and molecules. Following activation via α-GalCer-loaded CD1d-expressing APCs, NKT cells rapidly produce large quantities of IFN-γ [39]. As a result of their interaction with NKT cells, NKT cell-derived IFN-γ [40], and CD40-L [41], APCs such as DCs are reciprocally activated and begin secreting cytokines such as IL-12 [42,43] and enhancing their expression of the co-stimulatory molecules CD80, CD86, and CD40 [44–46]. The combination of NKT cell-derived IFN-γ and DC-derived factors leads to potent downstream activation of NK, CD8, and CD4 T cells [47–52]. As well as obvious increases in activation marker expression, NK and CD8 T cells become more effective producers of IFN-γ [36,38,47], which subsequently inhibits the growth of tumors by mechanisms that are not entirely clear, although inhibition of angiogenesis may be one mechanism [53]. These cells also increase their cytotoxic potential via up-regulation of effector molecules such as TRAIL [54] and perforin [36], which have been shown to be crucial to the anti-tumor effect of α-GalCer in some models. While α-GalCer elicits a potent immune response from NKT and downstream effector cells, it is important to clarify that for any given tumor model, not all of these cell types or effector mechanisms may be necessary for tumor rejection. Most models depict a crucial role for NKT and NK cells, IL-12, and IFN-γ; however, the importance of other effectors such as CD8 T cells, IL-18, perforin, and TRAIL in tumor clearance is more variable among studies [36, 54, 55].

4.2
Using Dendritic Cells to Enhance the Anti-tumor Efficacy of α-GalCer

While it is clear that treatment of mice with soluble α-GalCer is capable of stimulating potent protection from tumors in mice, the efficacy of this treatment has several important limitations. Firstly, treatment with soluble α-GalCer has only been demonstrated to be effective at the onset of disease, and it has now been demonstrated that treatment with soluble α-GalCer can induce long-term anergy in the NKT cell subset [56–58], an effect that may be due to the nature of the cell presenting α-GalCer to these NKT cells. In vitro studies have clearly depicted that DCs pulsed with α-GalCer are much more potent inducers of NKT cell activation than B cells, monocytes, or macrophages [59, 60]. However, these studies did not determine which APC subsets were important for α-GalCer-mediated anti-tumor immunity. Recent studies have shed some light on this question by showing that mice depleted of myeloid DCs display impaired production of IL-2 and IL-4, and an almost total abrogation of IFN-γ production following α-GalCer administration [61, 62]. Furthermore, α-GalCer treatment of mice lacking DCs failed to induce efficient downstream activation of NK cell functions [61, 62]. Interestingly, α-GalCer administration in μMT mice, which are deficient for B cells, leads to enhanced serum IL-2, IL-4, and IFN-γ and increased NK cell bystander activation, suggesting that B cells may actually inhibit the responsiveness of NKT cells to α-GalCer [61]. These data imply that in vivo, DCs may be essential mediators of α-GalCer-induced anti-tumor immunity; however, the ability of DC-deficient mice to reject tumors has not yet been formally tested. Nonetheless, adoptive transfer of α-GalCer-pulsed DCs is capable of inducing more potent anti-tumor effects than soluble α-GalCer when these treatments are tested in parallel [63]. This strategy for α-GalCer delivery prolongs the period of IFN-γ production [56] and allows for effective treatment of established experimental tumors [63] and chemically induced sarcomas [64]. Delivery of α-GalCer on DCs also prevents the induction of NKT cell anergy, thereby facilitating multiple treatment regimes [56].

These findings in preclinical animal models have been largely supported by early clinical trial data, which suggest that α-GalCer-pulsed autologous human DCs are the most efficient mechanism of reproducibly activating NKT cells (see 7. Clinical Trials Involving α-GalCer).

4.3
Induction of NKT Cell Anti-tumor Immunity by Cytokines

Activation of NKT cells following α-GalCer treatment involves TCR-dependent recognition of CD1d-antigen complexes; however, in some settings recombinant cytokine treatment can activate NKT cells to mediate anti-tumor effects in a seemingly TCR-independent manner. The best defined of these cytokines is IL-12, which when administered at a low dose is known to ameliorate the growth of tumors in an NKT and NK cell-dependent fashion [65–70]. Another DC-derived cytokine known to stimulate potent anti-tumor responses from NKT cells is IL-18. While IL-18 alone stimulates a Th2-biased response from NKT cells [71], in combination with IL-12, IL-18 effects potent NKT cell-dependent tumor rejection via IFN-γ and IL-2 production and enhances NK cell function [72]. More recently, therapy with a pegylated form of granulocyte-colony stimulating factor (G-CSF) was shown to mediate potent anti-leukemia responses in an NKT cell-dependent manner [73].

These studies imply that NKT cells are not solely under the control of the CD1d and glycolipid antigen pathway and may thus respond to tumors in a nonspecific manner. Intriguingly, findings that IL-12 only stimulates IFN-γ production by NKT cells in the presence of CD1d indicate that an endogenous ligand is present in CD1d, which when combined with IL-12 is a strong enough stimulus to provoke NKT cell responses [22]. It is thus important to understand that while NKT cells survey and reject tumors in a CD1d-dependent manner, this process may not necessarily involve the recognition of a tumor-specific antigen, but rather may involve stimulation via IL-12 in the presence of CD1d-expressing cells presenting an endogenous ligand.

5
Modulation of Tumor Immunity by Subsets of NKT Cells

5.1
NKT Cell Subsets

NKT cells, identified by staining with α-GalCer-loaded CD1d tetramers can be found in a number of primary and secondary lymphoid organs and divided into discreet subsets on the basis of their surface phenotype and functional properties [74, 75]. For example, mouse and human NKT cells may be separated on the basis of CD4 and CD8 expression. Approximately 70% of mouse NKT cells are $CD4^+8^-$ and the remainder are $CD4^-8^-$, whereas in humans, most NKT cells in the thymus express CD4, while a $CD4^-8^-$ population also resides in the periphery [76–78]. A subset of human NKT cells are also $CD4^-8^+$ [76,79], although this population does not exist in mice.

5.2
Functionally Distinct Subsets of NKT Cells

Adoptive transfer studies have clearly demonstrated that liver-derived NKT cells are capable of protecting NKT cell-deficient mice from the growth of MCA-1 sarcoma, and B16-F10 melanoma when treated with α-GalCer [20]. It was initially assumed that the ability of liver-derived NKT cells to protect against tumor growth in this model was representative of NKT cells from any organ. Surprisingly however, recent analysis of two different tumor models indicates that the ability of NKT cells to stimulate anti-tumor immunity upon transfer is dependent on their organ of origin. In contrast to their liver-derived equivalents, thymus- and spleen-derived NKT cells are relatively incapable of stimulating tumor rejection [23]. These results suggest that NKT cells may have distinct roles within the environment in which they are found. Furthermore, the CD4$^+$ and CD4$^-$ subsets of liver-derived NKT cells were also functionally distinct. Specifically, CD4$^-$ liver-derived NKT cells were much more potent suppressors of tumor growth than their CD4$^+$ counterparts [23]. It may be that CD4$^+$ liver NKT cells, and thymus and spleen NKT cells, are better suited to immunosuppressive roles such as prevention of autoimmune disease or graft rejection.

5.2.1
Functionally Distinct Subsets of NKT Cells: Cytokine Production

Reports on human NKT cells in the peripheral blood have shown that CD4$^+$ and CD4$^-$ NKT cells are capable of producing IFN-γ and TNF-α [76, 77]. However, only CD4$^+$ NKT cells in the blood are capable of producing Th2 cytokines such as IL-4, IL-13, and IL-10 [76, 77, 79]. Analysis of CD8$^+$ NKT cells has concluded that this subset behaves more like CD4$^-$ NKT cells in that they produce IFN-γ but very little IL-4, IL-13, or IL-10 [79]. These findings suggest that peripheral blood CD4$^+$ NKT cells may produce an inferior anti-tumor response compared to CD4$^-$ NKT cells [79–81]. Interestingly, analysis of human liver-derived cells has shown that NKT cells from this organ are quite distinct from peripheral blood NKT cells in terms of cytokine production. Specifically, NKT cells from the liver are quite potent producers of IFN-γ and TNF-α but produce very little IL-4 and IL-2 in response to α-GalCer [82]. This finding may result from the observed CD4$^+$:CD4$^-$ ratio of NKT cells in the liver, wherein most NKT cells are CD4$^-$ and may thus confer an inability to produce Th2 cytokines.

In mice, the cytokine-producing capability of different NKT cell subsets is less well defined. A number of studies have reported that CD4$^+$ NKT cells in the liver or spleen produce more IL-4, IL-5, and IL-13 than their CD4$^-$ counterparts [83]. However, this conflicts with other observations showing that IL-4 production, determined by intracellular cytokine staining following α-GalCer stimulation in vivo, is similar between CD4$^+$ and CD4$^-$ NKT cells, at least within hours of activation [23, 57, 84]. This discrepancy may stem from the mode of stimulation employed. While it has been suggested that thymus-derived NKT cells are refractory to stimulation [8], studies have shown that these cells are capable of being stimulated in vitro [23,75]. The difference may be due to local intrathymic environment in vivo, where thymocytes themselves may not act as efficient antigen-presenting cells to thymic NKT cells. NK cell receptor expression also influences the cytokine-producing capability of NKT cells. Functional analysis of splenic NKT cells has shown that the presence of inhibitory Ly-49 molecules can inhibit α-GalCer-induced cytokine production [85]. This implies that NKT cell cytokine responses and subsequent anti-tumor immunity may be under some control from NK cell receptors.

The broad range of cytokines that NKT cells produce make it unlikely that any single cytokine is responsible for the existence of functionally distinct NKT cell subsets. When IL-4-deficient NKT cells were transferred into TCR.Jα18$^{-/-}$ mice bearing B16-F10 melanoma, these cells showed improved anti-tumor activity compared to wild type NKT cells; however, this was not totally responsible for the difference in anti-tumor capability between liver- and thymus-derived NKT cells, and IL-10 blockade did not further enhance this activity [23]. The role of other factors such as IL-13 and TGF-β in adoptive transfer models requires investigation.

5.2.2
Migration

A very limited amount of research has investigated the migratory capability of NKT cells; however, evidence to date suggests the existence of NKT cell subsets with different homing properties. Thorough analysis of chemokine receptor expression has revealed quite distinct expression between CD4$^+$ and CD4$^-$ NKT cells from the peripheral blood of humans. While both of these subsets appear to express CCR2, CXCR3, and CXCR4, CD4$^-$ NKT cells appear to express higher levels of CCR5, CCR6, and CXCR6 than their CD4$^+$ counterparts, although the significance of this altered expression is unknown [77, 86, 87]. Mouse NKT cells express CXCR3, CXCR4, CXCR5, CXCR6, and CCR7 [88], and while different subsets were not extensively examined, there were no obvious differences in the migratory capability of CD4$^+$ and CD4$^-$ subsets from spleen that would be consistent with the different anti-tumor potential observed for these populations [23]. More recently, studies of mouse NKT cells have shown that DCs engineered to express OVA and CCL-21, the ligand for CCR7, and pulsed with α-GalCer, can lead to the enhanced rejection of OVA-expressing tumors compared with control DCs [89]. This study suggests that the expression of CCL-21 by DCs enhances the migration and subsequent activation of effector cells including NKT cells, and shows that NKT cell-mediated anti-tumor responses can be augmented by chemokines.

5.2.3
Activation of Downstream Effectors

Downstream effector cells such as NK and CD8 T cells play a crucial role in both natural and induced NKT cell anti-tumor responses [20, 36, 38, 55], and as such, the ability of different NKT cell subsets to trigger activation of these cells requires investigation. Recently, in vitro studies have shown that human $CD4^+8^-$ NKT cells induces more potent bystander activation of CD4 T, NK, and B cells compared with $CD4^-8^-$ or $CD8^+4^-$ NKT cells [90]. However $CD4^+$ NKT cells have also been shown to inhibit the generation of antigen-specific CTL in vitro [46]. In vitro experiments showed that NKT cells from the thymus, liver, or spleen of mice led to similar activation of NK cells and APCs [23]. However, these studies only show in vitro stimulation and the former study is complicated by the use of NKT cell lines, which may not represent the actual role of fresh peripheral blood NKT cells. A more comprehensive study of the effect of different NKT cell subsets on downstream effector cells is required in an in vivo setting.

Given that most NKT cells respond to α-GalCer, it remains puzzling that the administration of soluble α-GalCer, which stimulates a range of NKT cell subsets from a range of organs, is capable of mediating tumor rejection in some models and suppression of autoimmunity in others [91]. Thus, while functionally distinct NKT cell subsets may exist and mediate biased immune responses in isolation, it is still important to consider if or how these subsets may cooperate in vivo to stimulate a biased immune response.

6
NKT Cells and Human Cancer Patients

Alteration in NKT cell function or proportions have now been described in patients with a variety of malignancies, suggesting that either a deficiency in NKT cells is a risk factor for malignancy or that these cells are specifically influenced by the malignancy or the associated therapy. The functional status of NKT cells differs in a number of studies, and this may be the result of the different tumor types studied or in vitro experimental systems employed.

Early reports demonstrated that NKT cells activated by stimulation with α-GalCer-pulsed peripheral blood APCs were capable of killing a variety of tumor cell lines in vitro [92]. Tumor cell lysis was perforin mediated, and adoptive transfer of human NKT cells into nude mice was able to suppress the growth of an esophageal cancer xenograft [92]. In this study, it was also observed that patients with malignant melanoma have decreased numbers of circulating NKT cells [92]. Despite this finding, DCs derived from the blood of melanoma patients were able to stimulate NKT cell expansion, and NKT cells from cancer patients proliferated to a similar extent to those derived from healthy donors when stimulated with DCs from healthy donors. Prostate cancer patients also displayed diminished NKT cell proportion in the peripheral blood; however, in this setting, the ex vivo expansion of NKT cells from cancer patients was diminished, and their production of IFN-γ was compromised when compared to cells from healthy donors [93].

Several studies have now investigated NKT cell functions in leukemia. CD1d expression has been reported on acute myeloid leukemia (AML) cells and juvenile myelomonocytic leukemias, although expression levels are variable across samples [94]. In this study, pulsing CD1d⁺ tumor targets with α-GalCer resulted in efficient killing by NKT cells, and the degree of killing correlated with the level of CD1d expression by the target cells. CD1d expression has also been reported on B-chronic lymphocytic leukemia (B-CLL) [95], and while all tumors in this study were positive for CD1d, the level of expression was variable among different isolates. In agreement with the previous report on AML, CD1d-positive B-CLL cells pulsed with α-GalCer were efficiently lysed by NKT cells; however, no correlation between CD1d-expression levels and susceptibility to lysis by NKT cells was observed for B-CLL samples [95]. Similar data have also been reported for T-ALL, in which five of eight tumor lines tested expressed CD1d and could be recognized and lysed by NKT cells [96].

In patients with progressive multiple myeloma, NKT cells can be detected in the peripheral blood as well as in the tumor bed (i.e., the bone marrow) of patients, and functional analysis of these NKT cells demonstrated that they have an impaired ability to secrete IFN-γ in response to α-GalCer [97]. Interestingly, the diminished ability to secrete IFN-γ correlated with tumor progression, as NKT cells from donors with monoclonal gammopathy of undetermined significance (MGUS) or nonprogressive myeloma were able to secrete IFN-γ in a similar fashion to NKT cells from healthy donors. Importantly, in this study it was demonstrated that impaired NKT cell IFN-γ production could be overcome by stimulation of NKT cells with α-GalCer pulsed DCs. As has been reported for other hematological malignancies, primary multiple myeloma cells expressed CD1d, and when pulsed with α-GalCer, could again be lysed efficiently by NKT cells expanded by culture with α-GalCer pulsed DCs.

Other studies have also demonstrated the presence of NKT cells in cancerous tissues. Originally it was reported that NKT cells are increased in lung tumor samples when compared to normal lung tissue; however, the relevance of this finding to patient prognosis was not tested [98]. Interestingly, while in this study NKT cells were increased in tumor tissue, the proportion of NKT cells in the peripheral blood was diminished, suggesting a preferential accumulation of NKT cells within tumor tissue. The finding of diminished NKT cells in the peripheral blood of lung cancer patients was confirmed in a second study [99]; however, NKT cell proportions in the lung were not characterized in this report. More recently, intra-tumor NKT cell frequency has been identified as a prognostic factor in primary colorectal carcinomas [100]. In this study, the degree of NKT cell infiltration into colorectal carcinoma samples was quantitated by staining of sections with an anti-Vα24 antibody, and patients that exhibited high NKT cell infiltration had improved prognosis for both survival and disease-free survival. It was also shown that some of the NKT cells present in the tumor samples were activated, as Vα24$^+$ cells also stained positive for IFN-γ. It should be noted that in addition to this study, a previous report demonstrated that NKT cells are diminished in the liver of colon cancer patients with hepatic metastasis, but retain their functional properties [82]. These results suggest that NKT cells may be playing a natural role in tumor immunosurveillance in humans, similar to that seen in animal studies.

Overall, these studies provide strong evidence that NKT cell proportions and/or functions are significantly compromised in human cancer patients and provide a rationale for developing therapeutic strategies aimed at expanding and efficiently activating these cells, in the hope of stimulating anti-tumor immune responses.

7
Clinical Trials Involving α-GalCer

To date, four phase I clinical trials involving α-GalCer have been reported in the literature [101–104]. In the first reported trial, the ability of intravenous, soluble α-GalCer to stimulate NKT cell responses was tested in patients with solid tumors [101]. In this trial, α-GalCer was well tolerated, and some NKT cell expansion and cytokine production was observed. However, the response observed was highly variable between patients, and largely depended on the baseline proportion of NKT cells present at the time therapy commenced.

Subsequent to this initial trial, the ability of α-GalCer-pulsed autologous monocyte-derived DCs to stimulate NKT cell responses was tested in two individual trials, one involving patients with a variety of metastatic malignancies [102] and the other involving patients with non-small cell lung carcinoma (NSCLC) [103]. In both trials, the treatment was well tolerated, and this therapeutic regime was more successful at stimulating NKT cell responses than soluble α-GalCer. Activation of NKT cells and downstream effectors (T cells and NK cells), along with increases in serum IFN-γ levels were achieved in some patients. In both trials, the expansion of NKT cells observed was transient, and did not occur in all individuals treated.

In vitro findings showing that DCs matured with a cytokine cocktail were superior to immature DCs at activating NKT cells [59] led to the design of a third trial of α-GalCer-pulsed DCs [104]. Whereas in the two preceding studies, monocyte-derived DCs were not specifically matured, in this trial DCs were matured by incubation with IL-1β, IL-6, TNF-α, and PGE$_2$ at the time of pulsing with α-GalCer. Administration of mature, α-GalCer-pulsed DCs to patients with a variety of malignancies resulted in the long-term expansion of NKT cells in the blood of all patients tested, including patients in which no NKT cells could be detected before treatment. Interestingly, despite good expansion of NKT cells in vivo by this method, the NKT cells expanded in cancer patients after treatment displayed a diminished ability to secrete cytokines such as IFN-γ, when compared with NKT cells from healthy donors. In keeping with this finding, no reproducible increase in serum IFN-γ was detected during this study; however, increases in IL-12, macrophage inflammatory protein-1b (MIP-1b) and interferon-inducible protein 10 (IP-10) were observed in patient sera 24 h after treatment.

In summary, these results demonstrate that α-GalCer can be safely used to activate NKT cells in human cancer patients, although the efficacy of these approaches remains to be fully elucidated . It is not entirely clear that optimal activation of NKT cells has yet been achieved in these trials. In mouse studies, IFN-γ secretion is central to the anti-tumor efficacy of α-GalCer-based therapies, and to date the treatment that most reliably expands NKT cell numbers in cancer patients [104] fails to induce efficient IFN-γ secretion. This suggests that further optimization of this strategy by combination with other immunotherapeutic strategies may be required to stimulate effective anti-tumor responses, particularly in cancer patients where NKT cell function may be partially impaired [97].

8
Immunotherapeutic Strategies to Optimize α-GalCer Therapies

Several strategies to improve the efficacy of α-GalCer have been tested experimentally, including methods to enhance IFN-γ production and the function of downstream effectors. Figure 1 highlights some of the ways in which NKT cells may be implemented in immunotherapy against tumors.

One strategy involves the modification of α-GalCer itself to favor IFN-γ production over that of other cytokines. Two α-GalCer analogs, α-C-GalCer [105] and OCH [106] have been reported to bias the NKT cell-mediated response toward secretion of Th1 or Th2 cytokine profiles, respectively. Although it is unclear how these two compounds differentially induce cytokine secretion, it has been suggested that the affinity or length of binding of α-GalCer analogs for the NKT cell TCR may dictate the resulting cytokine secretion profile [107, 108]. Activation of NKT cells with α-C-GalCer has been shown to elicit a 100-fold more potent anti-tumor immune response against B16F10 lung metastases than α-GalCer, and this effect was attributed to a prolonged production of IFN-γ and IL-12, in combination with a reduced level of IL-4 [105]. The use of α-C-GalCer-pulsed matured DCs may therefore be more effective at inducing IFN-γ secretion by NKT cells in cancer patients.

An alternate strategy to enhance the anti-cancer capabilities of NKT cells may be to culture and polarize them toward a Th1 cytokine profile in vitro before transferring these cells back into patients. It has been noted that NKT cells stimulated with α-GalCer-pulsed mature monocyte-derived DCs can be expanded and polarized toward a cytokine profile by IL-15 treatment in vitro [60], and this strategy may overcome the functional deficiencies observed for in vivo activated NKT cells. It may also be possible to skew the cytokine profile of NKT cells in patients by the addition of recombinant IL-12 during therapy, and this approach can enhance the efficacy of α-GalCer in animal studies [109].

α-GalCer-pulsed mature DC therapy has also been found to stimulate very potent anti-tumor immune responses by combining this therapy with cytokine treatments aimed at enhancing the function of downstream effectors. In mice, the delayed administration of IL-21 following α-GalCer therapy enhances the anti-tumor response by maturing the NK cells expanded downstream of NKT cell activation and enhancing their perforin-dependent killing [64]. Interestingly, IL-21 treatment was a more potent adjuvant to therapy with α-GalCer-pulsed DCs than either IL-2 or IL-12, and was able to promote rejection of pre-established tumors.

The addition of α-GalCer to vaccination schedules has proven to be an effective way of boosting antigen-specific CD4[+] and CD8[+] T cell responses in mice [45, 110, 111], so the inclusion of NKT cell activation may represent a simple method to enhance the potency of tumor vaccines. Initial studies took advantage of the well-characterized antigen OVA to investigate the ability of α-GalCer to boost the efficacy of immunization with soluble and cell-associated antigen. Co-administration of α-GalCer and soluble OVA resulted in enhanced T cells priming when compared to OVA alone, and this effect was demonstrated to be dependent on the ability of NKT cells to stimulate DC maturation and cross-presentation [45, 111]. Critically, it was shown that for effective adjuvant activity, α-GalCer and protein antigen must be delivered simultaneously, and furthermore, experiments with α-GalCer- and peptide-pulsed DCs showed that both glycolipid and peptide antigen must be presented by the same APCs for effective enhancement of T cell responses [111]. Subsequent studies demonstrated that α-GalCer can also facilitate the induction of anti-tumor immune responses by vaccination with

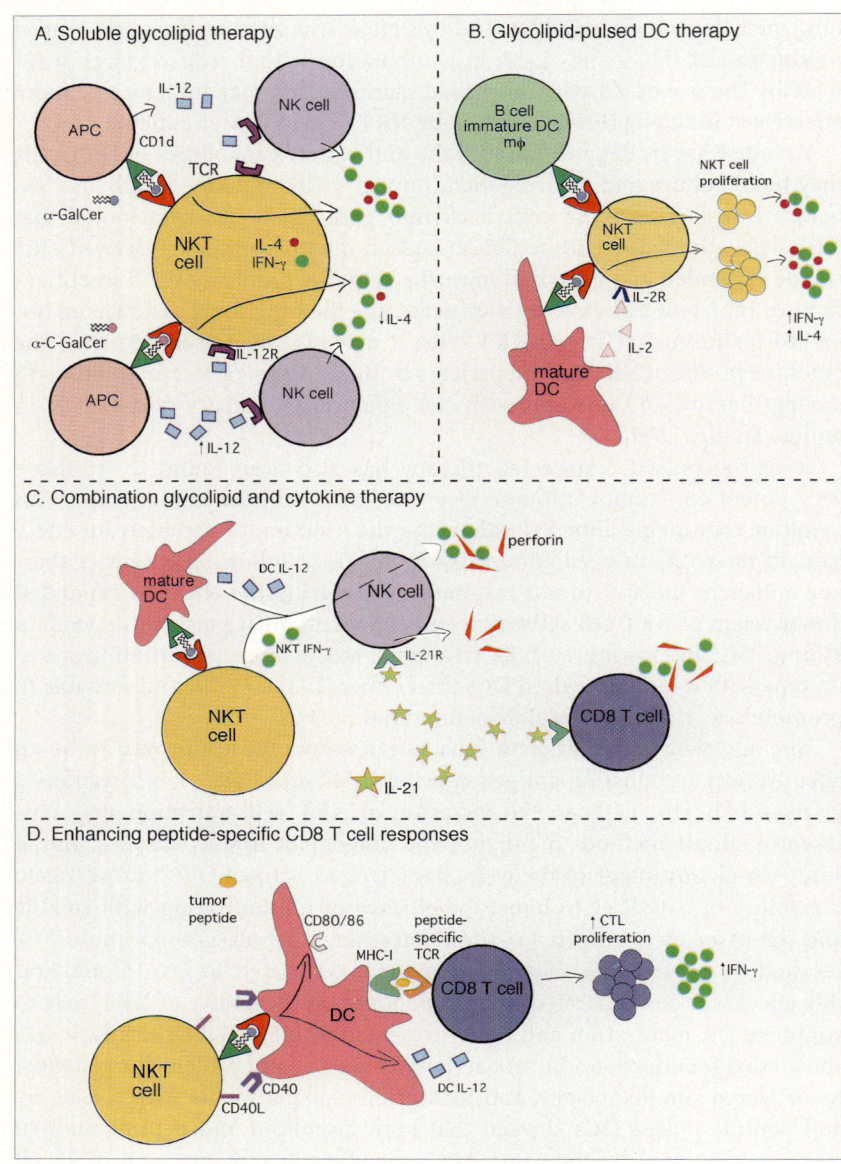

◀——

Fig. 1A–D Immunotherapeutic strategies comprising NKT cells. **A** Soluble glycolipid therapy comparing α-GalCer and α-C-GalCer. α-C-GalCer leads to enhanced serum IL-12 production, prolonged IFN-γ, and less IL-4 production than α-GalCer and an overall enhanced tumor rejection capability. More detailed diagrams depicting the exact mechanism of α-GalCer activity are in Hayakawa et al. [132] and Smyth et al. [133] **B** Therapy with in vitro matured α-GalCer-pulsed DCs enhances the proliferation and cytokine producing capability of NKT cells in an IL-2-dependent manner. Matured DCs enhance their expression of CD1d and are more potent inducers of NKT cell activation than other APCs. The ability of α-C-GalCer-pulsed DCs to mediate tumor rejection has not yet been determined. **C** Combined therapy of α-GalCer-pulsed DCs and delayed IL-21 enhances tumor rejection. α-GalCer activates NK cells to produce IFN-γ and perforin through NKT- and APC-derived factors, as depicted in **A**. Delayed therapy with a cytokine such as IL-21 enhances NK cell perforin-mediated killing, ultimately enhancing tumor rejection. Some evidence suggests that IL-21 therapy may also enhance the CD8 T cell response [134]. **D** NKT cells can enhance antigen-specific CD8 T cell responses by enhancing DC maturation and activation in a CD40/CD40-L dependent manner, leading to enhanced expression of CD80, CD86, IL-12, and CD40. This in turn enhances activation of conventional T cells, including tumor-specific CTL

irradiated tumor cells [110]. Vaccination with irradiated plasmacytoma or lymphoma cells failed to effectively prime anti-tumor immunity, but addition of α-GalCer to the vaccination resulted in potent tumor immunity mediated by both CD4$^+$ and CD8$^+$ T cells. Once again it was demonstrated that α-GalCer must be administered at the time of antigen challenge to successfully enhance immune priming. Interestingly, CMV-specific memory T cells were noted to expand in patients during a trial assessing the efficacy of α-GalCer pulsed mature DCs to activate NKT cells in cancer patients [104]. During the same trial, treatment also resulted in an apparent enhancement of a CD8 T cell response to flu vaccination in one patient. These intriguing findings suggest that a trial combining NKT cell activation and expansion via a glycolipid such as α-GalCer with tumor antigen vaccination is warranted.

Additionally, it should be noted that in animal models, α-GalCer treatment is most effective when administered early in disease and these studies provide an encouraging incentive for further trials in patients with less advanced tumors.

9
CD1d-Dependent Suppression of Tumor Immunity

9.1
The Role of Noninvariant NKT Cells in Suppressing Tumor Immunity

In addition to the evidence presented above for a role for NKT cells in promoting anti-tumor immunity, abundant evidence now suggests that CD1d can regulate immune responses independently of invariant NKT cells. A number of groups using a variety of tumor models have described CD1d-dependent suppression of tumor immunity. Evidence from three independent tumor models, the 15–12RM sarcoma model, the 4T1.2 metastatic mammary carcinoma model, and the Colo-26 colon carcinoma model all demonstrate that CD1d suppresses anti-tumor responses through incompletely understood, and apparently diverse, mechanisms.

Firstly, experiments using the 15–12RM tumor model demonstrated that CD1d suppresses anti-tumor immune responses by an effect on CTL quality [112]. In this model, 15–12RM grows, regresses due to an immune response toward a virus-derived surrogate tumor antigen (HIV gp160), and then subsequently relapses and grows progressively. T cell depletion studies demonstrated that the regression phase was mediated by gp160-specific CD8$^+$ T cells. Surprisingly, depletion of CD4$^+$ T cells prevented tumor relapse, indicating that a CD4$^+$ cell was influencing the quality of the anti-tumor immune response [112]. Further investigation revealed that CD1d-deficient mice were also resistant to tumor relapses, leading to the hypothesis that a CD4$^+$ CD1d-restricted T cell was responsible for altering the quality of the CTL response [113]. Experiments in STAT6-deficient mice demonstrated that a Th2-type cytokine was responsible for the suppression of the CTL response, and led to the discovery that neutralization of IL-13 through the use of a soluble receptor antagonist was able to prevent tumor recurrence [113]. These findings resulted in the elucidation of a complex immunosuppressive network, where CD4$^+$ CD1d-restricted T cells produce IL-13, which acts on CD11b$^+$Gr-1$^+$ cells, triggering them to secrete TGF-β, which in turn is responsible for inhibition of CTL function [114]. A similar immunosuppressive network functions in the Colo-26 tumor lung metastasis model [115].

After the initial report of CD1d-dependent suppression in the 15–12RM model, a related but distinct mechanism for controlling the anti-tumor immune response was reported in the 4T1.2 tumor model [116]. 4T1.2 is a metastatic mammary tumor line that metastasizes from the mammary fat pad to the lymph nodes, lung, bones, brain, and liver in WT mice. CD1d-deficient mice are resistant to 4T1.2 metastases [117], and this resistance is T cell-mediated [118]. Like the 15–12RM model, STAT6-dependent signaling was again implicated in suppression of anti-tumor immunity [117]. However, STAT6-deficient mice were more resistant to 4T1.2 tumor growth than CD1d-deficient mice, demonstrating that these pathways do not overlap completely [117]. In contrast to the 15–12RM model, neither CD4-depletion nor IL-13 neutralization were able to protect against 4T1.2 tumor metastasis [117]. These results demonstrate that while a role for CD1d-dependent regulation of tumor immunity is present in both the 15–12RM and 4T1.2 models, the mechanisms of suppression appear to differ for each tumor.

Following identification of a CD1d-dependent mechanism for regulation of tumor immunity, the role of NKT cells in suppression was subsequently investigated through the use of TCR.Jα18$^{-/-}$ mice, which specifically lack invariant but not noninvariant NKT cells, while still expressing CD1d. Surprisingly, in all cases, CD1d-dependent suppression of tumor immunity occurred independently of invariant NKT cells, as tumor growth in TCR.Jα18$^{-/-}$ mice was usually similar to that seen in WT mice [119]. These results, in combination with data demonstrating that CD4$^+$CD25$^+$Foxp3$^+$ Treg are not responsible for suppression in these models [115, 117, 119] suggest that noninvariant, but not Vα14-Jα18$^+$ NKT cells are responsible for the observed inhibition of tumor immunity.

Further evidence for a suppressive role for noninvariant CD1d-restricted T cells was provided when it was demonstrated that treatment of B16 melanomas by peritumoral injection of CpG oligodeoxynucleotides was more effective in CD1d$^{-/-}$ than in WT or TCR.Jα18$^{-/-}$ mice [120]. In this case, the enhanced tumor immunity observed in CD1d$^{-/-}$ mice correlated with an increased IFN-γ:IL-4 ratio. This is an interesting finding, given that rejection of B16F10 tumors in the GM-CSF vaccination model required the presence of NKT cells and CD1d, and tumor protection was associated with a Th2, and not a Th1 response [31]. These results demonstrate that there may be a complex interplay between invariant and noninvariant NKT cells in regulating tumor immunity, depending on the stimulus driving the anti-tumor response.

9.2
Candidate Immunoregulatory Noninvariant NKT Cell Populations

The identity of the noninvariant NKT cell responsible for suppression of tumor immunity and the glycolipid antigens they recognize remain elusive. Studies of CD1d-self reactive hybridomas has demonstrated that while CD1d-restricted T cells can express a more diverse range of T cell receptors [121], some specific TCR rearrangements appear repeatedly, suggesting the existence of other semi-invariant CD1d-restricted T cells in addition to the well characterized Vα14-Jα18$^+$ NKT cells [122]. It is worth noting that invariant and noninvariant NKT cells are suggested to have distinct antigen specificities: for example Vα14-Jα18$^+$ NKT cells fail to develop in mice expressing a version of CD1d that lacks the cytoplasmic tail. However, Vα3.2-Vβ8-expressing CD1d-restricted T cells develop in the usual proportions [123]. The antigen specificity of CD1d-restricted hybridomas has also demonstrated that antigens from distinct cellular compartments are differentially recognized by CD1d-restricted T cells depending on their TCR rearrangement [18].

Transgenic models have demonstrated that some noninvariant NKT cells are capable of immunomodulation in the setting of autoimmunity. For example, adoptive transfer of CD1d-restricted T cells expressing the Vα3.2-Vβ9 TCR combination protected NOD mice from diabetes [124]. These experiments provide proof of principal that noninvariant NKT cells can negatively regulate immune responses, and similar mechanisms may apply in tumor models. The existence of noninvariant NKT cells has also been described in humans: noninvariant NKT cells with a Th1 bias have been identified among the intrahepatic lymphocytes of hepatitis C-infected patients [125], while in the bone marrow noninvariant NKT cells make up a major proportion of the T cell population [126]. Bone marrow resident noninvariant NKT cells exhibit a Th2 cytokine bias and are capable of suppressing MLRs in vitro [126]. These findings may provide leads as to the identity of the noninvariant NKT cells that modulate anti-tumor immunity.

9.3
CD1d-Mediated, T Cell-Independent Modulation of Tumor Immunity

It should be noted that an alternate explanation for the CD1d-dependent suppressive mechanism may be that CD1d is capable of modulating tumor immunity independently of CD1d-restricted T cells. Some potential evidence for this hypothesis has been generated. Firstly, antibody mediated cross-linking of CD1d can stimulate cytokine secretion in vitro: cross-linking of CD1d on human monocytes triggers NF-κB activation and the secretion of IL-12 [127], while cross-linking CD1d on human epithelial cells results in the production of IL-10 [128]. In addition, CD1d appears to influence NK cell killing, as CD1d overexpressing NK cell targets are protected from lysis by LAK cells [129]. Further support for the existence of a molecule that interacts with CD1d was provided by the finding that a subset of NK cells binds to CD1d-coated latex beads [130], and more recently still it has been demonstrated that CD1d binds to CD160 [131]. Expression of CD160 on NK cells is regulated by CD1d expression, as NK cells in CD1d-deficient animals failed to express CD160 [131]. However, the implications of these findings are unclear at the present time.

Overall, in cases where a CD1d-dependent suppression of anti-tumor immunity has been observed, the effect is largely independent of $V\alpha14$-$J\alpha18^+$ NKT cells. However, the identity of the noninvariant NKT cell population (or other molecules interacting with CD1d) responsible for this effect remains an active area of research.

10
Conclusion

CD1d is a complex regulator of tumor immunity, on one hand capable of suppressing anti-tumor immunity through the action of noninvariant NKT cells and on the other enhancing immunity via invariant NKT cells. The mechanism by which noninvariant NKT cells suppress immunity remains ambiguous with no ligand as yet implicated in the activation of this subset, and a crucial role for IL-13 production by noninvariant NKT cells identified in some models but not others. Importantly, invariant NKT cells are also a potent source of IL-13, suggesting that the suppression of anti-tumor immunity mediated by noninvariant NKT cells may also rely on unique, as yet unidentified factors. The elucidation of ligands that specifically activate noninvariant NKT cells will greatly enhance our understanding of this NKT cell subset and their mode of action.

The ability of invariant NKT cells to protect against tumors in natural models of tumor immunosurveillance or through exogenous activation has now been well documented in a number of mouse models. The link to human malignancies is also well established with marked reductions in NKT cell numbers observed in cancer patients, and clear responses of NKT cells to CD1d-expressing tumors. As such, the use of α-GalCer or its analogs remains a tantalizing possibility for the treatment of cancer patients and is buoyed by constant improvements in techniques for the delivery of α-GalCer. It will be important to determine whether α-GalCer therapy can be best implemented in combination with exogenous cytokine administration, or as an adjuvant to tumor-peptide-specific vaccines. Importantly, the finding that functionally distinct NKT cell subsets exist within the NKT cell population has greatly enhanced our understanding of this multifunctional cell type. Further advances in the treatment of cancers in the clinic may well depend on our ability to harness the activity of favorable NKT cell subsets, without engaging responses from other, nonbeneficial NKT cells.

Acknowledgements The authors wish to thank Nadine Crowe and other members of the Godfrey and Smyth laboratories as well as Jay Berzofsky and Masaki Terabe for collaboration. This work was supported by a National Institutes of Health RO1

CA106377 an Association of International Cancer Research Grant, a National Health and Medical Research Council of Australia Program Grant and Research Fellowships to M. J. S. and D. I. G. J. M. C. C. is supported by a Cancer Research Institute (USA) Postgraduate Scholarship. J. B. S. is supported by an Australian Postgraduate Research Scholarship from the Department of Pathology, University of Melbourne.

References

1. Godfrey DI, MacDonald HR, Kronenberg M, Smyth MJ, Van Kaer L (2004) NKT cells: what's in a name? Nat Rev Immunol 4:231–237
2. Koseki H, Imai K, Nakayama F, Sado T, Moriwaki K, Taniguchi M (1990) Homogenous junctional sequence of the V14+ T-cell antigen receptor alpha chain expanded in unprimed mice. Proc Natl Acad Sci U S A 87:5248–5252
3. Bendelac A, Lantz O, Quimby ME, Yewdell JW, Bennink JR, Brutkiewicz RR (1995) CD1 recognition by mouse NK1+ T lymphocytes. Science 268:863–865
4. Smiley ST, Kaplan MH, Grusby MJ (1997) Immunoglobulin E production in the absence of interleukin-4-secreting CD1-dependent cells. Science 275:977–979
5. Chen YH, Chiu NM, Mandal M, Wang N, Wang CR (1997) Impaired NK1+ T cell development and early IL-4 production in CD1-deficient mice. Immunity 6:459–467
6. Mendiratta SK, Martin WD, Hong S, Boesteanu A, Joyce S, Van Kaer L (1997) CD1d1 mutant mice are deficient in natural T cells that promptly produce IL-4. Immunity 6:469–477
7. Kawano T, Cui J, Koezuka Y, Toura I, Kaneko Y, Motoki K, Ueno H, Nakagawa R, Sato H, Kondo E et al (1997) CD1d-restricted and TCR-mediated activation of valpha14. NKT cells by glycosylceramides. Science 278:1626–1629
8. Matsuda JL, Naidenko OV, Gapin L, Nakayama T, Taniguchi M, Wang CR, Koezuka Y, Kronenberg M (2000) Tracking the response of natural killer T cells to a glycolipid antigen using CD1d tetramers. J Exp Med 192:741–754
9. Benlagha K, Weiss A, Beavis A, Teyton L, Bendelac A (2000) In vivo identification of glycolipid antigen-specific T cells using fluorescent CD1d tetramers. J Exp Med 191:1895–1903
10. Brossay L, Chioda M, Burdin N, Koezuka Y, Casorati G, Dellabona P, Kronenberg M (1998) CD1d-mediated recognition of an alpha-galactosylceramide by natural killer T cells is highly conserved through mammalian evolution. J Exp Med 188:1521–1528
11. Wu DY, Segal NH, Sidobre S, Kronenberg M, Chapman PB (2003) Cross-presentation of disialoganglioside GD3 to natural killer T cells. J Exp Med 198:173–181
12. Rauch J, Gumperz J, Robinson C, Skold M, Roy C, Young DC, Lafleur M, Moody DB, Brenner MB, Costello CE et al (2003) Structural features of the acyl chain determine self-phospholipid antigen recognition by a CD1d-restricted invariant NKT (iNKT) cell. J Biol Chem 278:47508–47515
13. Ortaldo JR, Young HA, Winkler-Pickett RT, Bere EW Jr, Murphy WJ, Wiltrout RH (2004) Dissociation of NKT stimulation, cytokine induction, and NK activation in vivo by the use of distinct TCR-binding ceramides. J Immunol 172:943–953

14. Parekh VV, Singh AK, Wilson MT, Olivares-Villagomez D, Bezbradica JS, Inazawa H, Ehara H, Sakai T, Serizawa I, Wu L et al (2004) Quantitative and qualitative differences in the in vivo response of NKT cells to distinct alpha- and beta-anomeric glycolipids. J Immunol 173:3693–3706
15. Zhou D, Mattner J, Cantu C 3rd, Schrantz N, Yin N, Gao Y, Sagiv Y, Hudspeth K, Wu YP, Yamashita T et al (2004) Lysosomal glycosphingolipid recognition by NKT cells. Science 306:1786–1789
16. Mattner J, Debord KL, Ismail N, Goff RD, Cantu C 3rd, Zhou D, Saint-Mezard P, Wang V, Gao Y, Yin N et al (2005) Exogenous and endogenous glycolipid antigens activate NKT cells during microbial infections. Nature 434:525–529
17. Kinjo Y, Wu D, Kim G, Xing GW, Poles MA, Ho DD, Tsuji M, Kawahara K, Wong CH, Kronenberg M (2005) Recognition of bacterial glycosphingolipids by natural killer T cells. Nature 434:520–525
18. Chiu YH, Jayawardena J, Weiss A, Lee D, Park SH, Dautry-Varsat A, Bendelac A (1999) Distinct subsets of CD1d-restricted T cells recognize self-antigens loaded in different cellular compartments. J Exp Med 189:103–110
19. Smyth MJ, Thia KY, Street SE, Cretney E, Trapani JA, Taniguchi M, Kawano T, Pelikan SB, Crowe NY, Godfrey DI (2000) Differential tumor surveillance by natural killer (NK) and NKT cells. J Exp Med 191:661–668
20. Crowe NY, Smyth MJ, Godfrey DI (2002) A critical role for natural killer T cells in immunosurveillance of methylcholanthrene-induced sarcomas. J Exp Med 196:119–127
21. Gumperz JE, Roy C, Makowska A, Lum D, Sugita M, Podrebarac T, Koezuka Y, Porcelli SA, Cardell S, Brenner MB et al (2000) Murine CD1d-restricted T cell recognition of cellular lipids. Immunity 12:211–221
22. Brigl M, Bry L, Kent SC, Gumperz JE, Brenner MB (2003) Mechanism of CD1d-restricted natural killer T cell activation during microbial infection. Nat Immunol 4:1230–1237
23. Crowe NY, Coquet JM, Berzins SP, Kyparissoudis K, Keating R, Pellicci DG, Hayakawa Y, Godfrey DI, Smyth MJ (2005) Differential antitumor immunity mediated by NKT cell subsets in vivo. J Exp Med 202:1279–1288
24. Nishikawa H, Kato T, Tanida K, Hiasa A, Tawara I, Ikeda H, Ikarashi Y, Wakasugi H, Kronenberg M, Nakayama T et al (2003) CD4+ CD25+ T cells responding to serologically defined autoantigens suppress antitumor immune responses. Proc Natl Acad Sci U S A 100:10902–10906
25. Nishikawa H, Kato T, Tawara I, Takemitsu T, Saito K, Wang L, Ikarashi Y, Wakasugi H, Nakayama T, Taniguchi M et al (2005) Accelerated chemically induced tumor development mediated by CD4+CD25+ regulatory T cells in wild-type hosts. Proc Natl Acad Sci U S A 102:9253–9257
26. Azuma T, Takahashi T, Kunisato A, Kitamura T, Hirai H (2003) Human CD4+ CD25+ regulatory T cells suppress NKT cell functions. Cancer Res 63:4516–4520
27. Jiang S, Game DS, Davies D, Lombardi G, Lechler RI (2005) Activated CD1d-restricted natural killer T cells secrete IL-2: innate help for CD4+CD25+ regulatory T cells? Eur J Immunol 35:1193–1200
28. Crespo FA, Sun X, Cripps JG, Fernandez-Botran R (2006) The immunoregulatory effects of gangliosides involve immune deviation favoring type-2 T cell responses. J Leukoc Biol 79:586–595

29. Jaffee EM (1999) Immunotherapy of cancer. Ann N Y Acad Sci 886:67–72
30. Eager R, Nemunaitis J (2005) GM-CSF gene-transduced tumor vaccines. Mol Ther 12:18–27
31. Gillessen S, Naumov YN, Nieuwenhuis EE, Exley MA, Lee FS, Mach N, Luster AD, Blumberg RS, Taniguchi M, Balk SP et al (2003) CD1d-restricted T cells regulate dendritic cell function and antitumor immunity in a granulocyte-macrophage colony-stimulating factor-dependent fashion. Proc Natl Acad Sci U S A 100:8874–8879
32. Kobayashi E, Motoki K, Uchida T, Fukushima H, Koezuka Y (1995) KRN7000, a novel immunomodulator, and its antitumor activities. Oncol Res 7:529–534
33. Yamaguchi Y, Motoki K, Ueno H, Maeda K, Kobayashi E, Inoue H, Fukushima H, Koezuka Y (1996) Enhancing effects of (2S,3S,4R)-1-O-(alpha-D-galactopyranosyl)-2-(N-hexacosanoylamino)-1,3,4-octadecanetriol (KRN7000) on antigen-presenting function of antigen-presenting cells and antimetastatic activity of KRN7000-pretreated antigen-presenting cells. Oncol Res 8:399–407
34. Nakagawa R, Motoki K, Ueno H, Iijima R, Nakamura H, Kobayashi E, Shimosaka A, Koezuka Y (1998) Treatment of hepatic metastasis of the colon26 adenocarcinoma with an alpha-galactosylceramide KRN7000. Cancer Res 58:1202–1207
35. Nakagawa R, Motoki K, Nakamura H, Ueno H, Iijima R, Yamauchi A, Tsuyuki S, Inamoto T, Koezuka Y (1998) Antitumor activity of alpha-galactosylceramide KRN7000, in mice with EL-4 hepatic metastasis and its cytokine production. Oncol Res 10:561–568
36. Smyth MJ, Crowe NY, Pellicci DG, Kyparissoudis K, Kelly JM, Takeda K, Yagita H, Godfrey DI (2002) Sequential production of interferon-gamma by NK1.1(+) T cells and natural killer cells is essential for the antimetastatic effect of alpha-galactosylceramide. Blood 99:1259–1266
37. Hayakawa Y, Rovero S, Forni G, Smyth MJ (2003) Alpha-galactosylceramide (KRN7000) suppression of chemical- and oncogene-dependent carcinogenesis. Proc Natl Acad Sci U S A 100:9464–9469
38. Hayakawa Y, Takeda K, Yagita H, Kakuta S, Iwakura Y, Van Kaer L, Saiki I, Okumura K (2001) Critical contribution of IFN-gamma and NK cells, but not perforin-mediated cytotoxicity, to anti-metastatic effect of alpha-galactosylceramide. Eur J Immunol 31:1720–1727
39. Burdin N, Brossay L, Koezuka Y, Smiley ST, Grusby MJ, Gui M, Taniguchi M, Hayakawa K, Kronenberg M (1998) Selective ability of mouse CD1 to present glycolipids: alpha-galactosylceramide specifically stimulates V alpha 14+ NKT lymphocytes. J Immunol 161:3271–3281
40. Yang YF, Tomura M, Ono S, Hamaoka T, Fujiwara H (2000) Requirement for IFN-gamma in IL-12 production induced by collaboration between v(alpha)14(+) NKT cells and antigen-presenting cells. Int Immunol 12:1669–1675
41. Fujii S, Liu K, Smith C, Bonito AJ, Steinman RM (2004) The linkage of innate to adaptive immunity via maturing dendritic cells in vivo requires CD40 ligation in addition to antigen presentation and CD80/86 costimulation. J Exp Med 199:1607–1618

42. Kitamura H, Iwakabe K, Yahata T, Nishimura S, Ohta A, Ohmi Y, Sato M, Takeda K, Okumura K, Van Kaer L et al (1999) The natural killer T (NKT) cell ligand alpha-galactosylceramide demonstrates its immunopotentiating effect by inducing interleukin (IL)-12 production by dendritic cells and IL-12 receptor expression on NKT cells. J Exp Med 189:1121–1128

43. Fuji N, Ueda Y, Fujiwara H, Toh T, Yoshimura T, Yamagishi H (2000) Antitumor effect of alpha-galactosylceramide (KRN7000) on spontaneous hepatic metastases requires endogenous interleukin 12 in the liver. Clin Cancer Res 6:3380–3387

44. Tomura M, Yu WG, Ahn HJ, Yamashita M, Yang YF, Ono S, Hamaoka T, Kawano T, Taniguchi M, Koezuka Y et al (1999) A novel function of Valpha14+CD4+NKT cells: stimulation of IL-12 production by antigen-presenting cells in the innate immune system. J Immunol 163:93–101

45. Fujii S, Shimizu K, Smith C, Bonifaz L, Steinman RM (2003) Activation of natural killer T cells by alpha-galactosylceramide rapidly induces the full maturation of dendritic cells in vivo and thereby acts as an adjuvant for combined CD4 and CD8. T cell immunity to a coadministered protein. J Exp Med 198:267–279

46. Osada T, Morse MA, Lyerly HK, Clay TM (2005) Ex vivo expanded human CD4+ regulatory NKT cells suppress expansion of tumor antigen-specific CTLs. Int Immunol 17:1143–1155

47. Carnaud C, Lee D, Donnars O, Park SH, Beavis A, Koezuka Y, Bendelac A (1999) Cutting edge: cross-talk between cells of the innate immune system: NKT cells rapidly activate NK cells. J Immunol 163:4647–4650

48. Eberl G, MacDonald HR (2000) Selective induction of NK cell proliferation and cytotoxicity by activated NKT cells. Eur J Immunol 30:985–992

49. Eberl G, Brawand P, MacDonald HR (2000) Selective bystander proliferation of memory CD4+ and CD8+ T cells upon NKT or T cell activation. J Immunol 165:4305–4311

50. Nishimura T, Kitamura H, Iwakabe K, Yahata T, Ohta A, Sato M, Takeda K, Okumura K, Van Kaer L, Kawano T et al (2000) The interface between innate and acquired immunity: glycolipid antigen presentation by CD1d-expressing dendritic cells to NKT cells induces the differentiation of antigen-specific cytotoxic T lymphocytes. Int Immunol 12:987–994

51. Gonzalez-Aseguinolaza G, Van Kaer L, Bergmann CC, Wilson JM, Schmieg J, Kronenberg M, Nakayama T, Taniguchi M, Koezuka Y, Tsuji M (2002) Natural killer T cell ligand alpha-galactosylceramide enhances protective immunity induced by malaria vaccines. J Exp Med 195:617–624

52. Nakagawa R, Inui T, Nagafune I, Tazunoki Y, Motoki K, Yamauchi A, Hirashima M, Habu Y, Nakashima H, Seki S (2004) Essential role of bystander cytotoxic CD122+CD8+ T cells for the antitumor immunity induced in the liver of mice by alpha-galactosylceramide. J Immunol 172:6550–6557

53. Hayakawa Y, Takeda K, Yagita H, Smyth MJ, Van Kaer L, Okumura K, Saiki I (2002) IFN-gamma-mediated inhibition of tumor angiogenesis by natural killer T-cell ligand, alpha-galactosylceramide. Blood 100:1728–1733

54. Smyth MJ, Cretney E, Takeda K, Wiltrout RH, Sedger LM, Kayagaki N, Yagita H, Okumura K (2001) Tumor necrosis factor-related apoptosis-inducing ligand (TRAIL) contributes to interferon gamma-dependent natural killer cell protection from tumor metastasis. J Exp Med 193:661–670

55. Nakagawa R, Nagafune I, Tazunoki Y, Ehara H, Tomura H, Iijima R, Motoki K, Kamishohara M, Seki S (2001) Mechanisms of the antimetastatic effect in the liver and of the hepatocyte injury induced by alpha-galactosylceramide in mice. J Immunol 166:6578–6584

56. Fujii S, Shimizu K, Kronenberg M, Steinman RM (2002) Prolonged IFN-gamma-producing NKT response induced with alpha-galactosylceramide-loaded DCs. Nat Immunol 3:867–874

57. Uldrich AP, Crowe NY, Kyparissoudis K, Pellicci DG, Zhan Y, Lew AM, Bouillet P, Strasser A, Smyth MJ, Godfrey DI (2005) NKT cell stimulation with glycolipid antigen in vivo: costimulation-dependent expansion Bim-dependent contraction, and hyporesponsiveness to further antigenic challenge. J Immunol 175:3092–3101

58. Parekh VV, Wilson MT, Olivares-Villagomez D, Singh AK, Wu L, Wang CR, Joyce S, Van Kaer L (2005) Glycolipid antigen induces long-term natural killer T cell anergy in mice. J Clin Invest 115:2572–2583

59. Fujii S, Shimizu K, Steinman RM, Dhodapkar MV (2003) Detection and activation of human Valpha24+ natural killer T cells using alpha-galactosyl ceramide-pulsed dendritic cells. J Immunol Methods 272:147–159

60. Van der Vliet HJ, Nishi N, Koezuka Y, von Blomberg BM, van den Eertwegh AJ, Porcelli SA, Pinedo HM, Scheper RJ, Giaccone G (2001) Potent expansion of human natural killer T cells using alpha-galactosylceramide (KRN7000)-loaded monocyte-derived dendritic cells, cultured in the presence of IL-7 and IL-15. J Immunol Methods 247:61–72

61. Bezbradica JS, Stanic AK, Matsuki N, Bour-Jordan H, Bluestone JA, Thomas JW, Unutmaz D, Van Kaer L, Joyce S (2005) Distinct roles of dendritic cells and B cells in Va14Ja18 natural T cell activation in vivo. J Immunol 174:4696–4705

62. Schmieg J, Yang G, Franck RW, Van Rooijen N, Tsuji M (2005) Glycolipid presentation to natural killer T cells differs in an organ-dependent fashion. Proc Natl Acad Sci U S A 102:1127–1132

63. Toura I, Kawano T, Akutsu Y, Nakayama T, Ochiai T, Taniguchi M (1999) Cutting edge: inhibition of experimental tumor metastasis by dendritic cells pulsed with alpha-galactosylceramide. J Immunol 163:2387–2391

64. Smyth MJ, Wallace ME, Nutt SL, Yagita H, Godfrey DI, Hayakawa Y (2005) Sequential activation of NKT cells and NK cells provides effective innate immunotherapy of cancer. J Exp Med 201:1973–1985

65. Cui J, Shin T, Kawano T, Sato H, Kondo E, Toura I, Kaneko Y, Koseki H, Kanno M, Taniguchi M (1997) Requirement for Valpha14. NKT cells in IL-12-mediated rejection of tumors. Science 278:1623–1626

66. Takeda K, Seki S, Ogasawara K, Anzai R, Hashimoto W, Sugiura K, Takahashi M, Satoh M, Kumagai K (1996) Liver NK1.1+ CD4+ alpha beta T cells activated by IL-12 as a major effector in inhibition of experimental tumor metastasis. J Immunol 156:3366–3373

67. Kobayashi T, Shiiba K, Satoh M, Hashimoto W, Mizoi T, Matsuno S, Takeda K (2002) Interleukin-12 administration is more effective for preventing metastasis than for inhibiting primary established tumors in a murine model of spontaneous hepatic metastasis. Surg Today 32:236–242

68. Shin T, Nakayama T, Akutsu Y, Motohashi S, Shibata Y, Harada M, Kamada N, Shimizu C, Shimizu E, Saito T et al (2001) Inhibition of tumor metastasis by adoptive transfer of IL-12-activated Valpha14. NKT cells. Int J Cancer 91:523–528

69. Smyth MJ, Taniguchi M, Street SE (2000) The anti-tumor activity of IL-12: mechanisms of innate immunity that are model and dose dependent. J Immunol 165:2665–2670

70. Takeda K, Hayakawa Y, Atsuta M, Hong S, Van Kaer L, Kobayashi K, Ito M, Yagita H, Okumura K (2000) Relative contribution of NK and NKT cells to the anti-metastatic activities of IL-12. Int Immunol 12:909–914

71. Leite-De-Moraes MC, Hameg A, Pacilio M, Koezuka Y, Taniguchi M, Van Kaer L, Schneider E, Dy M, Herbelin A (2001) IL-18 enhances IL-4 production by ligand-activated NKT lymphocytes: a pro-Th2 effect of IL-18 exerted through NKT cells. J Immunol 166:945–951

72. Baxevanis CN, Gritzapis AD, Papamichail M (2003) In vivo antitumor activity of NKT cells activated by the combination of IL-12 and IL-18. J Immunol 171:2953–2959

73. Morris ES, MacDonald KP, Rowe V, Banovic T, Kuns RD, Don AL, Bofinger HM, Burman AC, Olver SD, Kienzle N et al (2005) NKT cell-dependent leukemia eradication following stem cell mobilization with potent G-CSF analogs. J Clin Invest 115:3093–3103

74. Eberl G, Lees R, Smiley ST, Taniguchi M, Grusby MJ, MacDonald HR (1999) Tissue-specific segregation of CD1d-dependent and CD1d-independent NKT cells. J Immunol 162:6410–6419

75. Hammond KJ, Pelikan SB, Crowe NY, Randle-Barrett E, Nakayama T, Taniguchi M, Smyth MJ, van Driel IR, Scollay R, Baxter AG et al (1999) NKT cells are phenotypically and functionally diverse. Eur J Immunol 29:3768–3781

76. Gumperz JE, Miyake S, Yamamura T, Brenner MB (2002) Functionally distinct subsets of CD1d-restricted natural killer T cells revealed by CD1d tetramer staining. J Exp Med 195:625–636

77. Lee PT, Benlagha K, Teyton L, Bendelac A (2002) Distinct functional lineages of human V(alpha)24 natural killer T cells. J Exp Med 195:637–641

78. Berzins SP, Cochrane AD, Pellicci DG, Smyth MJ, Godfrey DI (2005) Limited correlation between human thymus and blood NKT cell content revealed by an ontogeny study of paired tissue samples. Eur J Immunol 35:1399–1407

79. Takahashi T, Chiba S, Nieda M, Azuma T, Ishihara S, Shibata Y, Juji T, Hirai H (2002) Cutting edge: analysis of human V alpha 24+CD8+ NKT cells activated by alpha-galactosylceramide-pulsed monocyte-derived dendritic cells. J Immunol 168:3140–3144

80. Rogers PR, Matsumoto A, Naidenko O, Kronenberg M, Mikayama T, Kato S (2004) Expansion of human Valpha24+ NKT cells by repeated stimulation with KRN(7000). J Immunol Methods 285:197–214

81. Lin H, Nieda M, Nicol AJ (2004) Differential proliferative response of NKT cell subpopulations to in vitro stimulation in presence of different cytokines. Eur J Immunol 34:2664–2671

82. Kenna T, Golden-Mason L, Porcelli SA, Koezuka Y, Hegarty JE, O'Farrelly C, Doherty DG (2003) NKT cells from normal and tumor-bearing human livers are phenotypically and functionally distinct from murine NKT cells. J Immunol 171:1775–1779

83. Wang ZY, Kusam S, Munugalavadla V, Kapur R, Brutkiewicz RR, Dent AL (2006) Regulation of Th2 cytokine expression in NKT cells: unconventional use of Stat6, GATA-3, and NFAT2. J Immunol 176:880–888

84. Matsuda JL, Gapin L, Baron JL, Sidobre S, Stetson DB, Mohrs M, Locksley RM, Kronenberg M (2003) Mouse V alpha 14i natural killer T cells are resistant to cytokine polarization in vivo. Proc Natl Acad Sci U S A 100:8395–8400

85. Maeda M, Lohwasser S, Yamamura T, Takei F (2001) Regulation of NKT cells by Ly49: analysis of primary NKT cells and generation of NKT cell line. J Immunol 167:4180–4186

86. Kim CH, Butcher EC, Johnston B (2002) Distinct subsets of human Valpha24-invariant NKT cells: cytokine responses and chemokine receptor expression. Trends Immunol 23:516–519

87. Thomas SY, Hou R, Boyson JE, Means TK, Hess C, Olson DP, Strominger JL, Brenner MB, Gumperz JE, Wilson SB et al (2003) CD1d-restricted NKT cells express a chemokine receptor profile indicative of Th1-type inflammatory homing cells. J Immunol 171:2571–2580

88. Johnston B, Kim CH, Soler D, Emoto M, Butcher EC (2003) Differential chemokine responses and homing patterns of murine TCR alpha beta NKT cell subsets. J Immunol 171:2960–2969

89. Matsuyoshi H, Hirata S, Yoshitake Y, Motomura Y, Fukuma D, Kurisaki A, Nakatsura T, Nishimura Y, Senju S (2005) Therapeutic effect of alpha-galactosylceramide-loaded dendritic cells genetically engineered to express SLC/CCL21 along with tumor antigen against peritoneally disseminated tumor cells. Cancer Sci 96:889–896

90. Lin H, Nieda M, Rozenkov V, Nicol AJ (2006) Analysis of the effect of different NKT cell subpopulations on the activation of CD4 and CD8. T cells NK cells, and B cells. Exp Hematol 34:289–295

91. Van Kaer L (2005) Alpha-galactosylceramide therapy for autoimmune diseases: prospects and obstacles. Nat Rev Immunol 5:31–42

92. Kawano T, Nakayama T, Kamada N, Kaneko Y, Harada M, Ogura N, Akutsu Y, Motohashi S, Iizasa T, Endo H et al (1999) Antitumor cytotoxicity mediated by ligand-activated human V alpha24. NKT cells. Cancer Res 59:5102–5105

93. Tahir SM, Cheng O, Shaulov A, Koezuka Y, Bubley GJ, Wilson SB, Balk SP, Exley MA (2001) Loss of IFN-gamma production by invariant NKT cells in advanced cancer. J Immunol 167:4046–4050

94. Metelitsa LS, Weinberg KI, Emanuel PD, Seeger RC (2003) Expression of CD1d by myelomonocytic leukemias provides a target for cytotoxic NKT cells. Leukemia 17:1068–1077

95. Fais F, Morabito F, Stelitano C, Callea V, Zanardi S, Scudeletti M, Varese P, Ciccone E, Grossi CE (2004) CD1d is expressed on B-chronic lymphocytic leukemia cells and mediates alpha-galactosylceramide presentation to natural killer T lymphocytes. Int J Cancer 109:402–411

96. Takahashi T, Haraguchi K, Chiba S, Yasukawa M, Shibata Y, Hirai H (2003) Valpha24+ natural killer T-cell responses against T-acute lymphoblastic leukaemia cells: implications for immunotherapy. Br J Haematol 122:231–239

97. Dhodapkar MV, Geller MD, Chang DH, Shimizu K, Fujii S, Dhodapkar KM, Krasovsky J (2003) A reversible defect in natural killer T cell function characterizes the progression of premalignant to malignant multiple myeloma. J Exp Med 197:1667–1676

98. Motohashi S, Kobayashi S, Ito T, Magara KK, Mikuni O, Kamada N, Iizasa T, Nakayama T, Fujisawa T, Taniguchi M (2002) Preserved IFN-alpha production of circulating Valpha24. NKT cells in primary lung cancer patients. Int J Cancer 102:159–165

99. Konishi J, Yamazaki K, Yokouchi H, Shinagawa N, Iwabuchi K, Nishimura M (2004) The characteristics of human NKT cells in lung cancer–CD1d independent cytotoxicity against lung cancer cells by NKT cells and decreased human NKT cell response in lung cancer patients. Hum Immunol 65:1377–1388

100. Tachibana T, Onodera H, Tsuruyama T, Mori A, Nagayama S, Hiai H, Imamura M (2005) Increased intratumor Valpha24-positive natural killer T cells: a prognostic factor for primary colorectal carcinomas. Clin Cancer Res 11:7322–7327

101. Giaccone G, Punt CJ, Ando Y, Ruijter R, Nishi N, Peters M, von Blomberg BM, Scheper RJ, van der Vliet HJ, van den Eertwegh AJ et al (2002) A phase I study of the natural killer T-cell ligand alpha-galactosylceramide (KRN7000) in patients with solid tumors. Clin Cancer Res 8:3702–3709

102. Nieda M, Okai M, Tazbirkova A, Lin H, Yamaura A, Ide K, Abraham R, Juji T, Macfarlane DJ, Nicol AJ (2004) Therapeutic activation of Valpha24+Vbeta11+ NKT cells in human subjects results in highly coordinated secondary activation of acquired and innate immunity. Blood 103:383–389

103. Ishikawa A, Motohashi S, Ishikawa E, Fuchida H, Higashino K, Otsuji M, Iizasa T, Nakayama T, Taniguchi M, Fujisawa T (2005) A phase I study of alpha-galactosylceramide (KRN7000)-pulsed dendritic cells in patients with advanced and recurrent non-small cell lung cancer. Clin Cancer Res 11:1910–1917

104. Chang DH, Osman K, Connolly J, Kukreja A, Krasovsky J, Pack M, Hutchinson A, Geller M, Liu N, Annable R et al (2005) Sustained expansion of NKT cells and antigen-specific T cells after injection of alpha-galactosyl-ceramide loaded mature dendritic cells in cancer patients. J Exp Med 201:1503–1517

105. Schmieg J, Yang G, Franck RW, Tsuji M (2003) Superior protection against malaria and melanoma metastases by a C-glycoside analogue of the natural killer T cell ligand alpha-galactosylceramide. J Exp Med 198:1631–1641

106. Miyamoto K, Miyake S, Yamamura T (2001) A synthetic glycolipid prevents autoimmune encephalomyelitis by inducing TH2 bias of natural killer T cells. Nature 413:531–534

107. Oki S, Chiba A, Yamamura T, Miyake S (2004) The clinical implication and molecular mechanism of preferential IL-4 production by modified glycolipid-stimulated NKT cells. J Clin Invest 113:1631–1640

108. Stanic AK, Shashidharamurthy R, Bezbradica JS, Matsuki N, Yoshimura Y, Miyake S, Choi EY, Schell TD, Van Kaer L, Tevethia SS et al (2003) Another view of T cell antigen recognition: cooperative engagement of glycolipid antigens by Va14Ja18 natural T(iNKT) cell receptor [corrected]. J Immunol 171:4539–4551

109. Nakui M, Ohta A, Sekimoto M, Sato M, Iwakabe K, Yahata T, Kitamura H, Koda T, Kawano T, Makuuchi H et al (2000) Potentiation of antitumor effect of NKT cell ligand, alpha-galactosylceramide by combination with IL-12 on lung metastasis of malignant melanoma cells. Clin Exp Metastasis 18:147–153

110. Liu K, Idoyaga J, Charalambous A, Fujii S, Bonito A, Mordoh J, Wainstok R, Bai XF, Liu Y, Steinman RM (2005) Innate NKT lymphocytes confer superior adaptive immunity via tumor-capturing dendritic cells. J Exp Med 202:1507–1516

111. Hermans IF, Silk JD, Gileadi U, Salio M, Mathew B, Ritter G, Schmidt R, Harris AL, Old L, Cerundolo V (2003) NKT cells enhance CD4+ and CD8+ T cell responses to soluble antigen in vivo through direct interaction with dendritic cells. J Immunol 171:5140–5147

112. Matsui S, Ahlers JD, Vortmeyer AO, Terabe M, Tsukui T, Carbone DP, Liotta LA, Berzofsky JA (1999) A model for CD8+ CTL tumor immunosurveillance and regulation of tumor escape by CD4 T cells through an effect on quality of CTL. J Immunol 163:184–193

113. Terabe M, Matsui S, Noben-Trauth N, Chen H, Watson C, Donaldson DD, Carbone DP, Paul WE, Berzofsky JA (2000) NKT cell-mediated repression of tumor immunosurveillance by IL-13 and the IL-4R-STAT6 pathway. Nat Immunol 1:515–520

114. Terabe M, Matsui S, Park JM, Mamura M, Noben-Trauth N, Donaldson DD, Chen W, Wahl SM, Ledbetter S, Pratt B et al (2003) Transforming growth factor-beta production and myeloid cells are an effector mechanism through which CD1d-restricted T cells block cytotoxic T lymphocyte-mediated tumor immunosurveillance: abrogation prevents tumor recurrence. J Exp Med 198:1741–1752

115. Park JM, Terabe M, van den Broeke LT, Donaldson DD, Berzofsky JA (2005) Unmasking immunosurveillance against a syngeneic colon cancer by elimination of CD4+ NKT regulatory cells and IL-13. Int J Cancer 114:80–87

116. Ostrand-Rosenberg S, Clements VK, Terabe M, Park JM, Berzofsky JA, Dissanayake SK (2002) Resistance to metastatic disease in STAT6-deficient mice requires hemopoietic and nonhemopoietic cells and is IFN-gamma dependent. J Immunol 169:5796–5804

117. Ostrand-Rosenberg S, Grusby MJ, Clements VK (2000) Cutting edge: STAT6-deficient mice have enhanced tumor immunity to primary and metastatic mammary carcinoma. J Immunol 165:6015–6019

118. Sinha P, Clements VK, Ostrand-Rosenberg S (2005) Interleukin-13-regulated M2 macrophages in combination with myeloid suppressor cells block immune surveillance against metastasis. Cancer Res 65:11743–11751

119. Terabe M, Swann J, Ambrosino E, Sinha P, Takaku S, Hayakawa Y, Godfrey DI, Ostrand-Rosenberg S, Smyth MJ, Berzofsky JA (2005) A nonclassical non-Valpha14Jalpha18. CD1d-restricted (type II) NKT cell is sufficient for down-regulation of tumor immunosurveillance. J Exp Med 202:1627–1633

120. Sfondrini L, Besusso D, Zoia MT, Rodolfo M, Invernizzi AM, Taniguchi M, Nakayama T, Colombo MP, Menard S, Balsari A (2002) Absence of the CD1 molecule up-regulates antitumor activity induced by CpG oligodeoxynucleotides in mice. J Immunol 169:151–158

121. Behar SM, Podrebarac TA, Roy CJ, Wang CR, Brenner MB (1999) Diverse TCRs recognize murine CD1. J Immunol 162:161–167

122. Park SH, Weiss A, Benlagha K, Kyin T, Teyton L, Bendelac A (2001) The mouse CD1d-restricted repertoire is dominated by a few autoreactive T cell receptor families. J Exp Med 193:893–904

123. Chiu YH, Park SH, Benlagha K, Forestier C, Jayawardena-Wolf J, Savage PB, Teyton L, Bendelac A (2002) Multiple defects in antigen presentation and T cell development by mice expressing cytoplasmic tail-truncated CD1d. Nat Immunol 3:55–60

124. Duarte N, Stenstrom M, Campino S, Bergman ML, Lundholm M, Holmberg D, Cardell SL (2004) Prevention of diabetes in nonobese diabetic mice mediated by CD1d-restricted nonclassical NKT cells. J Immunol 173:3112–3118

125. Exley MA, He Q, Cheng O, Wang RJ, Cheney CP, Balk SP, Koziel MJ (2002) Cutting edge: compartmentalization of Th1-like noninvariant CD1d-reactive T cells in hepatitis C virus-infected liver. J Immunol 168:1519–1523

126. Exley MA, Tahir SM, Cheng O, Shaulov A, Joyce R, Avigan D, Sackstein R, Balk SP (2001) A major fraction of human bone marrow lymphocytes are Th2-like CD1d-reactive T cells that can suppress mixed lymphocyte responses. J Immunol 167:5531–5534

127. Yue SC, Shaulov A, Wang R, Balk SP, Exley MA (2005) CD1d ligation on human monocytes directly signals rapid NF-kappaB activation and production of bioactive IL-12. Proc Natl Acad Sci U S A 102:11811–11816

128. Colgan SP, Hershberg RM, Furuta GT, Blumberg RS (1999) Ligation of intestinal epithelial CD1d induces bioactive IL-10: critical role of the cytoplasmic tail in autocrine signaling. Proc Natl Acad Sci U S A 96:13938–13943

129. Chang CS, Brossay L, Kronenberg M, Kane KP (1999) The murine nonclassical class I major histocompatibility complex-like CD1.1 molecule protects target cells from lymphokine-activated killer cell cytolysis. J Exp Med 189:483–491

130. Huang MM, Borszcz P, Sidobre S, Kronenberg M, Kane KP (2004) CD1d1 displayed on cell size beads identifies and enriches an NK cell population negatively regulated by CD1d1. J Immunol 172:5304–5312

131. Maeda M, Carpenito C, Russell RC, Dasanjh J, Veinotte LL, Ohta H, Yamamura T, Tan R, Takei F (2005) Murine CD160, Ig-like receptor on NK cells and NKT cells, recognizes classical and nonclassical MHC class I and regulates NK cell activation. J Immunol 175:4426–4432

132. Hayakawa Y, Godfrey DI, Smyth MJ (2004) Alpha-galactosylceramide: potential immunomodulatory activity and future application. Curr Med Chem 11:241–252

133. Smyth MJ, Crowe NY, Hayakawa Y, Takeda K, Yagita H, Godfrey DI (2002) NKT cells—conductors of tumor immunity? Curr Opin Immunol 14:165–171

134. Zeng R, Spolski R, Finkelstein SE, Oh S, Kovanen PE, Hinrichs CS, Pise-Masison CA, Radonovich MF, Brady JN, Restifo NP et al (2005) Synergy of IL-21 and IL-15 in regulating CD8+ T cell expansion and function. J Exp Med 201:139–148

CTMI (2007) 314:325–338

Harnessing NKT Cells for Therapeutic Applications

V. Cerundolo (✉) · M. Salio

Cancer Research UK Tumour Immunology Group, The Weatherall Institute of
Molecular Medicine, Oxford OX3 9DS, UK
vincenzo.cerundolo@imm.ox.ac.uk

Abstract Activation of NKT cells leads to the maturation of dendritic cells and efficiently assists priming of antigen-specific immune responses. The lack of polymorphism of CD1d molecules and the evolutionary conservation of NKT cell responses
highlight the important role of these cells in bridging innate and adaptive immune
responses and advocate the value of harnessing this system in clinical settings. Compounds capable of fine tuning NKT cell activation should be actively exploited as
potent adjuvants in vaccination strategies or as immunomodulators of autoimmune
diseases.

1
Introduction

Current vaccination strategies based on the use of recombinant viruses are
failing to elicit T cell responses similar to those generated by natural infections. The limited success of recombinant viruses as backbone delivery
vectors in vaccine strategies is mainly due to their high immunogenicity
resulting in responses specific to the viral proteins, which out-number responses specific for recombinant protein antigens (Smith et al. 2005a, 2005b).
Although prime-boost vaccination strategies are designed to overcome the

immunodominance of virus-specific T cell responses (Schneider et al. 1999), current priming strategies, such as DNA priming, are failing in humans to generate large numbers of antigen-specific T cell responses (Donnelly et al. 2005).

Advances in molecular technology have permitted the design of synthetic protein vaccines, providing immunotherapy with a degree of specificity that has not been possible using traditional vaccines based on live attenuated pathogens or whole inactivated organisms. Such specificity is providing a platform for the design of T cell therapies for infectious diseases and cancer. It is therefore important to optimise vaccination strategies, using protocols capable of jump-starting immune responses specific to recombinant protein antigens. Optimisation of such vaccination protocols requires a deeper understanding of the signals that the immune system coordinates to respond to pathogenic infections. Compounds that mimic these signals, such as those capable of activating NKT cells, should therefore be exploited as adjuvants in current vaccination strategies. (For simplicity we are using the more general term "NKT" throughout the chapter unless functions of variable and invariant populations are specifically defined and contrasted.)

In the first part of this review we will summarise the results demonstrating that activation of human and mouse NKT cells leads to the maturation of dendritic cells (DC) and expansion of antigen-specific responses. The results of these experiments will then be discussed in the context of current and future clinical trials based on activation of NKT cells both as adjuvants in vaccination strategies and as immunomodulators of autoimmune diseases.

2
Immune Regulation by CD1d-Restricted NKT Cells

Following stimulation with α-galactosylceramide (α-GalCer), NKT cells rapidly release large amounts of both Th1 and Th2 cytokines, including TNF-α, IFN-γ and IL-4, and are capable of both enhancing and suppressing immune responses (Godfrey and Kronenberg 2004). The existence of functionally distinct subsets of CD1d-restricted T cells (Gumperz et al. 2002; Lee et al. 2002; Seino and Taniguchi 2005) may explain the different outcomes following their activation. The divergent roles of CD1d-restricted T cells in promoting both inflammatory and tolerogenic responses highlight the importance of being able to fine-tune their activation *in vivo* for therapeutic purposes.

2.1
NKT Cell-Dependent DC Maturation Results in the Expansion of Antigen-Specific Responses

It is becoming apparent that control of DC function during infection occurs via integration of a series of instructive signals from the pathogen itself, through pathogen-associated molecular pattern receptors, such as Toll-like receptors (TLRs), and also from other antigen-responsive cells in the environment that provide additional activating signals, such as through the ligation of CD40 (Reis e Sousa 2004). TLR and CD40 signalling appear to be highly coordinated, as triggering of CD40 in vivo with anti-CD40 antibodies in the absence of microbial stimulation results in only low levels of IL-12 p70 production (Schulz et al. 2000). Similarly, inflammatory factors in the absence of TLR stimulation fail to prime functional CD4$^+$ T cell responses (Sporri and Reis e Sousa 2005). Clearly, the timely provision of T cell signals is important for optimizing T cell responses.

A potential obstacle to the efficiency of DCs receiving appropriate T cell signals is the scarcity of T cells with reactivity to unique antigens presented by the DCs. However, in contrast to conventional, MHC-restricted CD4$^+$ and CD8$^+$ T cells, NKT cells are found in relative abundance (Porcelli and Modlin 1999). Since CD1d molecules are mainly expressed by professional antigen-presenting cells (such as DCs) and NKT cells express CD40L (Vincent et al. 2002), compounds which bind to CD1d molecules and are recognised by the NKT T cell receptor (TCR) should be capable of inducing NKT-dependent DC maturation.

This concept was first assessed in experiments which showed that CD1 reactive T lymphocytes, including NKT, can promote DC maturation (Vincent et al. 2002). This initial finding was further extended by experiments elegantly demonstrating a cross-talk between DCs and NKT cells (Brigl et al. 2003). Specifically, weak responses to CD1d-presented antigens were amplified by IL-12 secreted by DCs matured by microbial stimuli, supporting a model for the activation of NKT cells in the absence of direct recognition of microbial antigens (Fig. 1). Thus, DCs and NKT cells appear to communicate locally within cytokine circuits that promote one another's activation state.

These findings in turn suggest that this phenomenon could be exploited therapeutically by activating NKT cells that come into direct contact with DCs. For example, it was shown that when α-GalCer is selectively targeted to DCs, mice develop a more prolonged NKT cell response (Fujii et al. 2002). Interestingly, while repeated injections of α-GalCer led to NKT cell anergy (Parekh et al. 2005), repeated injections of α-GalCer pulsed DCs led to the expansion of NKT cells (Fujii et al. 2002). These results suggest that the quality

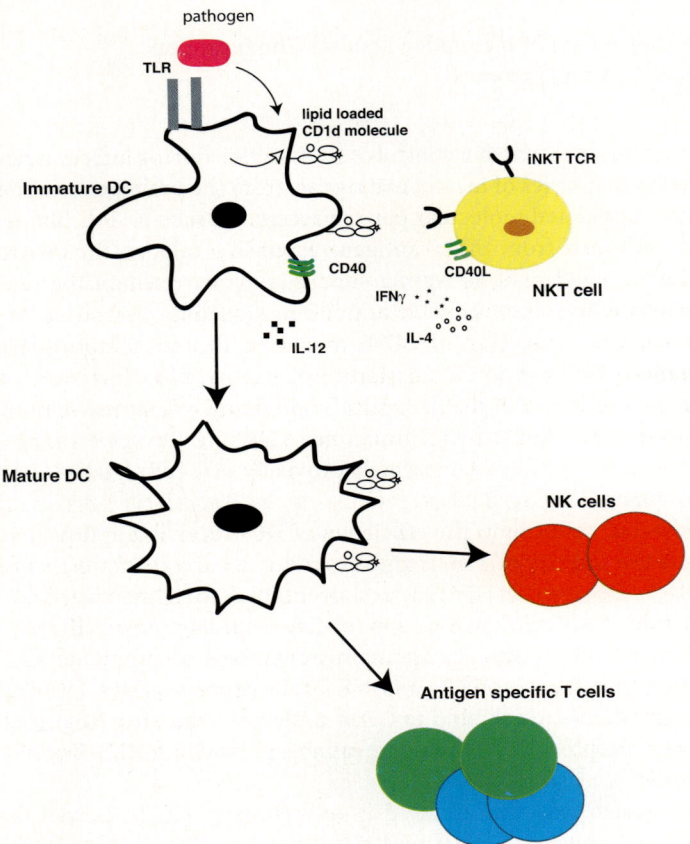

Fig. 1 NKT cell-dependent DC maturation. NKT cells recognise endogenous (Zhou et al. 2004) and exogenous (Kinjo et al. 2005; Mattner et al. 2005) CD1d-bound lipids on the surface of DCs. NKT cell activation results in cytokine secretion, induction of DC maturation via soluble factors and CD40L. Mature DCs are "licensed" by NKT to prime antigen-specific T cells and to activate NK cells. Recognition of CD1d–lipid complexes on the surface of B cells also results in B cell maturation and antibody secretion as shown by (Galli et al. 2003) (not shown)

and duration of the α-GalCer-dependent NKT cell response depend on the type of APC that acquires and presents α-GalCer. Follow-up papers have confirmed and extended this concept by demonstrating that α-GalCer pulsed B cells, unlike DCs, can anergise NKT cell responses (Bezbradica et al. 2005). NKT-dependent DC maturation and the subsequent cross-talk between DCs and NK cells (Zitvogel et al. 2006), resulting in sustained secretion of IFN-γ, also provide an explanation for the initial observation that injection of α-GalCer has a potent anti-tumour effect (Carnaud et al. 1999; Cui et al. 1997; Hayakawa et al. 2001; Smyth et al. 2002).

The finding that NKT cells can promote DC maturation highlighted the possibility that NKT cell activation could rapidly provide a source of help required to shape adaptive immune responses to defined antigens. Consistent with this hypothesis, NKT cell ligands have been shown to act as vaccine adjuvants for stimulating MHC-restricted T cells. For example, co-injection of α-GalCer with malaria sporozoites could lead to enhanced protection against malaria challenge (Gonzalez-Aseguinolaza et al. 2002). Subsequently it was shown that CD8$^+$ and CD4$^+$ T cell responses to tumour antigens could also be enhanced (Fujii et al. 2003; Hermans et al. 2003). This work demonstrated in vivo a link between innate and adaptive immune responses via NKT-dependent DC maturation. The importance of the adjuvant activity of NKT cells in the development of vaccines has been confirmed in the context of heterologous prime-boost protocols (Silk et al. 2004). NKT cell stimulation enhanced both the priming and boosting of CD4$^+$ and CD8$^+$ T cell responses to subunit vaccines incorporating peptide or protein antigens. Among the antigens assessed was a clinically relevant, HLA-A2-restricted epitope of the human tumour antigen NY-ESO-1 (J.L. Chen et al. 2005; Silk et al. 2004). More recently, it has been shown that intravenous injection of irradiated MHC class I negative tumour cells together with α-GalCer results in the capture of tumour debris by splenic DCs and generation of protective tumour-specific T cell responses (Liu et al. 2005), paving the way to rendering irradiated tumour cells more immunogenic.

2.1.1
Molecular Mechanisms of NKT-Dependent DC Maturation

It has been shown that DC maturation in response to *NKT* cell stimulation occurs via the release of TNF-α in concert with IFN-γ and other cytokines (Fujii et al. 2004). Further, activated NKT cells provide soluble factors, including both type I and II IFN, that can mature both DCs and B cells. Whereas maturation is mediated by soluble factors, there is compelling evidence indicating that enhancement of T cell responses by NKT cells is critically dependent on CD40 signalling (Fujii et al. 2004; Hermans et al. 2003). Thus, similar to the mechanism of cross-talk between CD4$^+$ T cells and DCs (Sporri and Reis e Sousa 2003), cell–cell interactions and release of soluble factors may be required to enable NKT cells to promote conventional T cell-mediated immunity.

These effects can be exploited in a practical way by injecting protein antigens together with agonists of NKT cells. For example, co-injecting protein and peptide vaccines with a combination of NKT cell-agonists and monophos-phoryl lipid A (MPL), a detoxified version of LPS that signals through TLR4, can augment MHC -restricted T cell responses (Silk et al. 2004). When α-GalCer treatment was combined with the TLR4 ligand MPL, DCs promoted antigen-specific T cell responses that were greater than those elicited with α-GalCer or MPL alone. In fact, a synergy addition of both an NKT cell ac-tivator and a TLR agonist was observed that resulted in a 60-fold increase in antigen-specific $CD8^+$ T cells over injection of protein antigen alone. This observation has been confirmed and extended in ongoing studies with a range of TLR ligands and human monocyte-derived DCs (Hermans et al. 2007). We extended these results to B cell responses by demonstrating that injection of α-GalCer in combination with MPL results in high OVA-specific IgG re-sponses. Thus, both cell-mediated and Ab-mediated immune responses are improved by provision of NKT cell-derived signals and TLR4 stimulation.

2.1.2
Route of Injection of NKT Cell Agonists

Therapeutic applications of glycolipids or glycolipid-treated DCs require that they efficiently contact NKT cells in vivo, so the trafficking of NKT cells introduces certain constraints in the route of injection of NKT cell agonists. The chemokine receptor and homing molecule profile of mouse and human NKT cells is similar to that of effector memory T cells and different from that of naïve T cells. It has been shown that a large proportion of human NKT cells express CCR5, CXCR3 and CXCR6, making them capable of being recruited rapidly into inflamed and infected tissues in vivo (Thomas et al. 2003). In contrast, a small proportion of NKT cells express CCR7 and no cells express CXCR5 and CD62L, limiting their ability to migrate into the T and B cell zones of lymphoid organs from the lymphatic vessels or from the high endothelial venules (Kim et al. 2002). It has been observed that effective activation of NKT cells in vivo is dependent on the route of administration of the activating ligand. Indeed, whereas intravenous (i.v.) and intraperitoneal (i.p.) injection of DCs loaded with α-GalCer leads to NKT cell activation and subsequent cytokine production (Hermans et al. 2003; Parekh et al. 2005), subcutaneous (s.c.) administration is less effective (Liu et al. 2005), presumably because of a low frequency of NKT cells in the region of injection (Fujii et al. 2002).

    The adjuvant effect of NKT cell stimulation was also observed after oral administration of protein vaccine and NKT cell ligand (Chung et al. 2004; Silk et al. 2004), a route considered to be most promising in terms of likely patient usage. These results were recently extended demonstrating that the adjuvant effect of NKT cell stimulation could also be exerted after nasal administration

(Ko et al. 2005). Interestingly, when protein was administered by the oral route, and α-GalCer was administered separately by i.v. injection, no adjuvant effect was observed (Silk et al. 2004). This most likely reflects a requirement for the glycolipid and peptide antigens to be presented simultaneously, presumably on the same APCs. Responses induced in the presence of NKT cell stimulation, by either the i.v. or the oral route, both elicited CTLs endowed with anti-tumour activity (Silk et al. 2004). These findings suggest that NKT cell ligands could be valuable compounds for use in T cell vaccines for the treatment of cancer and infectious agents.

2.2
Regulation of Immune Responses by NKT Cell Subsets

While invariant NKT cells represent an important subset of CD1d-restricted lymphocytes, compelling evidence in mouse models demonstrates the presence of suppressive CD1d-restricted T cells expressing TCR other than the invariant Vα14-Jα18 TCR. It has been shown that secretion of IL-13 by a population of CD1d-restricted lymphocytes may result in the activation of myeloid suppressor cells, which in turn contribute to the suppression of antigen specific T cell responses (Crowe et al. 2005; Terabe et al. 2003, 2004). The existence of functionally distinct subsets of CD1d-restricted T cells may explain the different outcomes following their activation and further highlights the importance of understanding these mechanisms so that it becomes possible to fine-tune their activation in vivo.

CD1d-reactive T cells with suppressive properties have been described in the bone marrow and are a major player in models of allograft survival (Exley et al. 2001; Zeng et al. 1999). It has also been shown that after ablation therapy, residual NKT cells present in the host reduce the severity of graft-versus-host disease (GVHD) via IL-4 production and Th2 polarisation of donor cells (Hashimoto et al. 2005). More recently it has been demonstrated that donor treatment with progenipoietin-1, a chimeric cytokine of G-CSF and FLT3L, expands splenic and hepatic NKT cells. In a model of allogeneic stem cell transplantation, progenipoietin-1-mediated expansion of donor NKT cells proved important to reduce GVHD and at the same time enhanced GVL effects, by inducing host DC activation (Morris et al. 2005). These results are consistent with the report that transplant patients with lower numbers of circulating NKT have more severe GVHD (Haraguchi et al. 2004).

There is also abundant evidence for the immunomodulatory role of NKT in the development of autoimmunity (Van Kaer 2005). Most of the results have been obtained in murine models of type I diabetes (NOD mice) and spontaneous autoimmune encephalitis (EAE), where the development of disease correlates with a Th1 type of infiltrate, while Th2 responses are protective (Ercolini and Miller 2006; Solomon and Sarvetnick 2004). As reviewed in Cardell (2006) and Miyake and Yamamura (2005), in some experimental systems, repeated injections of α-GalCer delayed the onset of both type I diabetes and EAE and reduced their incidence, an effect ascribed to an NKT-mediated switch to Th2 cellular and humoral responses. In addition, there may be an indirect effect via induction of tolerogenic APCs, which are also defective in NOD mice (Y.G. Chen et al. 2005; Naumov et al. 2001). Stronger protection against EAE has been observed with OCH, a sphingosine-truncated analogue of α-GalCer, which induces selective IL-4 production by NKT cells (Miyamoto et al. 2001), because of its faster rate of dissociation from CD1d molecules as compared to α-GalCer (Oki et al. 2004).

3
NKT Cells in Clinical Trials

Phase I clinical trials have compared safety and immunogenicity of i.v. injections of either α-GalCer alone (Giaccone 2002) or α-GalCer-loaded immature (Nieda et al. 2004; van der Vliet et al. 2003) and mature DCs (Chang et al. 2005). However, to date no clinical trials have been carried out by co-injecting NKT cell agonists with recombinant MHC-restricted protein or antigens. Consistent with mouse studies, delivery of α-GalCer on mature DCs has proven to be the best way to expand NKT cell numbers. It was shown that the NKT cells expressing the canonical and noncanonical TCR (Gadola et al. 2002, 2006) were expanded dramatically, more than 100-fold, after three immunisations with α-GalCer-loaded mature DCs (Chang et al. 2005). Of note, long-lasting NKT cell expansion was observed even in patients with severe NKT cell deficiencies at baseline, as is often the case in cancer patients (Chang et al. 2005).

It was of interest to observe that in myeloma patients who received repeated injections of α-GalCer-loaded mature DCs, expansion of NKT cell subsets was associated with an increase in the serum level of IL-12 p40, MIP-1β, IP-10 and an increase of cytomegalovirus (CMV)-specific CTL (Chang et al. 2005). The latter results were consistent with the presence of CMV in the treated patients, suggesting that NKT-dependent DC maturation in the presence of antigenic protein may result in the expansion of antigen-specific CTL responses.

Since a large number of NKT cells are resident in mouse liver, one of the concerns of clinical trials based on the i.v. injection of NKT cell agonists is the possibility of inducing liver damage. Consistent with this possibility, hepatotoxicity has been observed in murine models of NKT cell activation

(Osman et al. 2000). However, possibly because of lower numbers of NKT cells in human liver, abnormalities of liver function tests following i.v. injection of α-GalCer-loaded mature (Chang et al. 2005) and immature DCs has not been reported. It is of interest that hepatotoxicity has not even been observed in a dose escalation trial in patients injected intravenously with α-GalCer at doses up to 5 mg/m^2 (Giaccone 2002).

4
Future Directions

Overall, the capacity of NKT cells to rapidly activate both the innate and the adaptive components of the immune system, combined with their ability in promoting both inflammatory and tolerogenic responses highlight the importance of being able to fine-tune their activation in vivo for therapeutic purposes. Although the results of initial clinical trials are encouraging, to minimise any side effect due to lymphokines secreted by NKT cells, future clinical trials should be based on the use of NKT cell agonists which, unlike α-GalCer, would ensure optimal DC maturation without over-stimulating NKT cells. A better understanding of the biology of NKT cells and of factors capable of influencing NKT cell immunoregulatory properties is required. In particular, identification of compounds which can modulate the lymphokine profile secreted by NKT cells may contribute to promoting either inflammatory or tolerogenic responses.

Recently the x-ray crystal structures of CD1d proteins in complex with α-GalCer (Koch et al. 2005; Zajonc et al. 2005) have been solved. Separately, the three-dimensional crystal structures of both canonical and noncanonical NKT T cell receptors (TCRs) have been solved (Gadola et al. 2006; Kjer-Nielsen et al. 2006). Although a ternary co-crystal of α-GalCer-CD1d bound to the NKT TCR has not yet been solved, the existing crystal structures predict a TCR binding mode that is similar to that of conventional αβ T cells. The knowledge derived from these structural studies combined with kinetic and functional analyses of the mechanisms which control lipid presentation by CD1d molecules will aid the design of novel synthetic NKT cell agonists useful in immunotherapeutic applications.

An important parameter to consider in evaluating the biological effects of NKT agonists is the affinity of TCR binding to the glycolipid–CD1d complex and the stability of glycolipid ligands bound to CD1d molecules. It has been shown that the compound OCH, an analogue of α-GalCer with a truncated-sphingosine chain, binds less stably to CD1d compared to α-GalCer, resulting in a less sustained TCR stimulation and secretion of higher amounts of IL-

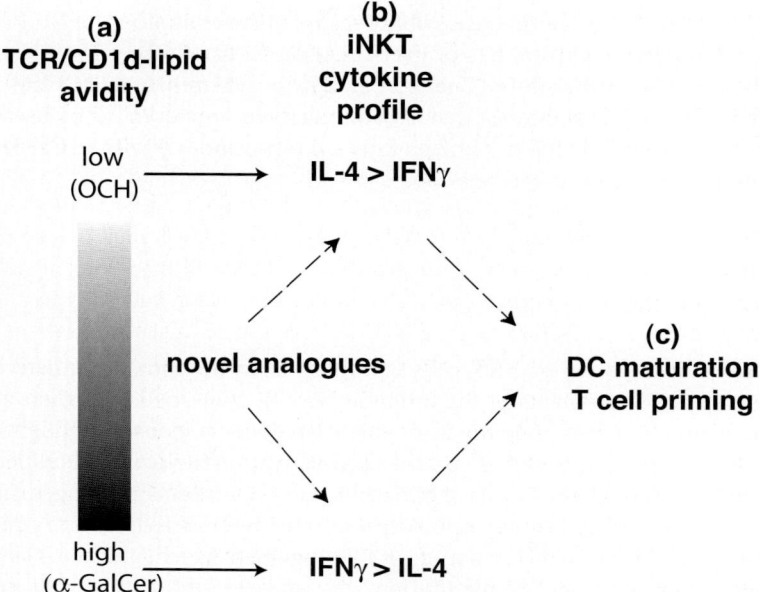

Fig. 2a–c The avidity of TCR–CD1-lipid interactions influences the type of immune response (**a**). Lipids that bind strongly to CD1d molecules elicit sustained NKT cell IFN-γ secretion. Lipids with a weaker binding affinity elicit higher levels of IL-4 by NKT cells (**b**). Both sets of lipids, however, are capable of inducing DC maturation and T cell priming (**c**). Novel α-GalCer analogues with a range of binding affinities resulting in different degrees of NKT cell stimulation need to be carefully chosen to control autoimmune diseases and in vaccination strategies

4 than IFN-γ by NKT cells (Oki et al. 2004). It is of interest, however, that despite marked differences in CD1d affinities between α-GalCer and OCH, both compounds were shown to induce comparable DC maturation and when co-injected with soluble OVA, they were capable of eliciting equally protective CTL responses (Silk et al. 2004). These results suggest that NKT cell agonists with lower CD1d affinities, which maintain a full spectrum of biological activities, may be more desirable in clinical settings to avoid immunopathology, due to a NKT cell-driven cytokine storm (Fig. 2). Furthermore, since it has recently been shown that over-stimulation of NKT cells by repeated α-GalCer injections results in NKT cell anergy, expansion of regulatory DCs and unresponsiveness to subsequent stimulations (Kojo et al. 2005; Parekh et al. 2005), it will be interesting to see whether analogues with weaker CD1d binding affinities will overcome NKT cell anergy.

It is possible that targeting different APC populations in vivo may influence the biological outcome of therapeutic applications of NKT cell activation protocols. This is consistent with the observation that multiple i.v. injections of mature DCs pulsed with α-GalCer in humans led to the expansion of NKT cells (Chang et al. 2005), as compared to trials based on the i.v. injection of α-GalCer alone. It has been suggested that the use of NKT cell agonists with an increased ability to be loaded onto surface-bound CD1d molecules could favor presentation by nonprofessional or unactivated APCs such as gastrointestinal epithelia or even resting B cells. This contrasts with NKT cell agonists requiring endosome loading onto CD1d molecules, which could be preferentially presented by professional APCs that have the cellular mechanisms for antigen internalisation. Consistent with this hypothesis, it has been shown that α-GalCer variants with shorter and unsaturated acyl chains can be presented by nonprofessional APCs, resulting in higher levels of IL-4 secretion (Yu et al. 2005). In contrast, α-GalCer analogues with saturated acyl chains are preferentially presented by professional APCs, resulting in the secretion of larger amounts of γ-IFN. These results highlight the possibility that modifications of the α-GalCer alkyl chains to produce analogues with high stringency loading requirements for presentation by DCs and other professional APCs could be considered in future therapeutic strategies to induce type 1 (in cancer and infectious diseases) or type 2 (in autoimmune diseases) responses by targeting professional or nonprofessional APCs.

Finally, modulating the activity of different NKT cell subsets might also be of great clinical relevance. For example, it has been shown that only hepatic NKT cells, rather than splenic or thymic NKT cells, are capable of mediating tumour rejection (Crowe et al. 2005), highlighting the importance of selectively targeting NKT cells resident in different organs.

In conclusion, the use of NKT cell agonists as adjuvants in vaccination strategies and modulators in autoimmune diseases is on a solid conceptual and technical footing. The challenge remains to translate the preclinical results into clinical uses. The success of such strategies will require careful optimisation of a range of glycolipid agonists in phase I clinical trials and it will depend on the timing and dose of administration, on the stage of disease and possibly the existing cytokine milieu. In vivo targeting of NKT cells should also be combined with other strategies known to alter the Th1/Th2 balance, such as the use of TLR ligands (Marschner et al. 2005; Silk et al. 2004). Since in cancer patients and in some autoimmune disorders there are fewer numbers of NKT cells, an attractive possibility is to expand in vitro NKT cells and then adoptively transfer them in the presence of cytokines (such as IL-2, IL-15, and IL-7). Lastly, understanding the identity of natural ligands recognised by CD1-restricted T cells, such as sulfatide in murine models of EAE (Jahng et al.

2004), and the mechanisms that control their expression in different tissues and tumours may also be of tremendous importance to modulate NKT cell function in autoimmune diseases and cancer.

References

Bezbradica JS, Stanic AK, Matsuki N, Bour-Jordan H, Bluestone JA, Thomas JW, Unutmaz D, Van Kaer L, Joyce S (2005) Distinct roles of dendritic cells and B cells in Va14Ja18 natural T cell activation in vivo. J Immunol 174:4696–4705

Brigl M, Bry L, Kent SC, Gumperz JE, Brenner MB (2003) Mechanism of CD1d-restricted natural killer T cell activation during microbial infection. Nat Immunol 4:1230–1237

Cardell SL (2006) The natural killer T lymphocyte: a player in the complex regulation of autoimmune diabetes in non-obese diabetic mice. Clin Exp Immunol 143:194–202

Carnaud C, Lee D, Donnars O, Park SH, Beavis A, Koezuka Y, Bendelac A (1999) Cutting edge: cross-talk between cells of the innate immune system: NKT cells rapidly activate NK cells. J Immunol 163:4647–4650

Chang DH, Osman K, Connolly J, Kukreja A, Krasovsky J, Pack M, Hutchinson A, Geller M, Liu N, Annable R et al (2005) Sustained expansion of NKT cells and antigen-specific T cells after injection of alpha-galactosyl-ceramide loaded mature dendritic cells in cancer patients. J Exp Med 201:1503–1517

Chen JL, Stewart-Jones G, Bossi G, Lissin NM, Wooldridge L, Choi EM, Held G, Dunbar PR, Esnouf RM, Sami M et al (2005) Structural and kinetic basis for heightened immunogenicity of T cell vaccines. J Exp Med 201:1243–1255

Chen YG, Choisy-Rossi CM, Holl TM, Chapman HD, Besra GS, Porcelli SA, Shaffer DJ, Roopenian D, Wilson SB, Serreze DV (2005) Activated NKT cells inhibit autoimmune diabetes through tolerogenic recruitment of dendritic cells to pancreatic lymph nodes. J Immunol 174:1196–1204

Chung Y, Chang WS, Kim S, Kang CY (2004) NKT cell ligand alpha-galactosylceramide blocks the induction of oral tolerance by triggering dendritic cell maturation. Eur J Immunol 34:2471–2479

Crowe NY, Coquet JM, Berzins SP, Kyparissoudis K, Keating R, Pellicci DG, Hayakawa Y, Godfrey DI, Smyth MJ (2005) Differential antitumor immunity mediated by NKT cell subsets in vivo. J Exp Med 202:1279–1288

Cui J, Shin T, Kawano T, Sato H, Kondo E, Toura I, Kaneko Y, Koseki H, Kanno M, Taniguchi M (1997) Requirement for Valpha14. NKT cells in IL-12-mediated rejection of tumors. Science 278:1623–1626

Donnelly JJ, Wahren B, Liu MA (2005) DNA vaccines: progress and challenges. J Immunol 175:633–639

Ercolini AM, Miller SD (2006) Mechanisms of immunopathology in murine models of central nervous system demyelinating disease. J Immunol 176:3293–3298

Exley MA, Tahir SM, Cheng O, Shaulov A, Joyce R, Avigan D, Sackstein R, Balk SP (2001) A major fraction of human bone marrow lymphocytes are Th2-like CD1d-reactive T cells that can suppress mixed lymphocyte responses. J Immunol 167:5531–5534

Fujii S, Shimizu K, Kronenberg M, Steinman RM (2002) Prolonged IFN-gamma-producing NKT response induced with alpha-galactosylceramide-loaded DCs. Nat Immunol 3:867–874

Fujii S, Shimizu K, Smith C, Bonifaz L, Steinman RM (2003) Activation of natural killer T cells by alpha-galactosylceramide rapidly induces the full maturation of dendritic cells in vivo and thereby acts as an adjuvant for combined CD4 and CD8. T cell immunity to a coadministered protein. J Exp Med 198:267–279

Fujii S, Liu K, Smith C, Bonito AJ, Steinman RM (2004) The linkage of innate to adaptive immunity via maturing dendritic cells in vivo requires CD40 ligation in addition to antigen presentation and CD80/86 costimulation. J Exp Med 199:1607–1618

Gadola SD, Dulphy N, Salio M, Cerundolo V (2002) Valpha24-JalphaQ-independent CD1d-restricted recognition of alpha-galactosylceramide by human CD4(+) and CD8alphabeta(+) T lymphocytes. J Immunol 168:5514–5520

Gadola SD, Koch M, Marles-Wright J, Lissin NM, Shepherd D, Matulis G, Harlos K, Villiger PM, Stuart DI, Jakobsen BK et al (2006) Structure and binding kinetics of three different human CD1d-alpha-galactosylceramide-specific T cell receptors. J Exp Med 203:699–710

Galli G, Nuti S, Tavarini S, Galli-Stampino L, De Lalla C, Casorati G, Dellabona P, Abrignani S (2003) CD1d-restricted help to B cells by human invariant natural killer T lymphocytes. J Exp Med 197:1051–1057

Giaccone G (2002) A phase I study of the natural killer T-cell ligand alpha-galactosylceramide in patients with solid tumors. Clin Cancer Res 8:3702–3709

Godfrey DI, Kronenberg M (2004) Going both ways: immune regulation via CD1d-dependent NKT cells. J Clin Invest 114:1379–1388

Gonzalez-Aseguinolaza G, Van Kaer L, Bergmann CC, Wilson JM, Schmieg J, Kronenberg M, Nakayama T, Taniguchi M, Koezuka Y, Tsuji M (2002) Natural killer T cell ligand alpha-galactosylceramide enhances protective immunity induced by malaria vaccines. J Exp Med 195:617–624

Gumperz JE, Miyake S, Yamamura T, Brenner MB (2002) Functionally distinct subsets of CD1d-restricted natural killer T cells revealed by CD1d tetramer staining. J Exp Med 195:625–636

Haraguchi K, Takahashi T, Hiruma K, Kanda Y, Tanaka Y, Ogawa S, Chiba S, Miura O, Sakamaki H, Hirai H (2004) Recovery of Valpha24+ NKT cells after hematopoietic stem cell transplantation. Bone Marrow Transplant 34:595–602

Hashimoto D, Asakura S, Miyake S, Yamamura T, Van Kaer L, Liu C, Tanimoto M, Teshima T (2005) Stimulation of host NKT cells by synthetic glycolipid regulates acute graft-versus-host disease by inducing Th2 polarization of donor T cells. J Immunol 174:551–556

Hayakawa Y, Takeda K, Yagita H, Kakuta S, Iwakura Y, Van Kaer L, Saiki I, Okumura K (2001) Critical contribution of IFN-gamma and NK cells, but not perforin-mediated cytotoxicity, to anti-metastatic effect of alpha-galactosylceramide. Eur J Immunol 31:1720–1727

Hermans IF, Silk JD, Gileadi U, Salio M, Mathew B, Ritter G, Schmidt R, Harris AL, Old L, Cerundolo V (2003) NKT cells enhance CD4+ and CD8+ T cell responses to soluble antigen in vivo through direct interaction with dendritic cells. J Immunol 171:5140–5147

Hermans IF, Silk JD, Gileadi U, Masri SH, Shepherd D, Farrand KJ, Salio M, Cerundolo V (2007) Dendritic cell function can be modulated through cooperatve actions of TLR ligands and invariant NKT cells. J Immunol 178:2721–2729

Jahng A, Maricic I, Aguilera C, Cardell S, Halder RC, Kumar V (2004) Prevention of autoimmunity by targeting a distinct, noninvariant CD1d-reactive T cell population reactive to sulfatide. J Exp Med 199:947–957

Kim CH, Johnston B, Butcher EC (2002) Trafficking machinery of NKT cells: shared and differential chemokine receptor expression among V alpha 24(+)V beta 11(+) NKT cell subsets with distinct cytokine-producing capacity. Blood 100:11–16

Kinjo Y, Wu D, Kim G, Xing GW, Poles MA, Ho DD, Tsuji M, Kawahara K, Wong CH, Kronenberg M (2005) Recognition of bacterial glycosphingolipids by natural killer T cells. Nature 434:520–525

Kjer-Nielsen L, Borg NA, Pellicci DG, Beddoe T, Kostenko L, Clements CS, Williamson NA, Smyth MJ, Besra GS, Reid HH et al (2006) A structural basis for selection and cross-species reactivity of the semi-invariant NKT cell receptor in CD1d/glycolipid recognition. J Exp Med 203:661–673

Ko SY, Ko HJ, Chang WS, Park SH, Kweon MN, Kang CY (2005) Alpha-galactosylceramide can act as a nasal vaccine adjuvant inducing protective immune responses against viral infection and tumor. J Immunol 175:3309–3317

Koch M, Stronge VS, Shepherd D, Gadola SD, Mathew B, Ritter G, Fersht AR, Besra GS, Schmidt RR, Jones EY, Cerundolo V (2005) The crystal structure of human CD1d with and without alpha-galactosylceramide. Nat Immunol 6:819–826

Kojo S, Seino K, Harada M, Watarai H, Wakao H, Uchida T, Nakayama T, Taniguchi M (2005) Induction of regulatory properties in dendritic cells by Valpha14. NKT cells. J Immunol 175:3648–3655

Lee PT, Benlagha K, Teyton L, Bendelac A (2002) Distinct functional lineages of human V(alpha)24 natural killer T cells. J Exp Med 195:637–641

Liu K, Idoyaga J, Charalambous A, Fujii S, Bonito A, Mordoh J, Wainstok R, Bai XF, Liu Y, Steinman RM (2005) Innate NKT lymphocytes confer superior adaptive immunity via tumor-capturing dendritic cells. J Exp Med 202:1507–1516

Marschner A, Rothenfusser S, Hornung V, Prell D, Krug A, Kerkmann M, Wellisch D, Poeck H, Greinacher A, Giese T et al (2005) CpGODN enhance antigen-specific NKT cell activation via plasmacytoid dendritic cells. Eur J Immunol 35:2347–2357

Mattner J, Debord KL, Ismail N, Goff RD, Cantu C 3rd, Zhou D, Saint-Mezard P, Wang V, Gao Y, Yin N et al (2005) Exogenous and endogenous glycolipid antigens activate NKT cells during microbial infections. Nature 434:525–529

Miyake S, Yamamura T (2005) Therapeutic potential of glycolipid ligands for natural killer (NK) T cells in the suppression of autoimmune diseases. Curr Drug Targets Immune Endocr Metabol Disord 5:315–322

Miyamoto K, Miyake S, Yamamura T (2001) A synthetic glycolipid prevents autoimmune encephalomyelitis by inducing TH2 bias of natural killer T cells. Nature 413:531–534

Morris ES, MacDonald KP, Rowe V, Banovic T, Kuns RD, Don AL, Bofinger HM, Burman AC, Olver SD, Kienzle N et al (2005) NKT cell-dependent leukemia eradication following stem cell mobilization with potent G-CSF analogs. J Clin Invest 115:3093–3103

Naumov YN, Bahjat KS, Gausling R, Abraham R, Exley MA, Koezuka Y, Balk SB, Strominger JL, Clare-Salzer M, Wilson SB (2001) Activation of CD1d-restricted T cells protects NOD mice from developing diabetes by regulating dendritic cell subsets. Proc Natl Acad Sci U S A 98:13838–13843

Nieda M, Okai M, Tazbirkova A, Lin H, Yamaura A, Ide K, Abraham R, Juji T, Macfarlane DJ, Nicol AJ (2004) Therapeutic activation of Valpha24+Vbeta11+ NKT cells in human subjects results in highly coordinated secondary activation of acquired and innate immunity. Blood 103:383–389

Oki S, Chiba A, Yamamura T, Miyake S (2004) The clinical implication and molecular mechanism of preferential IL-4 production by modified glycolipid-stimulated NKT cells. J Clin Invest 113:1631–1640

Osman Y, Kawamura T, Naito T, Takeda K, Van Kaer L, Okumura K, Abo T (2000) Activation of hepatic NKT cells and subsequent liver injury following administration of alpha-galactosylceramide. Eur J Immunol 30:1919–1928

Parekh VV, Wilson MT, Olivares-Villagomez D, Singh AK, Wu L, Wang CR, Joyce S, Van Kaer L (2005) Glycolipid antigen induces long-term natural killer T cell anergy in mice. J Clin Invest 115:2572–2583

Porcelli SA, Modlin RL (1999) The CD1 system: antigen-presenting molecules for T cell recognition of lipids and glycolipids. Annu Rev Immunol 17:297–329

Reis e Sousa C (2004) Toll-like receptors and dendritic cells: for whom the bug tolls. Semin Immunol 16:27–34

Schneider J, Gilbert SC, Hannan CM, Degano P, Prieur E, Sheu EG, Plebanski M, Hill AV (1999) Induction of CD8+ T cells using heterologous prime-boost immunisation strategies. Immunol Rev 170:29–38

Schulz O, Edwards AD, Schito M, Aliberti J, Manickasingham S, Sher A, Reis e Sousa C (2000) CD40 triggering of heterodimeric IL-12 p70 production by dendritic cells in vivo requires a microbial priming signal. Immunity 13:453–462

Seino K, Taniguchi M (2005) Functionally distinct NKT cell subsets and subtypes. J Exp Med 202:1623–1626

Silk JD, Hermans IF, Gileadi U, Chong TW, Shepherd D, Salio M, Mathew B, Schmidt RR, Lunt SJ, Williams KJ et al (2004) Utilizing the adjuvant properties of CD1d-dependent NKT cells in T cell-mediated immunotherapy. J Clin Invest 114:1800–1811

Smith CL, Dunbar PR, Mirza F, Palmowski MJ, Shepherd D, Gilbert SC, Coulie P, Schneider J, Hoffman E, Hawkins R et al (2005a) Recombinant modified vaccinia Ankara primes functionally activated CTL specific for a melanoma tumor antigen epitope in melanoma patients with a high risk of disease recurrence. Int J Cancer 113:259–266

Smith CL, Mirza F, Pasquetto V, Tscharke DC, Palmowski MJ, Dunbar PR, Sette A, Harris AL, Cerundolo V (2005b) Immunodominance of poxviral-specific CTL in a human trial of recombinant-modified vaccinia Ankara. J Immunol 175:8431–8437

Smyth MJ, Crowe NY, Pellicci DG, Kyparissoudis K, Kelly JM, Takeda K, Yagita H, Godfrey DI (2002) Sequential production of interferon-gamma by NK1.1(+) T cells and natural killer cells is essential for the antimetastatic effect of alpha-galactosylceramide. Blood 99:1259–1266

Solomon M, Sarvetnick N (2004) The pathogenesis of diabetes in the NOD mouse. Adv Immunol 84:239–264

Sporri R, Reis e Sousa C (2003) Newly activated T cells promote maturation of bystander dendritic cells but not IL-12 production. J Immunol 171:6406–6413

Sporri R, Reis e Sousa C (2005) Inflammatory mediators are insufficient for full dendritic cell activation and promote expansion of CD4+ T cell populations lacking helper function. Nat Immunol 6:163–170

Stober D, Jomantaite I, Schirmbeck R, Reimann J (2003) NKT cells provide help for dendritic cell-dependent priming of MHC class I-restricted CD8+ T cells in vivo. J Immunol 170:2540–2548

Terabe M, Matsui S, Park JM, Mamura M, Noben-Trauth N, Donaldson DD, Chen W, Wahl SM, Ledbetter S, Pratt B et al (2003) Transforming growth factor-beta production and myeloid cells are an effector mechanism through which CD1d-restricted T cells block cytotoxic T lymphocyte-mediated tumor immunosurveillance: abrogation prevents tumor recurrence. J Exp Med 198:1741–1752

Terabe M, Park JM, Berzofsky JA (2004) Role of IL-13 in regulation of anti-tumor immunity and tumor growth. Cancer Immunol Immunother 53:79–85

Thomas SY, Hou R, Boyson JE, Means TK, Hess C, Olson DP, Strominger JL, Brenner MB, Gumperz JE, Wilson SB, Luster AD (2003) CD1d-restricted NKT cells express a chemokine receptor profile indicative of Th1-type inflammatory homing cells. J Immunol 171:2571–2580

Van der Vliet HJ, Molling JW, Nishi N, Masterson AJ, Kolgen W, Porcelli SA, van den Eertwegh AJ, von Blomberg BM, Pinedo HM, Giaccone G, Scheper RJ (2003) Polarization of Valpha24+ Vbeta11+ natural killer T cells of healthy volunteers and cancer patients using alpha-galactosylceramide-loaded and environmentally instructed dendritic cells. Cancer Res 63:4101–4106

Van Kaer L (2005) Alpha-galactosylceramide therapy for autoimmune diseases: prospects and obstacles. Nat Rev Immunol 5:31–42

Vincent M, Leslie DS, Gumperz JE, Xiong X, Grant EP, Brenner MB (2002) CD1-dependent dendritic cell instruction. Nat Immunol 3:1163–1168

Yu KO, Im JS, Molano A, Dutronc Y, Illarionov PA, Forestier C, Fujiwara N, Arias I, Miyake S, Yamamura T et al (2005) Modulation of CD1d-restricted NKT cell responses by using N-acyl variants of alpha-galactosylceramides. Proc Natl Acad Sci U S A 102:3383–3388

Zajonc DM, Cantu C 3rd, Mattner J, Zhou D, Savage PB, Bendelac A, Wilson IA, Teyton L (2005) Structure and function of a potent agonist for the semi-invariant natural killer T cell receptor. Nat Immunol 6:810–818

Zeng D, Lewis D, Dejbakhsh-Jones S, Lan F, Garcia-Ojeda M, Sibley R, Strober S (1999) Bone marrow NK1.1(–) and NK1.1(+) T cells reciprocally regulate acute graft versus host disease. J Exp Med 189:1073–1081

Zhou D, Mattner J, Cantu C 3rd, Schrantz N, Yin N, Gao Y, Sagiv Y, Hudspeth K, Wu YP, Yamashita T et al (2004) Lysosomal glycosphingolipid recognition by NKT cells. Science 306:1786–1789

Zitvogel L, Terme M, Borg C, Trinchieri G (2006) Dendritic cell-NK cell cross-talk: regulation and physiopathology. Curr Top Microbiol Immunol 298:157–174

Subject Index

Current Topics in Microbiology and Immunology

Volumes published since 1989 (and still available)

Vol. 291: **Boquet, Patrice; Lemichez Emmanuel (Eds.)** Bacterial Virulence Factors and Rho GTPases. 2005. 28 figs., IX, 196 pp. ISBN 3-540-23865-4

Vol. 292: **Fu, Zhen F (Ed.):** The World of Rhabdoviruses. 2005. 27 figs., X, 210 pp. ISBN 3-540-24011-X

Vol. 293: **Kyewski, Bruno; Suri-Payer, Elisabeth (Eds.):** CD4+CD25+ Regulatory T Cells: Origin, Function and Therapeutic Potential. 2005. 22 figs., XII, 332 pp. ISBN 3-540-24444-1

Vol. 294: **Caligaris-Cappio, Federico, Dalla Favera, Ricardo (Eds.):** Chronic Lymphocytic Leukemia. 2005. 25 figs., VIII, 187 pp. ISBN 3-540-25279-7

Vol. 295: **Sullivan, David J.; Krishna Sanjeew (Eds.):** Malaria: Drugs, Disease and Post-genomic Biology. 2005. 40 figs., XI, 446 pp. ISBN 3-540-25363-7

Vol. 296: **Oldstone, Michael B. A. (Ed.):** Molecular Mimicry: Infection Induced
Autoimmune Disease. 2005. 28 figs., VIII, 167 pp. ISBN 3-540-25597-4

Vol. 297: **Langhorne, Jean (Ed.):** Immunology and Immunopathogenesis of Malaria. 2005. 8 figs., XII, 236 pp. ISBN 3-540-25718-7

Vol. 298: **Vivier, Eric; Colonna, Marco (Eds.):** Immunobiology of Natural Killer Cell Receptors. 2005. 27 figs., VIII, 286 pp. ISBN 3-540-26083-8

Vol. 299: **Domingo, Esteban (Ed.):** Quasispecies: Concept and Implications. 2006. 44 figs., XII, 401 pp. ISBN 3-540-26395-0

Vol. 300: **Wiertz, Emmanuel J.H.J.; Kikkert, Marjolein (Eds.):** Dislocation and Degradation of Proteins from the Endoplasmic Reticulum. 2006. 19 figs., VIII, 168 pp. ISBN 3-540-28006-5

Vol. 301: **Doerfler, Walter; Böhm, Petra (Eds.):** DNA Methylation: Basic Mechanisms. 2006. 24 figs., VIII, 324 pp. ISBN 3-540-29114-8

Vol. 302: **Robert N. Eisenman (Ed.):** The Myc/Max/Mad Transcription Factor Network. 2006. 28 figs. XII, 278 pp. ISBN 3-540-23968-5

Vol. 303: **Thomas E. Lane (Ed.):** Chemokines and Viral Infection. 2006. 14 figs. XII, 154 pp. ISBN 3-540-29207-1

Vol. 304: **Stanley A. Plotkin (Ed.):** Mass Vaccination: Global Aspects -- Progress and Obstacles. 2006. 40 figs. X, 270 pp. ISBN 3-540-29382-5

Vol. 305: **Radbruch, Andreas; Lipsky, Peter E. (Eds.):** Current Concepts in Autoimmunity. 2006. 29 figs. IIX, 276 pp. ISBN 3-540-29713-8

Vol. 306: **William M. Shafer (Ed.):** Antimicrobial Peptides and Human Disease. 2006. 12 figs. XII, 262 pp. ISBN 3-540-29915-7

Vol. 307: **John L. Casey (Ed.):** Hepatitis Delta Virus. 2006. 22 figs. XII, 228 pp. ISBN 3-540-29801-0

Vol. 308: **Honjo, Tasuku; Melchers, Fritz (Eds.):** Gut-Associated Lymphoid Tissues. 2006. 24 figs. XII, 204 pp. ISBN 3-540-30656-0

Vol. 309: **Polly Roy (Ed.):** Reoviruses: Entry, Assembly and Morphogenesis. 2006. 43 figs. XX, 261 pp. ISBN 3-540-30772-9

Vol. 310: **Doerfler, Walter; Böhm, Petra (Eds.):** DNA Methylation: Development, Genetic Disease and Cancer. 2006. 25 figs. X, 284 pp. ISBN 3-540-31180-7

Vol. 311: **Pulendran, Bali; Ahmed, Rafi (Eds.):** From Innate Immunity to Immunological Memory. 2006. 13 figs. X, 177 pp. ISBN 3-540-32635-9

Vol. 312: **Boshoff, Chris; Weiss, Robin A. (Eds.):** Kaposi Sarcoma Herpesvirus: New Perspectives. 2006. 29 figs. XVI, 330 pp. ISBN 3-540-34343-1

Vol. 313: **Pandolfi, Pier P.; Vogt, Peter K. (Eds.):** Acute Promyelocytic Leukemia. 2007. 16 figs. VIII, 273 pp. ISBN 3-540-34592-2